Advances in Drug Research

Volume 12

Advances in Drug Research

Series Editors

N. J. HARPER

Weddel Pharmaceuticals Ltd
St Albans, Hertfordshire, England

and

ALMA B. SIMMONDS

Chelsea College
University of London, England

Volume 12

edited by Alma B. Simmonds

1977

ACADEMIC PRESS
LONDON   NEW YORK   SAN FRANCISCO

A Subsidiary of Harcourt Brace Jovanovich, Publishers

ACADEMIC PRESS INC. (LONDON) LTD.
24–28 Oval Road
London NW1

US edition published by
ACADEMIC PRESS INC.
111 Fifth Avenue,
New York, New York 10003

Library of Congress Catalog Card Number: 64-24672
ISBN: 0-12-013312

PRINTED IN GREAT BRITAIN AT THE SPOTTISWOODE BALLANTYNE PRESS BY
WILLIAM CLOWES & SONS LIMITED, LONDON, COLCHESTER AND BECCLES

Contributors to Volume 12

*M. SAMIR AMER, MS, PhD, Diploma in Hospital Pharmacy
Mead Johnson Research Center, Evansville, Indiana 47721, USA

NORMAN O. CROSSLAND, BSc
*Shell Research Limited, Shell Toxicology Laboratory (Tunstall),
Sittingbourne, Kent, England*

WINIFRED G. NAYLER, DSc
*Cardiothoracic Institute, University of London, 2 Beaumont Street,
London W1N 2DX, England*

DAVID PARKES, MD, FRCP
*University Department of Neurology, Institute of Psychiatry and
King's College Hospital, London SE5, England*

TSUNG-YING SHEN, PhD
*Merck Sharp and Dohme Research Laboratories, Rahway, New Jersey 07065,
USA*

CHARLES A. WINTER, PhD
8540 S.E. 78th Street, Mercer Island, Washington 98040, USA

* *Present address: Bristol Myers Co., International Division, New York, N.Y. 10022, USA*

Contents

Cyclic Nucleotides as Targets for Drug Design[1]

M. SAMIR AMER, BPharm, Dipl. Hosp. Pharm., MS, PhD[2]

Mead Johnson Research Center, Evansville, Indiana, USA

1 Introduction

It is apparent to those involved in drug research and development that it is increasingly difficult to discover new drugs. The traditional approaches to drug development based primarily on mass synthesis and screening are slowly giving way to more deliberate and targeted approaches where the chances for drug discovery are maximized. One approach involves detailed study, at the cellular molecular levels, of the diseases for which drugs are to be designed. Such studies could uncover specific processes or reactions crucial to the disease process yet amenable to modulation by specific chemical entities. This could narrow both compound and target selection and enhance the prospects for drug discovery. The cyclic nucleotide system provides a powerful tool for the study of the biochemical abnormalities in disease and could provide a useful stimulus to enhance and upgrade drug design.

[1] An expanded version of a talk given at the symposium "Cyclic Nucleotide Systems: Targets for Drug Design", Society for Drug Research, London, September 8, 1976.

[2] Present address: Bristol Myers Co., International Division, New York, N.Y. 10022, USA.

[3] The references in this article are by no means exhaustive but only illustrative. Preference was given to those recent references that could lead the reader to the bulk of the original observations.

The explosive growth of cyclic nucleotide research over the past two decades is significantly advancing our understanding of a variety of diseases and of the mechanisms of action of both new and old drugs. It is creating important new opportunities for the development of new agents designed to act primarily via regulation of these important messengers. This is becoming more so as evidence of the apparent involvement of the cyclic nucleotides in an ever-expanding number of disease states accumulates (Amer, 1975; Weiss, 1975) and greater understanding of the factors responsible for controlling their intracellular levels is achieved (Greengard and Robison, 1971–6).

The cyclic nucleotides provide the biologist with a heretofore unavailable intracellular vantage point to view the interplay between the abnormal cellular conditions in disease and the changes effected by drugs. This makes it possible to examine both diseases and drugs from the point of view of the involved cells themselves.

The role that the cyclic nucleotides may play in the etiology and/or maintenance of disease is a natural consequence of their apparent involvement in the control of almost all facets of cellular activity and metabolism. The intracellular synthesis of the cyclic nucleotides represents the net biochemical translation of the combined hormonal, neural and other control mechanisms. Abnormal levels of these second messengers in disease, by necessity, indicate abnormal responsiveness of the tissues in question to biological control.

The importance of the disease-associated alterations in cyclic nucleotide metabolism in the etiology and/or maintenance of the various disease conditions is basic to their possible treatment by correcting the associated cyclic nucleotide abnormalities via the development of agents with specific effects on cyclic nucleotide metabolism (Amer and McKinney, 1973, 1974).

This chapter concentrates primarily on the sites which could be used to develop useful drug entities based on actions involving the cyclic nucleotide system. Special emphasis will be placed on those areas where the probability for the development of disease-corrective agents exists.

Any discussion of the cyclic nucleotides should include both cyclic AMP[1] and cyclic GMP[2]. Although other cyclic nucleotides have been shown to occur in biological materials, their role in disease or drug development is not sufficiently developed at this time.

The reciprocal association between the two main naturally occurring cyclic nucleotides, cyclic AMP and cyclic GMP, in a variety of disease states, is indeed impressive. However, there are important exceptions to the "Yin-Yang" hypothesis (Goldberg, 1973) reaffirming the belief that the two cyclic nucleotides probably act independently of each other in most systems. This is based on the facts that: (a) the two cyclic nucleotides appear to exist in different

---

[1] Cyclic 3′,5′-adenosine monophosphate.
[2] Cyclic 3′,5′-guanosine monophosphate.

compartments of the same cells (Fallon *et al.*, 1974) and may be under separate genetic control (Russell and Pastan, 1974); (b) in most cell-free systems the two messengers promote similar rather than dissimilar effects; (c) the time course of the reciprocal changes in their levels is rarely similar, and in many systems their levels change in the same, rather than in the opposite, direction as would be expected if a strict Yin-Yang relationship holds. In addition, there is evidence in rat heart that both adenylyl and guanylyl cyclases may be interchangeable, in parallel with the interchangeability of the adrenergic receptors, and that the availability of metabolic energy determines which cyclic nucleotide is synthesized under any particular set of conditions (Amer and Byrne, 1975).

2   Possible sites in the cyclic nucleotide system as targets for drug design

The sites at which appropriately designed drugs could act to alter cyclic nucleotide-mediated events are shown in Fig. 1 and will be discussed in the same order as they appear therein. These sites include:
  i. Modulation of the intracellular levels of the cyclic nucleotides by action on their:
     a. synthesis via stimulation, inhibition and/or blockage of the hormonal stimulation of the nucleotidyl cyclases (sites 1, 2 and 3, respectively);
     b. loss to extracellular fluids (site 4);
     c. degradation via stimulation, inhibition and/or blockade of the hormonal effects on the phosphodiesterases (sites 5, 6 and 7, respectively).
  ii. Alteration in the intracellular activity of the cyclic nucleotides by changing:
     a. the size of their free pool (site 8);
     b. mimicking their actions, (site 9); and
     c. antagonizing their intracellular effects (site 10).
  iii. Indirect effects on the cyclic nucleotide system due to effects on allied systems such as:
     a. the prostaglandins (site 11, 12 and 13); or
     b. cations.

3   Effects on intracellular levels

3.1   SYNTHESIS

The synthesis of each of the two naturally occurring cyclic nucleotides is catalyzed by a specific cyclase that uses the corresponding nucleotide triphosphate (ATP or GTP) as its substrate. The activity of these cyclases, to a

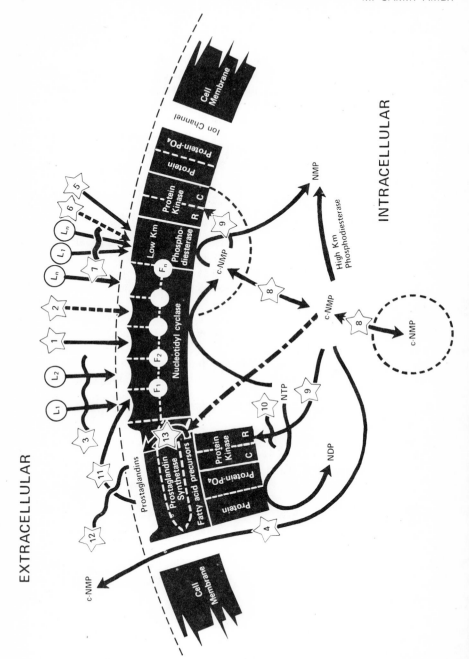

great extent, determines the intracellular levels of these important messengers. Consequently, modulation of the activity of these cyclases represents an important site for possible drug effects on this system.

Stimulation of the cyclases has long been limited to hormones and their immediate derivatives only. This is not surprising since the cyclases appear to represent the membrane sites for hormonal regulation and have consistently demonstrated marked specificity to certain hormones in target tissues. Although some drugs, e.g. isoproterenol, are known to stimulate the cyclase enzymes, these for the most part have represented only minor modifications in the structures of the parent hormones. Compounds less closely related to the natural hormones now appear capable of cyclase stimulation in a variety of tissues thus enlarging the possibilities for drug discovery. Among these are a group of insecticides including DDT, α-chlordane and heptachlor on liver adenylate cyclase (AC) (Tsant et al., 1976; Dacew and Singhal, 1973) tolbutamide and ethanol on pancreatic islet AC (Kuo et al., 1973) and the long-described effects of fluoride ions. Fatty acids were reported to stimulate GC activity in fibroblasts (Wallach and Pastan, 1976). Hydrazine may mediate the carcinogenic effects of tobacco via stimulation of GC from a variety of tissues (Vesely and Levey, 1977).

Direct inhibition of the activity of the cyclases is also an important site for the control of the intracellular cyclic nucleotide levels. This may be the mechanism for the central effects of at least some antipsychotic drugs (Roufogalis, 1976). Lithium ions were reported to directly inhibit AC in brain, platelets and thyroid. Valinomycin and possibly other antibiotics as well also appear to act via the inhibition of AC (Dorigo et al., 1973). Adenosine acts at least partially via a similar mechanism (Weinryb et al., 1973). The β-adrenergic blocker propranolol also inhibited AC in cat myocardium and turkey erythrocytes (Bilezikian and Aurbach, 1973). This suggested that AC inhibition may underlie the membrane stabilizing effects of propranolol which appear unrelated to its β-adrenergic receptor blocking activity. Sotalol, a β-adrenergic receptor blocker devoid of these membrane effects, did not inhibit AC under similar conditions. Alloxan and ethacrynic acid selectively inhibited AC in the pancreas and kidney, respectively (Cohen et al., 1969; Ferrendelli et al., 1973). The mercurial diuretics also inhibited AC from rat liver (Mavier and

FIG. 1. Possible sites of drug activity on the cyclic nucleotide systems c-NMP, cyclic nucleotide-3′,5′ monophosphate (either cyclic AMP or cyclic GMP); NTP, nucleotide triphosphate; NDP, nucleotide diphosphate; NMP, nucleotide monophosphate; F, cofactor, e.g. Mg^{++} and Mn^{++}; L, ligand, e.g. norepinephrine or acetylcholine; ☆, possible drug action site; →, stimulation; ---→, inhibition; —→, modulation; ⌒, blockade; ͟͟͟, bound c-NMP; R, regulatory unit; C, catalytic unit; K_m, Michaelis–Menten constant. Note the multiple receptor sites on nucleotidyl cyclase and the membranous location of the low K_m phosphodiesterase. Two bound (one membrane-associated) and one free pools of the cyclic nucleotides are also shown.

Hanoune, 1975). There are indications from studies with brain tissue *in vitro* that cobalt ions may inhibit guanylate cyclase (GC) activity.

In addition to either stimulating or inhibiting cyclase activity, blockade of enzyme stimulation by hormones represents a major site for the action of potential drugs. Hormone antagonists and β-adrenergic (Murad, 1973), as well as α-adrenergic (Amer, 1974), blockers probably act at this site. In general, compounds that are capable of antagonizing hormone-induced effects in intact systems are also capable of antagonizing the effects of the same hormones on the cyclic nucleotide system. This applies equally well to those derivatives of peptide, steroid and other hormone antagonists. Frequently, hormonal derivatives devoid of hormone-like actions fail to induce responses similar to those induced by the active hormones on the cyclic nucleotide system. This re-emphasizes the value of the cyclic nucleotide system as a faithful indicator of target tissue sensitivity to hormonal effects.

3.1.1   *Mechanisms of adenylate cyclase stimulation and/or inhibition*

Studies continue to advance our understanding of the mechanisms involved in cyclase activation and/or inhibition. Studies by Najjar and Constantonopoulos (1973) suggested that net AC activity may represent an equilibrium between two forms of the enzyme, a phosphorylated-inactive and a dephosphorylated-active form. Phosphorylation of AC is catalyzed by a cyclase kinase, the properties of which are presently unknown and could hold the answer to many questions related to the actions of drugs on AC activity (Walton *et al.*, 1974). It appears, for example, that fluoride ions (Schmidt and Najjar, 1976) and the prostaglandins of the E type activate AC by shifting the cyclase kinase reaction toward the active, dephospho-form. Other drugs stimulating or inhibiting cyclase activity might well be expected to act on the cyclase kinase shifting the reaction toward the dephospho- or the phospho-forms, respectively. It is conceivable that GC could be similarly regulated.

Many models of adenylate cyclase were proposed. Most results can, however, be explained by a simple hypothetical, three component model (Birnbaumer *et al.*, 1973). According to this model the enzyme is composed of discriminator, transducer and amplifier subunits (Fig. 2). The discriminator subunit is that part exposed on the exterior surface of the cell and may be indistinguishable from the long sought hormonal receptor. It embodies the specific structural features necessary for the recognition of, and binding with, the natural hormone. The catalytic unit is that part facing the interior of the cell and catalyzes the conversion of ATP to cyclic AMP. The discriminator or receptor unit is coupled to the catalytic unit via the transducer or coupling unit. This subunit transmits the information from the receptor after hormonal inter-action to the catalytic subunit leading to increased or decreased catalytic activity. Although the structural requirements for interaction with the receptor

EXTRACELLULAR

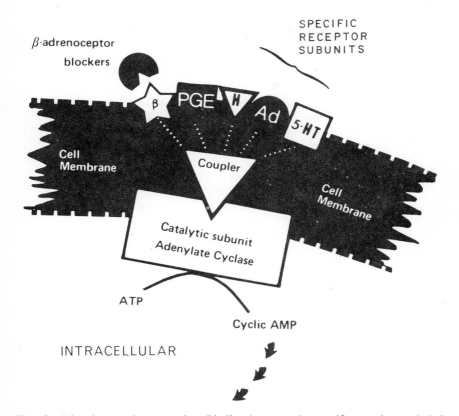

FIG. 2. Adenylate cyclase complex. Binding between the specific agonists and their specific receptor subunits (β, β-adrenergic; PGE, prostaglandin E; H, histamine; Ad, adenosine; and 5-HT, 5-hydroxytryptamine (serotonin)) activates the coupler subunit which in turn activates the catalytic subunit that catalyzes the conversion of ATP to cyclic AMP. β-Adrenoceptor blockers block the β-adrenergic receptor without blocking the effect of other hormones on the system.

subunit are well defined in many systems and the cofactor and other requirements for optimal activity of the catalytic subunit are also known, little, if any, information is available about the structure and/or function of the transducer or coupling subunit. It, thus far, remains a conceptual component of the AC complex. The coupling subunit appears to be the locus where cation interactions with the AC system occur. Furthermore, most disease-related aberrations in the cyclic AMP system seem to be closely related to abnormal function of this subunit (defective coupling), since it appears to have the major role of regulating the overall responsiveness or sensitivity of the entire system to hormones.

Several receptor subunits appear to be coupled to the same catalytic unit in many systems probably through a single coupler subunit. This conclusion is based primarily on the lack of additivity on cyclic AMP synthesis of maximal concentrations of several hormones (Fig. 2). This arrangement could at least theoretically represent a safety device to guard against excessive cyclic nucleotide synthesis when the cell is bombarded simultaneously with several hormones or drugs. The situation with GC could be similar but is probably more complex since its activity is not limited to cellular membranes (Sulakhe *et al.*, 1976; 1976a). Soluble GC activity appears to exist in a number of tissues.

3.1.2   *Cyclase sensitivity in disease*

By far the most common cyclic nucleotide abnormality in disease is the abnormal sensitivity of the nucleotidyl cyclase enzymes to the appropriate hormonal stimuli (Table 1). This is not unexpected since these cyclases represent the interface at which these stimuli induce biochemical responses in target cells. Examples are the reduced adenylyl cyclase (AC) sensitivity to

TABLE 1

Loss of cyclase sensitivity in disease

Disease	Hormone(s) involved	Hormone binding	NaF-Response	References
Aging	epinephrine, others	normal	normal	Cooper and Gregeman (1976)
Asthma	epinephrine, glucagon	normal	normal	Parker and Smith (1973), Haddock *et al.* (1975) Trembath and Shaw (1976)
Cancer	epinephrine, PGE, glucagon	?	normal	Martin *et al.* (1976)
Diabetes	insulin	normal or reduced		Cuatrecasas (1974)
Hyper-tension	epinephrine, glucagon	normal	normal	Amer (1975)
Obesity	epinephrine, ACTH	normal or reduced	normal	Laudat and Pairault (1975)
Psoriasis	epinephrine, PGE, glucagon	normal	normal	Aso *et al.* (1975)

Other diseases: eczema, cirrhosis, dwarfism (Kemp *et al.*, 1973), hypothyroidism (Grill and Rosenquist, 1975), nephrogenic diabetes insipidus (Dousa *et al.*, 1975) etc.

catecholamines in asthma (Fireman, 1973), hypertension (Amer, 1975), muscle dystrophy (Mawatari et al., 1974) and psoriasis (Mui et al., 1975), to ADH in diabetes insipidus (Fishman and Brooker, 1972), to epinephrine in immunodeficiency (Kemp et al., 1973), and to a variety of stimuli in tumor cells. Reduction in hepatic binding and in hepatic cyclic AMP responsiveness to glucagon may also occur in periods of sustained endogenous hyper-glucagonemia (Zenser et al., 1974). The factors responsible for the control of cyclase sensitivity are therefore of utmost importance to the disease process as a whole and may represent sites at which curative drugs may be required to act. Correction of the disease-related abnormality in the cyclase responsiveness is an extremely important site for drug development. If that were possible, tissue-specific and disease-specific drugs relatively free of possible side effects could be produced since the disease-associated loss of AC-sensitivity is both tissue and disease specific.

The disease-related loss of AC sensitivity, in addition, could lend itself to the development of new diagnostic techniques based on the measurement of AC sensitivity in tissue samples or in blood-formed elements. Similar techniques would also be valuable in monitoring the development of the disease process and the progress of drug treatment.

Acute and reversible decreases in cyclase sensitivity have been demonstrated in response to high levels of stimulating ligands in a number of systems in vitro (e.g. Remold-O'Donnell, 1974; Roy et al., 1976). Increased sensitivity of the cyclases in response to decreased levels of hormones are also expected (e.g. Sporn et al., 1976). Whether the loss of sensitivity of AC can become irreversible on prolonged exposure to the activating ligands in vivo and whether the mechanisms involved in vitro are similar to the disease-associated changes in AC sensitivity remains to be seen. Similar changes are frequently seen also in vivo (e.g. in brain ACs, Dismukes and Daly, 1976, and vas deferens GC, Hsu et al., 1976). From preliminary indications it appears that the loss of AC sensitivity following excessive hormonal exposure in vitro may be different in certain respects from the disease-associated sensitivity loss since the former is usually more selective to the specific hormones used to stimulate the enzyme and is normally associated with a reduction in the number of hormonal receptors (e.g. Mickey et al., 1975). In disease, the defect appears to occur primarily at the level of the coupling of the receptor to the catalytic subunit of AC with minimal agonist selectivity or receptor loss. This appears to be the case in at least some in vitro systems (Johnson and Perkins, 1976).

It is conceivable that excessive hormonal secretion (involving multiple hormones) and/or nervous tone at some early stage in disease development, possibly in an effort to control a deteriorating situation, results in the ultimate loss of hormonal sensitivity of the particular cyclase in the target tissue in question resulting in the loss of hormonal control. This may represent a primary biochemical lesion, at least in diseases where loss of AC-sensitivity has been documented. A hypothesis was proposed that uses this exact mechanism as the biochemical basis for the development of hypertension (Amer, 1975). It is therefore very important to understand the mechanisms involved in the control of cyclase sensitivity and the modalities essential for the maintenance of that sensitivity. Since excessive hormonal stimulation may trigger the disease-related hormonal AC subsensitivity, a possible corrective treatment of disease could involve reducing hormone levels and thus permitting the AC sensitivity to recover. Such an approach may in fact underlie the beneficial effects of β-blockers in hypertension (Amer, 1977) and of diet therapy in diabetes. The latter presumably acts via the associated decrease in the circulating blood levels of insulin (Maugh, 1976).

Several additional factors may also contribute to the disease-associated loss of AC sensitivity, e.g. increased calcium ion influx into the affected cells. Excess of Ca^{++} inhibits AC from a number of tissues and appears to play an important regulatory role in the response of the cyclase enzymes to hormones (Steer et al., 1974). Another factor is increased phosphodiesterase (PDE) activity which could result from the increased ionized Ca^{++} levels as well as from other factors (Amer and Kreighbaum, 1975). This does not appear to be the case in at least some systems (Su et al., 1976). Cyclic AMP and the catecholamines can, in addition, induce the synthesis of PDE (Pawlson et al., 1974) which could abort the AC catalyzed increase in cyclic AMP levels. Increased PDE activity characterizes a number of diseases including hypertension (Amer et al., 1974, 1975), psoriasis (Vorhees et al., 1975), hypothyroidism (Stouffer et al., 1974), and obesity (Lovell-Smith and Sneyd, 1974).

A number of mechanisms appear to be involved in the AC sensitivity loss following excessive agonist exposure. Protein synthesis is not consistently involved (Lauzon et al., 1976). Increased PDE activity was shown to occur following norepinephrine addition to astrocytoma cells (Browning et al., 1976), although this was not observed with Glioma cells (Franklin and Twose, 1976). Loss of binding sites (Mickey et al., 1976) were shown to occur in frog erythrocytes following excessive agonist exposure (Mukherjee et al., 1975). Protection of the receptors from agonist interaction, e.g. β-blockade in the case of β-stimulants, can protect AC from the loss of hormonal sensitivity (Mukherjee, 1975). Since, in the case of the β-receptors, antagonists bind at least as well as the agonists to the receptor, hormonal subsensitivity could not be only a function of receptor occupancy but must be related to agonist triggered events, e.g. the elevated cyclic AMP contents. Dibutyryl cyclic AMP caused unspecific desensitization of AC in human astrocytoma cells (Su et al., 1976a). Studies with glioma cells and Graafian follicle membranes tend to minimize the role that cyclic AMP could play in this process (Franklin and Twose, 1976;

Bockaert *et al.*, 1976). This should shed doubt on the value of binding techniques in the study of this phenomenon. Loss of hormone binding may be *only* a reflection of other more primary events.

Changes in the structure of the AC complex could also play an important role in the hormonal sensitivity of AC and could occur on at least three levels:

i. The receptor unit. Binding between the agonist and receptor could serve as an indicator of changes in receptor integrity.

ii. The coupler unit. Changes in the structure of this subunit could result in a change in the transmission of the signal resulting from the hormone–receptor interaction to the catalytic subunit. This could lead to either increased or decreased AC sensitivity.

iii. The catalytic unit. The involvement of this subunit in disease is uncommon since in most disease states examined the susceptibility of AC to stimulation by sodium fluoride is usually preserved. Thus, changes in AC sensitivity are probably not related to the changed catalytic ability of the enzyme to form cyclic AMP.

3.1.3   *Factors influencing cyclase sensitivity*

What are the factors that control AC sensitivity? Are these factors involved in the disease-associated loss of AC sensitivity? The answer to these questions may contain important information pertinent to the development of drugs designed to correct the disease related abnormalities in the cyclic nucleotide system. Some of the factors that appear to affect the hormonal AC sensitivity include:

3.1.3.1   *Nucleotides.* GTP and its nonhydrolysable analogues "guanylyl-imido diphosphate, Gpp(NH)p" and "guanylylmethylene diphosphate, Gpp(CH$_2$)p" have been found to greatly influence AC sensitivity in a large number of systems (Rodbell *et al.*, 1974). These systems include rat liver (Flores and Sharp, 1975) and fat cells (Ebert and Schwabe, 1974), adrenal cortex, heart (Lefkowitz, 1975), avian erythrocytes, thyroid, anterior pituitary and platelets. GTP appears to bind to specific receptors and induce a more stimulated state of the enzyme AC in a manner similar in many respects to that of cholera toxin (Sevilla *et al.*, 1976). In fact GTP may be acting on the same site as cholera toxin since the effect of GTP and cholera toxin on the enzyme are not additive. GTP enhanced the sensitivity of the AC to a variety of hormones and hormone-like substances including prostaglandins (Zenser et al., 1974), glucagon (Sweat and Wincek, 1973), luteinizing hormone (Deery and Howell, 1973), thyroid-stimulating hormone (Sato *et al.*, 1974), catecholamines, calcitonin, parathyroid hormone, vasopressin and secretin. It was proposed that GTP acts by enhancing the dissociation of the bound hormone from its binding site, thus allowing for more frequent interaction of the receptor with the hormone molecules (Lacombe and Hanoune, 1974). The reverse situation may prevail, however, in fat cell membranes (Cooper et al., 1976). There is now some doubt that ATP in extremely high concentration can take over the functions of GTP (Kimura et al., 1976). It is interesting to note that F⁻, GTP, and cholera toxin can inhibit AC activity when added to a maximally stimulated system (Rodbell, 1975). Fully stimulated solubilized AC–GTP complex is generally not sensitive to hormones and AC stimulants, e.g. in fat cell membranes (Cooper et al., 1976). GTP–AC complex also displays characteristics different from unstimulated AC including temperature stability (Harwood et al., 1973).

The binding site for GTP is believed by many to be on the coupler unit of the AC complex, to modulate the response to all hormones (Dalton et al., 1973). GTP may, by binding with the coupler unit, produce an active coupler-GTP-catalytic unit complex that is maximally stimulated and fixed in the fully active state.

3.1.3.2 *Phospholipids*. The studies of Levey (1972) with solubilized cat myocardial AC have generated great interest in the role of phospholipids in modulating and coupling the receptor to catalytic activity of AC. Levey has shown a differential effect of different phospholipids in restoring specific hormonal sensitivity to the hormonally insensitive soluble cat myocardial AC. Phosphatidylserine restored histamine and glucagon sensivity and phosphatidylinositol restored the norepinephrine-sensitivity. Gangliosides were also shown by Mullin et al. (1976) to interact with thyrotropin and cholera toxin in a similar manner resulting in conformational changes in the thyrotropin and the cholera β-chains essential for AC activation by the α-chains. Addition of phosphatidylserine selectively increases the stimulation of rat pancreas AC by pancreozymin-octapeptide (Kempen et al., 1974). Significant differences between the different phospholipids were also observed in the response to different hormones since the enhancement of the response to pancreozymin was not true for secretin. Phospholipids have strong effects on AC hormonal sensitivity both from liver (Rubalcava and Rodbell, 1973) and thyroid plasma membranes (Yamashita and Field, 1973). Fatty acids and membrane lipid-perturbing agents were also reported to have strong effects on AC coupling (Limbird and Lefkowitz, 1976; Orly and Schramm, 1975). Most of these effects do not appear to involve the catalytic unit of AC.

3.1.3.3 *Maintenance hormones*. The permissive effects of several "maintenance hormones" on the action of other "information transferring hormones" is well known. This permissive effect appears to be translated, at least in the systems examined so far, primarily into maintaining a state of hormonal sensitivity of the cyclase enzymes (e.g. growth hormone and glucagon sensitivity, August and Hung, 1976; thyroid hormones and epinephrine sensitivity, Armstrong and Stouffer, 1974). Although some of the maintenance hormones, particularly the steroids, may act at sites other than cyclic nucleotide generation, a major site of their activity remains at the cell membrane.

Estrogen pretreatment enhanced the cyclic AMP response of uteri (Cheu and Rinard, 1974). Adrenal steroids also appear to have a dual influence on vasopressin sensitivity of AC in the kidney. Studies in the laboratories of Jard (Rajerison et al., 1974) showed that adrenalectomy in rats reduced the kidney medulla AC sensitivity to vasopressin with only minimal loss of hormone binding. It is interesting to note that the loss of sensitivity to vasopressin was selective in that it was not observed with parathyroid hormone. Aldosterone treatment enhanced vasopressin-binding but did not restore the AC coupling loss. Dexamethasone enhanced both the AC coupling and the membrane binding of vasopressin. Adrenal steroids therefore appear to exert a dual action on the vasopressin-sensitive AC cyclase of the rat kidney:

a. modulation of the number of receptor sites (mineral- and corticosteroids);
b. control of synthesis of a component enhancing receptor-enzyme coupling (only corticosteroids).

It is interesting to note that in normal animals, the coupling efficiency of AC is not maximal, since the response of normal kidney cyclase to vasopressin can be increased by dexamethasone with little, if any, effect on the binding of the hormone.

Glucocorticoids potentiated the plasma rise in cyclic AMP in response to norepinephrine in dogs (Issekutz, 1975). They also stimulated the cyclic AMP response to norepinephrine in glial tumor cells in culture (Brostrom et al., 1974). Similar effects on AC sensitivity may also underlie the effects of progesterone in synergizing the effects of epinephrine on intraoccular pressure (Chang and Thomas, 1973), and those of dexamethasone on the stimulation by glucagon of ion fluxes in adrenalectomized rats (Friedman and Dambach, 1973) and the induction of amino acid transport (Kletzien et al., 1975). Effects on AC coupling may also underlie the potentiation by testosterone (Greenberg et al., 1974) and prolactin (Manku et al., 1973) of the pressor responses to norepinephrine and tyramine, e.g. the diminished pressor response to norepinephrine in pregnant rats. Androgens may act via similar mechanisms in diabetes, where estrogens and corticoids may have the opposite effects (Houssay et al., 1954). Similar mechanisms may underlie the steroid mediated excessive responsiveness to the pressor effects of the catecholamines (Dagett and Franks, 1977), and the restoration of their bronchiodilator effects in asthma (Parker et al., 1973).

3.1.3.4 *Prostaglandins.* These important and very active lipids appear to play a very important role in the regulation of cyclase sensitivity. In some systems they appear as obligatory intermediates in cyclase activation. In general, the role that prostaglandins play in biology is not well understood, but their effects on cyclic nucleotide metabolism are very significant. In fact, the cyclic nucleotides may represent the only system via which the effects of the prostaglandins are translated into biological events. Prostaglandins enhance the hormonal sensitivity of many AC systems. Among these are isoproterenol and secretin sensitivity of pancreatic islet AC (Thompson *et al.*, 1976) and bradykinin sensitivity of normal fibroblasts (Ishikawa *et al.*, 1976). Indomethacin treatment completely abolishes cyclic AMP response to bradykinin in normal fibroblasts which become similar to transformed fibroblasts. The latter are unresponsive to bradykinin.

A role for prostaglandins and their endoperoxides as feedback regulators in adipose ghosts has been proposed (Gorman *et al.*, 1975). A similar role was also proposed to explain their excessive production in obesity. The prostaglandins are clearly involved in the generation and maintenance of spontaneous activity in a number of tissues and have been shown to modulate the responses of a number of tissues to hormones, e.g. the responses of vascular smooth muscles to the catecholamines (Goldyne and Winkelmann, 1973).

3.1.3.5   *Ions.* The effects of fluoride ions on AC are well known (Manganiello and Vaughan, 1976). In many respects, the effects are similar to, and in others different from, those of cholera toxin, GTP or its analogues. Chloride, bromide and iodide also have significant stimulant effects. The stimulant effects of azide ions on GC from a number of tissues have also been described. NaN_3 also appears capable of stimulating AC from rat liver (Johnson *et al.*, 1975). Polycations, apparently acting unspecifically via charge effects, produce general stimulation of AC from beef thyroid membranes (Wolff and Cook, 1975). Mg^{++} may play an important role in the process of desensitization of LH-dependent AC in Graafian follicle membranes (Bockaert *et al.*, 1976).

Activation of AC by hormones was postulated (Steer and Levitzki, 1975, 1975a) to involve the release of enzyme bound Ca^{++} and thus removing the AC inhibition generally observed with Ca^{++}. This is supported by the facts that (a) Ca^{++} release is the first observed event of hormonal stimulation in many systems; (b) although Ca^{++} addition frequently does not inhibit hormonal stimulation, it does so in presence of calcium ionophores that equilibrate intra- with extracellular Ca^{++}, and (c) Ca^{++} also stimulates phosphodiesterase and thus lowers the rate of cyclic nucleotide accumulation. Furthermore, Ca^{++} appears to be essential for the activity of GC and plays a very important role in the actions of cyclic GMP (Wallachand Pastan, 1976).

3.1.3.6   *Feedback modulators.* A number of factors have been described both with large and small molecular weights that appear to be involved in feedback regulation of AC sensitivity. Among the small molecular weight candidates are adenosine (Schwabe, 1973), lactate, cyclic AMP (Lehotay and Murphy, 1975), Ca^{++} and others. A number of protein factors were also described by Ho and Sutherland (1975) and Cheung et al. (1975). The latter is apparently the same Ca^{++} dependent PDE activator (Huang et al., 1975) also described by Breckenridge's group (Brostrom et al., 1975) and by Izumi et al. (1975). Production of protein feedback regulators may account for the effects of protein synthesis inhibitors on the AC-sensitivity loss following excessive agonist exposure (Vellis and Brooker, 1974; Ciosek et al., 1975; Franklin et al., 1975).

The problem of the specificity of hormonal subsensitivity loss previously discussed is important not only from the point of view of similarity or dissimilarity to the disease process, but also from the view of the possible mediating factors. Specific phospholipids appear involved in specific coupling of certain specific hormonal receptors to the catalytic subunit. Specific hormonal sensitivity loss may indicate that such mediators are involved. Ho and Sutherland's feedback modulator (1975) appears to mediate a nonspecific hormonal sensitivity loss in adipocytes. AC sensitivity is uniformly lost to a number of hormones including epinephrine, ACTH and glucagon. Such factors are likely to be involved in disease where uniform hormonal sensitivity loss is observed. Loss of AC sensitivity in many systems, although unspecific, may occur on different time scales for the different agonists (Haslam and Goldstein, 1974), e.g. growth fibroblasts in vitro (epinephrine and PGE) and the loss of sensitivity with age to epinephrine and glucagon in rat liver (Christoffersen, 1973). This could imply the involvement of a number of specific factors.

From the point of view of developing new drugs, one should also be interested in conditions where enhanced AC sensitivity occurs and in the factors involved. Cold exposure (Muirhead and Himms-Hagen, 1974) and muscular exercise (Yakovlev, 1974) produce greater increases in AC response to epinephrine over and above that seen in basal and fluoride stimulated enzyme. The factors involved are unknown. Enrichment of cell membranes with unsaturated fatty acids also enhanced the response of adipose tissue cell membranes to norepinephrine (Coumis, 1973). Addition of fatty acids (Orly and Schramm, 1975), endotoxin (Spitzer, 1974) and cholera toxin (Ganguly and Greenough, 1975), in vitro, also enhanced the isoproterenol response of AC.

3.1.3.7 *Adenylate and guanylate cyclase interactions.* Adenylate and guanylate cyclases appear to be coupled together in more than one way. Changes in the hormonal sensitivity of one may be associated with opposite changes in the sensitivity of the other, e.g. the effects of lysolecithin (Shier et al., 1976) and in most disease states (Amer, 1975). Energy availability (Amer and Byrne, 1975) appears to determine which cyclase is to be involved and subsequently what metabolic machinery will be brought into action in response to hormones. α-Adrenergic receptors blockers which presumably inhibit cyclic GMP generation are capable, at least in some systems, of preventing the development of AC subsensitivity to excessive hormonal stimulation (see Fleisch and Titus, 1972). Corticosteroids enhance the response and coupling of AC and decrease the response and coupling of GC. Cortisone is a classic agent causing insulin resistance which may involve loss of GC insulin sensitivity. Progestins also cause insulin resistance which is easily demonstrated in pregnancy.

3.1.3.8 *Drugs.* A number of drugs appear to influence hormonal cyclase sensitivity. Amphetamine was reported to decrease the AC sensitivity to norepinephrine in mouse brain, which may be secondary to excessive stimulation of norepinephrine receptors (Martres *et al.*, 1975). Lithium was also reported to inhibit AC sensitivity to norepinephrine and prostaglandin E_1 in a number of systems (Murphy *et al.*, 1973). More importantly α-adrenocepter blocking agents were reported capable of reversing the reduced AC sensitivity to iso-proterenol in asthmatics (Alston *et al.*, 1974; Assem and Paterson, 1974).

3.2 LOSS TO EXTRACELLULAR FLUID

The loss of the cyclic nucleotides from cells is an important factor in the control of their intracellular levels. Released cyclic nucleotides can be valuable indicators of hormonal activity (Catt *et al.*, 1972) since they reflect the "free", metabolically active pool(s) (Kuster *et al.*, 1973). The system regulating cyclic nucleotide leakage represents an important site for drugs that can act by stimulating or inhibiting the release of cyclic nucleotides to the extracellular fluids and thus indirectly affecting the size of their free intracellularly active pools. Whether the same factors are involved in the transport of the cyclic nucleotide into the cells are also involved in their leakage out of the cells (Ryan and Durick, 1972) is not at all clear. Present evidence appears to indicate that loss of cyclic nucleotides to extracellular fluid accounts for the readily assayable levels of these nucleotides in plasma. This led some investigators to consider a possible primary messenger function for these nucleotides. However, this consideration is complicated by the notorious inability of these nucleotides to cross cellular membranes necessitating extremely high extra-cellular levels, above those normally encountered *in vivo* probably due to extracellular metabolism (Gorin and Brenner, 1976).

Loss of cyclic nucleotides to the outside of cells may at least partly explain the rapid decay of the hormonally induced rises in intracellular cyclic nucleo-tides in some systems even in the continued presence of the stimulating hormones. This complicates studies designed to correlate cyclic nucleotide levels with hormonal effects.

Leakage of cyclic nucleotides to the extracellular fluid appears sensitive to drug effects. In man, probenecid caused a substantial increase in the cyclic AMP level in lumbar spinal fluid (Cramer *et al.*, 1973). Adenosine also enhances the release of cyclic AMP from cortical tissue, an effect sensitive to inhibition by Ca^{++} (Pull and McIlwain, 1973). The loss of cyclic AMP into the cerebrospinal fluid also appears to increase in coma or head trauma (Rudman *et al.*, 1976) and thus could serve as a valuable indicator of the progression of that condition.

3.3 DEGRADATION

Stimulation and inhibition of cyclic nucleotide degradation, via effects on cyclic nucleotide phosphodiesterases, (PDEs), are very important mechanisms for controlling their intracellular levels, and historically represented the most fertile sources of prototype drugs. The central importance of cyclic nucleotide PDEs in drug design stems from the significant role that they must play in the control of intracellular cyclic nucleotide levels coupled with their apparent sensitivity to a large variety of chemical structures (Amer and Kreighbaum, 1975).

Abnormal levels or forms of PDEs are associated with, and appear to contribute to, the cyclic nucleotide abnormalities in a number of disease states. Furthermore, various hormones may act by modulating the activity of the PDEs in their target tissues. In a number of situations, the intracellular levels of the cyclic nucleotides and their related effects appear to be correlated closely with the level of PDE activity. It appears that the PDEs represent more than just an off-switch for the cyclic nucleotide system and that they share with the cyclases the important function of the delicate control of the intracellular cyclic nucleotide levels and consequently their myriad of important effects.

Although the cyclases, at least theoretically, present a possibly superior locus for the modulation of intracellular cyclic nucleotide levels, they presently occupy a position secondary to the PDEs as a target for drug development. This limitation may not include, however, the compounds that can specifically block the stimulatory effects of the natural hormones on the cyclase enzymes where a slightly wider selection of chemical entities allows for the development of still better and possibly more selective blockers of hormonal effects on the cyclase enzymes (Murad, 1973). Conversely, PDEs, owing to their apparent sensitivity (both stimulation and inhibition) to a wider selection of chemical structures, present a more fertile field for development of new drugs with wider ranges of actions and selectivity. Because of the wide involvement of the cyclic nucleotides in nearly all facets of cellular activity there is no limit to the range of pharmacological effects that PDE modifiers may produce, hence the central importance of PDEs for modern drug development.

Several factors play important roles in the use of PDEs for drug development. These factors include:

3.3.1 Different forms of PDEs in the same cell lines

Multiple forms of PDEs have been shown to exist under a wide variety of conditions and from a large number of sources (for review see Amer and Kreighbaum, 1975). These forms appear to differ mainly in their substrate affinities, heat and cation sensitivities, substrate specificities, chromatographic and electrophoretic mobilities, subcellular localization, and, possibly, function. The presence of multiple forms may explain the frequently anomalous kinetic behavior of these enzymes. It also allows for speculation as to the mode and manner in which these forms may be involved in the moment-to-moment control of PDE activity and, consequently, the moment-to-moment control of the basal cyclic nucleotide levels.

Most investigators in this area agree that only two main forms of the enzyme exist in any homologous tissue preparation; multiple forms could only be an artifact of the heterogeneity of the tissues used (e.g. Thompson *et al.*, 1976). A case in point is the work of Uzunov and Weiss (1972) who found at least six forms of the enzyme in rat brain. However, when homologous preparations of rat astrocytoma cells were examined, only two forms were found (Uzunov *et al.*, 1973).

3.3.1.1 *High and low K_m forms.* The two forms of PDE differ in a number of aspects, and in particular in affinity for their substrates. Since there are two naturally occurring substrates for these enzymes, cyclic 3',5'-adenosine monophosphate (cyclic AMP) and cyclic guanosine-3',5' monophosphate (cyclic GMP), two forms of the enzyme may exist for each substrate. Some tissues, however, appear to contain only one substrate-specific form of the enzyme. For example, human blood platelets (Amer and Mayol, 1973), and rat brain seem to contain one cyclic GMP–PDE (Brooker *et al.*, 1968).

The resolution of the two forms is best achieved by kinetic analysis at a wide range of substrate concentrations (Amer and McKinney, 1972), particularly if coupled by physical separation. Table 2 summarizes the kinetic parameters of the enzyme forms present in a number of tissues obtained by kinetic analysis combined with chromatography. The methods used are quite simple and can easily detect the presence of two forms of the enzyme.

The presence of multiple forms of the PDE enzymes stimulated speculation as to which, if either, of the two forms is more important in the control of the intracellular cyclic nucleotide levels. Since the intracellular levels of the cyclic nucleotide are in the micromolar range or lower, the low K_m, high affinity PDE (Form II) is favored for this role. In most tissues, Form II has a K_m value close

TABLE 2

Cyclic AMP and cyclic GMP phosphodiesterases from a number of tissues[a]

Tissue	Cyclic AMP (cAMP)				Cyclic GMP (cGMP)				Total V_m cAMP / Total V_m cGMP
	$K_m I^b$	$K_m II^b$	V_m^c	$\%V_m II^d$	$K_m I^b$	$K_m II^b$	V_m^c	$\%V_m II^d$	
Human blood platelets[e]	$6\cdot1 \times 10^{-4}$	$3\cdot2 \times 10^{-6}$	$0\cdot025$	$4\cdot2$	$1\cdot6 \times 10^{-5}$		$0\cdot009$	—	$2\cdot84$
Monkey brain (sediment)	$1\cdot7 \times 10^{-2}$	$1\cdot7 \times 10^{-5}$	$0\cdot081$	$30\cdot3$	$1\cdot4 \times 10^{-4}$		$0\cdot019$	—	$4\cdot20$
Monkey brain (supernate)	$3\cdot0 \times 10^{-4}$		$0\cdot282$	—	$3\cdot2 \times 10^{-4}$		$0\cdot478$	—	$0\cdot59$
Rabbit brain (sediment)	$6\cdot6 \times 10^{-3}$	$5\cdot6 \times 10^{-5}$	$0\cdot130$	$21\cdot1$	$1\cdot7 \times 10^{-4}$	$3\cdot7 \times 10^{-6}$	$0\cdot073$	$19\cdot4$	$1\cdot78$
Rabbit brain (supernate)	$1\cdot9 \times 10^{-3}$	$9\cdot8 \times 10^{-5}$	$0\cdot390$	$8\cdot7$	$6\cdot6 \times 10^{-5}$	$2\cdot9 \times 10^{-6}$	$0\cdot122$	$7\cdot8$	$3\cdot20$
Rabbit fundic mucosa	$4\cdot7 \times 10^{-4}$	$1\cdot2 \times 10^{-6}$	$0\cdot139$	$14\cdot3$	$2\cdot7 \times 10^{-4}$	$5\cdot4 \times 10^{-7}$	$0\cdot185$	$13\cdot7$	$0\cdot75$
Rabbit gallbladder	$4\cdot0 \times 10^{-3}$	$6\cdot0 \times 10^{-6}$	$0\cdot059$	$14\cdot6$	$4\cdot0 \times 10^{-3}$	$3\cdot0 \times 10^{-7}$	$0\cdot028$	$12\cdot6$	$2\cdot10$
Rabbit heart	$1\cdot7 \times 10^{-2}$	$4\cdot1 \times 10^{-6}$	$0\cdot104$	$13\cdot0$	$2\cdot0 \times 10^{-4}$	$3\cdot3 \times 10^{-6}$	$0\cdot023$	$21\cdot4$	$4\cdot47$
Rabbit intestines	$5\cdot9 \times 10^{-5}$	$1\cdot0 \times 10^{-6}$	$0\cdot048$	$26\cdot6$	$4\cdot6 \times 10^{-4}$	$3\cdot4 \times 10^{-6}$	$0\cdot137$	$4\cdot5$	$0\cdot35$
Rabbit kidneys	$5\cdot1 \times 10^{-4}$	$5\cdot5 \times 10^{-6}$	$0\cdot456$	$5\cdot7$	$2\cdot2 \times 10^{-3}$	$2\cdot0 \times 10^{-5}$	$0\cdot328$	$5\cdot9$	$1\cdot39$
Rabbit liver	$6\cdot9 \times 10^{-5}$	$4\cdot0 \times 10^{-7}$	$0\cdot358$	$3\cdot1$	$7\cdot2 \times 10^{-5}$	$4\cdot0 \times 10^{-6}$	$0\cdot416$	$19\cdot5$	$0\cdot86$
Rabbit pyloric mucosa	$2\cdot7 \times 10^{-3}$	$8\cdot7 \times 10^{-6}$	$0\cdot117$	$24\cdot3$	$1\cdot1 \times 10^{-5}$	$1\cdot2 \times 10^{-6}$	$0\cdot041$	$17\cdot2$	$2\cdot85$

[a] Cyclic AMP and cyclic GMP phosphodiesterase activities were determined in $4000 \times g$ supernates at 15 substrate concentrations. The incubation mixture contained ³H-cyclic AMP or ³H-cyclic GMP ($2 \times 10^{-11} - 2 \times 10^{-6}$ mol), $0\cdot9$ μmol MgSO$_4$, and 25 μmol tris buffer at pH 7·5 in a total volume of 0·5 ml.

[b] Michaelis–Menten constant.

[c] Enzyme maximal velocity, μmol hydrolyzed per 30 min at 30° per 20 mg wet tissue.

[d] Per cent of total V_m as form II.

[e] $10\,000 \times g$ supernate of platelet homogenates was used. Platelets from 6·3 ml of blood were used per assay.

to 10^{-6} M, at least two orders of magnitude lower than that of the high K_m, low affinity Form I.

Only recently has the importance of Form II in the control of intracellular cyclic nucleotide levels in intact cells become more apparent. In tissues from a variety of hypertensive rats, the intracellular levels of cyclic nucleotides are inversely correlated with the Form II activity present. No such correlation existed with Form I activity, which was also measured in these same studies (Amer, 1973; Amer et al., 1974, 1975). The role, if any, played by Form I is open to question; studies utilizing high substrate concentrations that would preferably measure Form I activity are, therefore, of questionable significance. At the present time, studies utilizing low substrate concentrations, in the micromolar range, that would preferentially reflect Form II activity appear to be more valuable since such studies would reflect the activity of the enzyme most probably involved in the *in vivo* control of intracellular cyclic nucleotide levels.

Most of the reported PDE activity in different tissues was determined at relatively high substrate concentrations and would, under most experimental conditions, represent the form that is probably less important *in vivo*. This led to the somewhat misleading conclusion that PDE activity may be 100 times the adenylate cyclase activity in some tissues (Bucher and Sutherland, 1962).

The structural relationships between the two main forms of the enzyme are far from clear. Studies on the molecular structure of the two forms must await further purification of the different PDEs. Furthermore, it is not completely clear whether cyclic AMP hydrolysis is carried out by the same set of enzymes that also catalyzes the hydrolysis of other cyclic nucleotides. There are some indications in certain tissues that one of the two forms of the enzyme may be an artifact of the isolation procedures employed.

From the point of view of drug development, the sensitivities of the two forms of PDEs to activators or inhibitors appear to be different. This is a very important point, since it is doubtful that agents acting on only the high K_m forms of the enzymes would be useful. It appears that screening compounds for possible activity against PDEs should stress the importance of the low K_m forms, since these are likely to be the more critical. An impressive example of drug selectivity for the low K_m PDE is that of adenosine on the enzymes from human blood platelets. As can be seen in Fig. 3, adenosine inhibited the Form II activity with no effect on the Form I activity present in the platelet homogenates (Amer and Marquis, 1971).

3.3.1.2 *Particulate and soluble forms.* In a number of studies, the particulate nature of Form II was clearly stressed. Its presence on the external surface of cells has been well documented. This, in combination with its apparent calcium and hormonal sensitivity, supports the possible role of Form II as a hormonal

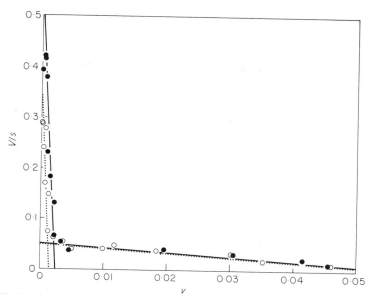

FIG. 3. Eadie plots for the effects of adenosine (10^{-4} M) on phosphodiesterase activity from human blood platelet membrane-supplemented whole homogenates. Note the selective inhibition by adenosine on Form II (vertical trace) while no effect is evident on Form I (lower trace). Control, ●; adenosine 10^{-4} M, ○.

receptor. In addition, there are some reports supporting an inhibitory effect of calcium ions on PDE activity in certain tissues.

The presence of soluble and particulate forms of PDE should lead to a reconsideration of the role of the enzyme in the control of cyclic nucleotide levels. The occurrence of soluble and particulate forms of the same enzyme differing in kinetic parameters is not unknown. For example, malate dehydrogenase occurs in both soluble and particulate forms in Neurospora (Benveniste and Munkres, 1970). It could be hypothesized that the active form of PDE is membrane bound and is in equilibrium with a soluble, low affinity form. Association or dissociation from the membranes would represent activation or inactivation of the enzyme, respectively. The membranous site for the attachment of the enzyme could then represent a receptor site for the action of ligands affecting intracellular cyclic nucleotide levels via activating or inactivating PDE. More gentle methods for the preparation and assay of PDE should be used to avoid the transfer of activity to the soluble fraction and the consequent obliteration of induced effects. Some recent studies with insulin support such a hypothesis (Manganiello and Vaughan, 1973).

3.3.1.3 *Interchangeability of different forms.* The significance of the presence of two main enzymes with two widely varying affinities for the hydrolysis of either cyclic nucleotide is not entirely clear. There are indications that the two forms are interconvertible (Amer and McKinney, 1972; Amer and Marquis, 1972; Pichard and Cheung, 1976; Pichard and Kaplan, 1975). This makes it possible to speculate that the two dimorphs of PDE could provide adequate means of controlling PDE activity *in vivo*. Form I may represent a large store of the enzyme which is quickly convertible to the higher affinity Form II when the need arises (Song and Cheung, 1971). It may also serve the function of handling sudden surges of cyclic nucleotide concentrations. Form II would be the form normally concerned with the control of the *in vivo* cyclic nucleotide levels.

3.3.2   *Different forms in different cell lines*

One prime requirement in drug development is the tissue specificity of the drug in question. The differences between the PDEs from different tissues appear to be large enough to support the use of this enzyme as a target for the development of new drugs. There appear to be both structural and kinetic differences among the PDEs isolated from different tissues. These differences are reflected in the differential sensitivities to drugs of the enzymes from different sources and even from neighboring areas of the brain (Uzunov and Weiss, 1971). Therefore, testing the responses of PDEs from different tissues may provide preliminary clues to the possible tissue selectivity of the drug in question.

3.3.3   *Cyclic GMP versus cyclic AMP PDEs*

Although several pyrimidine and purine cyclic nucleotides are hydrolyzed by different tissue preparations, the significance of this observation is presently unclear since only two main cyclic nucleotides appear to occur in nature both of which are purines. The hydrolysis of the two naturally occurring cyclic nucleotides was thought at one time to be catalyzed by the same set of enzymes. Present evidence, however, points to the possible existence of two different sets of enzymes with widely different affinities for the two naturally occurring cyclic nucleotides.

Recent studies seem to emphasize the differences between cyclic AMP and cyclic GMP PDEs in subcellular localization, cation requirements, and response to drugs. Since the two naturally occurring cyclic nucleotides appear to mediate different, if not antagonistic, events in many systems, it is significant to recognize the functionally different natures of the cyclic AMP and cyclic GMP PDEs. The selective effects of drugs on these enzymes will greatly determine their biological effects on the tissues examined. This is exemplified by the effects of theophylline on PDE preparations from the guinea pig stomach and lung, using each cyclic nucleotide as a substrate (Table 3).

TABLE 3

Inhibitor constants $(K_i)^a$ of theophylline on form II activity from guinea pig lung and stomach using cyclic AMP or cyclic GMP as substrate[b]

Substrate	Lung	Stomach
Cyclic AMP	4×10^{-4}	4×10^{-4}
Cyclic GMP	2×10^{-3}	$1 \cdot 3 \times 10^{-4}$

[a] Molar, determined as described by Dixon (1964).
[b] Assayed according to Thompson and Appleman (1971) at substrate concentrations of 1 and 2 μM and six drug concentrations.

Theophylline shows greater selectivity for cyclic AMP phosphodiesterase than for cyclic GMP PDE in the lung than in the stomach. This may at least partially explain the effects of theophylline in the two tissues.

Not only do the selective effects of a drug on cyclic AMP and cyclic GMP PDEs vary from tissue to tissue but also the effects in the same tissue vary with different drugs. The effects of the three PDE inhibitors, theophylline, papaverine, and glycyrrhetinic acid, on the enzymes from the fundic mucosa of three species serve to illustrate the latter point (Table 4). Greater selectivity for cyclic AMP PDE is correlated with greater inhibitory effect on gastric acid secretion. The three compounds have profoundly different selectivities for the specific PDEs and produce different effects on the output of the system.

The realization of the possible importance of substrate selectivity in the use of phosphodiesterases as targets for the development of new drugs is quite recent. Little screening work has been reported where different substrates for the enzymes were used. This matter will probably attract more and more attention.

One important point to stress in this respect is the ability of each naturally occurring cyclic nucleotide to influence the rate of hydrolysis of the other. Thus, compounds selectively affecting the specific PDE for either nucleotide will have indirect effects on the activity of the other. This is complicated by the ability of either cyclic nucleotide to both stimulate and inhibit the rate of hydrolysis of the other, depending on its concentration. This may provide an explanation for the nonconforming effects of exogenously applied cyclic nucleotides in some systems, as in the stimulatory effects of cyclic AMP on the contraction of some smooth muscles. It also may explain the antagonistic effects of some drugs on the levels of the two cyclic nucleotides.

A model enzyme system composed of specific subunits with affinity for cyclic AMP and others for cyclic GMP has been proposed (Appelman et al., 1973). It is quite apparent that cyclic GMP may be involved as an in vivo regulator of PDE activity. The greater sensitivity of the cyclic GMP–PDE to

TABLE 4

Selectivity of theophylline, papaverine hydrochloride, and glycyrrhetinic acid for low K_m cyclic AMP and cyclic GMP phosphodiesterase from the fundic mucosa of three species and their effects on acid secretion[a]

	Dog			Rat			Rabbit			Effect of gastric acid
Substrate	Cyclic AMP	Cyclic GMP	G/A[b]	Cyclic AMP	Cyclic GMP	G/A[b]	Cyclic AMP	Cyclic GMP	G/A[b]	
Theophylline	50[c]	26[c]	0.5	38[c]	17[c]	0.5	44[c]	17[c]	0.4	potentiates
Papaverine	2	2·6	1·3	2·5	2·8	1·1	2·5	3	1·2	no effect
Glycyrrhetinic acid	7	13	1·9	4·0	10	2·5	7·5	15	2·0	inhibits

[a] Enzyme activity was determined by a radioactive assay technique.

[b] G/A = K_i (cyclic GMP as substrate)/K_i (cyclic AMP as substrate) M; higher numbers indicate greater selectivity for cyclic AMP phosphodiesterase.

[c] Inhibitor constants (K_i), Molar $\times 10^{-5}$. Determined at two substrate (0·8 and 1 $\times 10^{-6}$ M cyclic AMP and 1 and 2 $\times 10^{-6}$ M cyclic GMP) and six drug concentrations bracketing the K_i value.

calcium ions (Kakiuchi *et al.*, 1971) strongly emphasizes this possibly important role.

In general, there is greater affinity of PDE for cyclic GMP than for cyclic AMP. This may be related to the generally lower *in vivo* concentrations of cyclic GMP.

The previously unsuspected selectivity of PDE inhibitors for either cyclic AMP or cyclic GMP enzymes may provide an explanation for the anomalous behavior of some of these compounds *in vivo*. For example, papaverine, although far more potent than theophylline as an inhibitor of cyclic AMP PDE, is less potent than expected in elevating plasma free fatty acids and blood glucose.

3.3.4   *Natural modulators of PDE activity*

Protein activators for PDE were isolated from a number of tissues (Cheung, 1971). These activators appear to mediate the stimulatory effects of calcium ions on the enzyme activity from the brain and possibly other tissues as well (Ho *et al.*, 1977). The protein PDE activators may prove important as natural regulators of the enzyme activity and in the mechanism of action of drugs in PDE activity (Donelly, 1976). Natural protein inhibitors for PDE have also been described which in some systems may also have other functions (Staniel *et al.*, 1973). A heat-stable, nondialyzable PDE inhibitor was also isolated from soybeans (Brewin and Northcote, 1973) and slime mold (Cheung, 1970).

ATP, pyrophosphate, adenosine, citrate, isocitrate, pyruvate, oxalate, malate, and tartrate were reported to inhibit the enzyme activity. The possible role of any or all of these intermediates in the control of PDE activity *in vivo* remains to be determined. The possible physiological role, if any, of these inhibitors in the control of the enzyme activity has not been established.

Whether interference with the effects of these activators or inhibitors can present a mechanism for possible drug effects on PDE remains to be seen. Also it is not clear whether these activators or inhibitors are collectively similar or different.

Cyclic nucleotides appear to be capable of inducing PDE synthesis. Evidence obtained primarily from studies with tissue cultures and bacteria strongly supports a role for cyclic AMP in the control of PDE synthesis, probably via a cyclic nucleotide-dependent protein kinase mechanism (Bourne *et al.*, 1973).

3.3.5   *Effects of hormones*

Several hormones, including insulin, ACTH, growth hormone, cholecystokinin, gastrin, aldosterone, histamine, epinephrine, prostaglandins, corticoids, thyroxine, and plant cytokinesins have been reported to change PDE activities in their target issues (Amer and Kreighbaum, 1975). In most of these situations, the forms of the enzyme affected appear to be the particulate low K_m, high affinity forms. These effects tend to bolster the possible hormonal receptor function of PDE and particularly its low K_m forms (Tria *et al.*, 1976; Selstam and Rosenberg, 1976).

In none of these situations, however, has the importance of the PDE effects been unequivocally established in the mechanisms of action of these hormones. It is not clear whether the hormonal effects on PDE are primary or secondary since similar effects are produced by cyclic GMP or its hydrolysis product GMP. In addition, it is not clear whether these hormonal effects could lend themselves to modulation via the use of drugs. The hormonal effects on PDE remain potentially important.

3.3.6 *Activators*

Compounds reported to stimulate phosphodiesterase are not as numerous as those that can inhibit it. Since the most common abnormalities in cyclic nucleotide metabolism usually result in lower levels of these important mediators, inhibition of their degradation is the more desirable therapeutic target. Nevertheless, activators are of interest in diseases associated with elevated cyclic nucleotide levels, e.g. cyclic AMP in diabetes, cholera, alcoholism, and mania and cyclic GMP in psoriasis and hypertension (Amer and Kreighbaum, 1975).

Several compounds of widely different structures were reported to activate phosphodiesterase from a variety of tissues (Amer and Kreighbaum, 1975). These activators include nitroglycerin, papaverine and a vitamin E derivative (Sakai *et al.*, 1976). The effects of these compounds on phosphodiesterase could be indirect. In most systems, crude preparations of the enzyme were used and effects on cyclic GMP synthesis and/or metabolism cannot be ruled out. Cyclic GMP has repeatedly been shown to have significant effects on cyclic AMP phosphodiesterase activity.

3.3.7 *PDE in disease*

In some diseases as in hypertension, cancer (Singer *et al.*, 1976), diabetes, hyperthyroidism, psoriasis and obesity, increased activity of the low K_m, high affinity phosphodiesterase may be an important part of the etiology of the disease state (Amer, 1975; Nagasaka and Hidaka, 1976). In these conditions, the use of appropriate PDE inhibitors could alleviate the deficiency in intracellular cyclic AMP by the most desired mechanism for any drug, namely, by correcting a basic biological defect, e.g. RO-1724 in psoriasis (Stawiski *et al.*,

1976). There is also evidence that PDE activity may be decreased in diabetes and hepatomas.

In some diseases, the lowered cyclic AMP levels in target tissues are associated with decreased sensitivity of adenylyl cyclase to hormonal stimulation. The most feasible approach to correct the cyclic AMP deficiency under these circumstances would be the inhibition of PDE. Examples of these conditions are hypertension, asthma, psoriasis and, possibly, cancer.

3.3.8   General comments

Many compounds thought to act via PDE inhibition and the consequent cyclic nucleotide accumulation are weak inhibitors of the enzyme, with K_i values often in the millimolar range. In most of these situations, it is doubtful that the compounds could attain high enough concentrations *in vivo* for effective PDE inhibition. Often, insignificant or only marginal *in vivo* PDE inhibition could be demonstrated; yet some accumulation of the cyclic nucleotides may occur. The latter may become evident only if accompanied with cyclase stimulation.

A popular example of this is theophylline, a weak PDE inhibitor with a K_i value of about 1 mmol or greater in most systems. It is doubtful that it reaches this high concentration *in vivo* when administered in the usual therapeutic doses. No *in vivo* PDE inhibition by theophylline could be demonstrated in most systems, yet theophylline by itself sometimes produces small elevations of cyclic nucleotide tissue levels when administered *in vivo*. It is widely believed, however, that PDE inhibition and the consequent cyclic nucleotide elevations represent the main mechanism for its biological effects. The potentiation of hormonal effects by theophylline is one main criterion stipulated by Sutherland to verify the possible mediator role of cyclic nucleotides in the mechanism or action of the hormones.

Most PDE inhibitors, including the more active ones, cause relatively small accumulations of cyclic nucleotides when compared with the amounts generally produced via adenylate or guanylate cyclase stimulation. In many systems, small cyclic nucleotide elevations is all that is needed for maximal stimulation of the specific physiological response studied. Often it is not clear what role, if any, the extremely high cyclic nucleotide levels, which are sometimes produced via cyclase stimulation, play in the physiological effects observed since, in most instances, these effects are usually essentially complete at much lower intracellular levels of the cyclic nucleotides.

It should always be remembered that PDE inhibition may represent only one of several effects that PDE inhibitors can produce. Some of these other effects may be totally independent of the cyclic nucleotide system and may, in certain instances, be the major contributors to the drug's pharmacological effects of these agents. Other properties of these agents may also play a role in determining their effects on the cyclic nucleotide system *in vivo*, e.g. the ability of the drug to reach the enzyme. Membrane permeability may have been important in the case of xanthine derivative, where striking differences between its *ex vivo* and *in vitro* potency on phosphodiesterase were demonstrated (Iwangoff and Enz, 1973).

A negative feedback role for the PDE activator has been proposed where stimulation of cAMP synthesis activates protein kinase to phosphorylate a binding protein that usually binds the activator. Phosphorylation releases the activator which then activates PDE and gets rid of the excess cyclic AMP (Gnegy *et al.*, 1976). This somewhat agrees with the hypothesized translocation of the activated and inactive forms of the kinase.

Are the abnormal and new PDE activities in disease different enough to allow for specific drug development? Can one inhibit the allosteric modulation of the PDE system? These are very important questions, the answer to which may contain clues to specific drug design.

The PDEs have stimulated the development of many new drugs. A good illustration of the use of the cyclic nucleotide system for the development of useful drugs is in the development of the antihypertensive agent, prazosin (Hess, 1975). Here, structure–activity relationships of the two PDE inhibitors papaverine and theophylline were studied and the important structural features of both molecules were combined. This led to the synthesis of prazosin (Hess, 1974). Prazosin is interesting as a PDE inhibitor, since it demonstrates greater activity on cyclic AMP–PDE in the vasculature and on cyclic GMP–PDE in the heart. This confers an additional advantage to its profile as an antihypertensive agent, i.e. myocardial inhibition to counter the reflex cardiostimulation generally associated with vasodilator antihypertensive agents.

4   Effects on intracellular activity

4.1   BOUND AND FREE POOLS

Several lines of evidence strongly indicate the existence of at least two pools of cyclic AMP: one free, and the other bound (Schultz and Daley, 1973; Zakarija and McKenzie, 1973; Khac *et al.*, 1973) mirroring the different pool of the precursor ATP (Rapaport and Zamecnik, 1976). A similar situation may also prevail for cyclic GMP. Bound cyclic nucleotides are apparently unavailable for PDE hydrolysis and there is evidence to support the existence of at least one membrane-bound pool. Methods of measuring both bound and free pools are becoming available and cyclic nucleotide effects appear to be related to the size of the free pools. Although no drugs are yet known that can change the sizes of these pools, this remains an important potential mechanism for drug action.

4.2 PROTEIN KINASES

The relative inability of the natural cyclic nucleotides to cross cellular membranes limits to a great extent their utility as drugs in cyclic nucleotide-deficiency diseases. This has stimulated a search for cyclic nucleotide derivatives that can penetrate cellular membranes with greater ease, while retaining the ability to activate the cyclic nucleotide-dependent protein kinases which are thought to translate the effects of the cyclic nucleotides into meaningful biochemical events. The importance of this potential mechanism is underscored by the possible involvement of protein kinase in disease (e.g. cardiac hypertrophy (Byus et al., 1976), atherosclerosis (Davies et al., 1975), and hypertension (Kuo et al., 1976)) and in the mechanism of action of at least some hormones. Several cyclic nucleotide derivatives have been prepared and tested for activity against protein kinases from a variety of sources with excellent drug possibilities (Simon et al., 1973). Some of these do reproduce the effects of hormones independant of the hormonal receptors (for an example see Evans et al., 1976). Some well-known drugs, including tolbutamide Kanamori et al., 1974), furosemide, and mefenamic acid and phenylbutazone (Dinnendahl et al., 1973), were shown to directly affect protein kinase activity. Thus, the possibilities of this site for drug development appear promising.

Agents capable of antagonizing the intracellular effects of the cyclic nucleotide also present a potential approach that would be particularly useful in situations where excessive cyclic nucleotide synthesis may represent a disease-related defect, e.g. cyclic AMP in diabetes, alcoholism, cholera, and mania, and cyclic GMP in psoriasis and hypertension.

5 Indirect effects

5.1 PROSTAGLANDINS

The cyclic nucleotides appear to be obligatory intermediates in the action of the prostaglandins (Kuehl et al., 1971; Braun and Shiozawa, 1973; Kahn and Lands, 1973). The latter thus represent an important target for modulation of the cyclic nucleotide system via effects on prostaglandin metabolism, e.g. prostaglandin antagonists and prostaglandin synthesis inhibitors. The prostaglandins also appear to be obligatory intermediates in the actions of at least some hormones and drugs on the cyclic nucleotide system. Some exceptions to this are also known (Süsskand et al., 1976). It is of interest to note that the cyclic nucleotides can also modulate the synthesis of prostaglandins, suggesting a complex system involving both prostaglandins and cyclic nucleotides in the regulation of tissue responses to hormones. When applied exogenously, prostaglandins of the E type appear to stimulate the synthesis of cyclic AMP, whereas those of the F type appear to act via increased cyclic GMP. Thus, there are reasonable grounds for the assumption of strict coupling between the prostaglandin system on the one hand and the cyclic nucleotide system on the other.

5.2   IONS

Since several enzymes with varying cofactor requirements are involved in the cyclic nucleotide system, it is at least theoretically possible to modulate the system significantly by controlling the availability of the essential co-factors. Of these factors, Ca^{++} occupies a commanding position. Ca^{++} generally inhibits AC activity, is essential for GC activity, modulates PDE activity and its efflux may be controlled by the prostaglandins (see Rodan and Feinstein, 1976, for an example). Furthermore, activation of protein kinase by cyclic AMP seems to enhance Ca^{++} uptake. The importance of Ca^{++} to the functioning of cyclic nucleotide system is indicated by the lack of hormonal response in Ca^{++}-free media in many systems despite the observed accumulation of the cyclic nucleotides.

6   Cyclic nucleotides and drug actions

The cyclic nucleotides now appear to be involved in the mechanisms of action of a large variety of drugs, both old (e.g. morphine (Askew and Charalampous, 1976)) and new, encompassing nearly all pharmacology (Amer and McKinney, 1975). In fact, it is exceptional to find a drug that does not invoke, in the responsive tissues, a change in intracellular cyclic nucleotide levels which appear to mediate at least part of the activity of almost all classes of drugs including those thought to act primarily via other mechanisms, e.g. the non-steroidal anti-inflammatory agents that are supposed to act via inhibition of prostaglandin synthesis (Peters *et al.*, 1975). This is not unexpected since the cyclic nucleotides appear to function primarily as universal messengers that translate changes in the extracellular milieu into intracellular biochemical, and hence functional, responses. For this reason, in many instances, the relationship between the cyclic nucleotide changes and the pharmacologic effects of drugs may only be incidental and not causally related. Care must therefore be exercised in drawing the conclusion that cyclic nucleotides mediate the pharmacologic effects of any particular drug.

That a drug may influence the intracellular metabolism of the cyclic nucleotides in a particular *in vitro* system is not by itself sufficient to implicate these messengers in mediating its effects on that system under normal therapeutic circumstances. Other criteria similar to those established for the hormones must be satisfied before it can be concluded that the drug in question acts via the cyclic nucleotide system. Such criteria may require that the drug effects on the cyclic nucleotide system:

a. precede its pharmacological actions;
b. be shown to occur in the appropriate intact organ system in a dose related manner;
c. occur at *in vivo* therapeutic concentrations;
d. be modified in a predictable way by other compounds with known activity on the cyclic nucleotide system;
e. be blocked under the same conditions that result in blockade of the drug-induced pharmacologic effects;
f. be mimicked by the appropriate cyclic nucleotides or their derivatives.

It should also be recognized that actions on the cyclic nucleotide system may represent only one of several effects a particular drug may produce and hence may not account for all the activities of a compound in a particular system. This has been shown to be the case for a number of PDE inhibitors. In addition, the cyclic nucleotides not only mediate the activities of a large variety of drugs but they also appear to mediate some of their well-known side effects, e.g. salivary gland enlargement following isoproterenol therapy appears to be mediated by cyclic AMP.

A final complication in understanding the role that cyclic nucleotides may play in the mechanism of action of drugs is the present sparsity of data on the involvement of cyclic GMP. Most of the reported studies deal primarily with cyclic AMP which represents only part of the total picture. It is hoped that the availability of better and simpler methods for the study of cyclic GMP will expedite fuller characterization of its role in the actions of drugs. This is expected to result in better correlations between cyclic nucleotide metabolism and drug action.

7 Summary

There are a number of sites at which drugs can affect the cyclic nucleotide system. Some of these sites are more attractive for drug development where tissue selectivity, specificity of desirable actions and minimal side effects are of paramount importance. Greater understanding of the factors operating at these sites and their susceptibility to drug effects must be achieved before successful and deliberate design of useful drug entities can be made. The involvement of cyclic nucleotides in disease makes it, at least theoretically, possible to produce agents that could correct the basic metabolic disease-associated abnormalities and thus could be more curative than presently available drugs. Possibilities for prophylactic approaches designed to minimize or even circumvent the disease-associated changes in cyclic nucleotide metabolism can also be explored. The close association and collaboration between the biochemical pharmacologists, chemists and other biologists and the long-term commitment of the pharmaceutical industry can move these considerations from the realm of possibility into the realm of reality.

References

Alston, W. C., Patel, K. R. and Kerr, J. W. (1974). *British Medical Journal*, i, 90.

Amer, M. S. (1973). *Science*, **179**, 807.

Amer, M. S. (1974). *Gastroenterology*, **67**, 333.

Amer, M. S. (1975). *Life Sciences*, **17**, 1021.

Amer, M. S. (1977). *Biochemical Pharmacology*, **26**, 171.

Amer, M. S. and Byrne, J. E. (1975). *Nature*, **256**, 421.

Amer, M. S. and Kreighbaum, W. E. (1975). *Journal of Pharmacological Science*, **64**, 1.

Amer, M. S. and Marquis, N. R. (1971). *In* "Prostaglandins in Cellular Biology" (Eds P. W. Ramwell and B. B. Pharriss), p. 93. Academic Press, New York and London.

Amer, M. S. and Mayol, R. F. (1973). *Biochemica et Biophysica Acta*, **309**, 149.

Amer, M. S. and McKinney, G. R. (1972). *Journal of Pharmacology and Experimental Therapeutics*, **183**, 535.

Amer, M. S. and McKinney, G. R. (1973). *Life Sciences*, **13**, 753.

Amer, M. S. and McKinney, G. R. (1974). *Annual Reports in Medicinal Chemistry*, **9**, 203.

Amer, M. S. and McKinney, G. R. (1975). *Annual Reports in Medicinal Chemistry*, **10**, 192.

Amer, M. S., Gomoll, A. W., Perhach, Jr., J. L., Ferguson, H. C. and McKinney, G. R. (1974). *Proceedings of the National Academy of Sciences, USA*, **71**, 4930.

Amer, M. S., Doba, N. and Reis, D. J. (1975). *Proceedings of the National Academy of Sciences, USA*, **72**, 2135.

Appleman, M. M., Thompson, W. J. and Russell, T. R. (1973). *In* "Advances in Cyclic Nucleotide Research" (Eds P. Greengard and G. A. Robison) p. 65. Raven Press, New York.

Armstrong, K. J. and Stouffer, J. E. (1974). *Journal of Biological Chemistry*, **249**, 4226.

Askew, W. E. and Charalampous, K. D. (1976). *Experientia*, **32**, 1454.

Aso, K., Deneau, D. G., Krulic, L., Wilkinson, D. I. and Farber, E. M. (1975). *Journal of Investigative Dermatology*, **64**, 326.

Assem, E. S. K. and Paterson, S. (1974). *British Medical Journal*, i, 457.

August, G. P. and Hung, W. (1976). *Journal of Clinical Endocrinology and Metabolism*, **43**, 1029.

Benveniste, K. and Munkres, K. D. (1970). *Biochimica et Biophysica Acta*, **220**, 161.

Bilezikian, J. P. and Aurbach, G. D. (1973). *Journal of Biological Chemistry*, **248**, 5577.

Birnbaumer, L., Pohl, S. L., Kraus, M. L. and Rodbell, M. (1970). *Psychopharmacology*, **3**, 185.

Bockaert, J., Hunzicker-Dunn, M. and Birnbaumer, L. (1976). *Journal of Biological Chemistry*, **251**, 2653.

Bourne, H. R., Tomkins, G. M. and Dion, S. (1973). *Science*, **181**, 952.

Braun, W. and Shiozawa, C. (1973). *In* "Prostaglandins and Cyclic AMP" (Eds R. H. Khan and W. E. M. Lands), p. 21. Academic Press, New York and London.

Brewin, N. J. and Northcote, D. H. (1973). *Biochimica et Biophysica Acta*, **320**, 104.

Brooker, G., Thomas, L. J. and Appleman, M. M. (1968). *Biochemistry*, **7**, 4177.

Brostrom, M. A., Kon, C., Olson, D. R. and Breckenridge, B. M. (1974). *Molecular Pharmacology*, **10**, 711.

Brostrom, C. O., Huang, Y-C., Breckenridge, B. M. and Wolff, D. J. (1975). *Proceedings of the National Academy of Sciences, USA*, **72**, 64.

Browning, E. T., Brostrom, C. O. and Groppi, Jr., V. E. (1976). *Molecular Pharmacology*, **12**, 32.

Butcher, R. W. and Sutherland, E. W. (1962). *Journal of Biological Chemistry*, **237**, 1244.

Byus, C. V., Chubb, J. M., Huxtable, R. J. and Russell, D. H. (1976). *Biochemical and Biophysical Research Communications*, **73**, 694.

Catt, K. J., Watanabe, K. and Dufae, M. L. (1972). *Nature*, **239**, 280.

Cheung, W. Y. (1970). *Biochemical and Biophysical Research Communications*, **38**, 533.

Cheung, W. Y. (1971). *Journal of Biological Chemistry*, **246**, 2859.

Cheung, W. Y., Bradham, L. S., Lynch, T. J., Lin, Y. M. and Tallant, E. A. (1975). *Biochemical and Biophysical Research Communications*, **66**, 1055.

Chew, C. S. and Rinard, G. A. (1974). *Biochimica et Biophysica Acta*, **362**, 493.

Chiang, T. S. and Thomas, R. P. (1973). *European Journal of Pharmacology*, **22**, 304.

Christoffersen, T., Osnes, J. B. and Oye, I. (1973). *Acta Physiologica*, **5**, 9.

Ciosek, Jr., C. P., Fahey, J. V., Ishikawa, Y. and Newcombe, D. S. (1975). *Journal of Cyclic Nucleotide Research*, **1**, 229.

Cohen, K. L. and Bitensky, M. W. (1969). *Journal of Pharmacology and Experimental Therapeutics*, **169**, 80.

Cooper, B. and Gregerman, R. I. (1976). *Journal of Clinical Investigation*, **57**, 161.

Cooper, B., Partilla, J. S. and Gregerman, R. I. (1976). *Biochimica et Biophysica Acta*, **445**, 246.

Counis, R. (1973). *Biochimica et Biophysica Acta*, **306**, 391.

Cramer, H., Ng, L. K. Y. and Chase, T. N. (1973). *Archives de Neurologie*, **29**, 197.

Cuatrecasas, P. (1974). *Biochemical Pharmacology*, **23**, 2353.

Daggett, P. and Franks, S. (1976). *British Medical Journal*, i, 84.

Dalton, C., Hope, H. and Sheppard, H. (1973). *Federation Proceedings*, **32**, 3290.

Davis, C. W., Murthy, V. V. and Kuo, J. F. (1975). *Federation Proceedings*, **32**, 3290.

Deery, D. and Howell, S. L. (1973). *Biochimica et Biophysica Acta*, **329**, 17.

DeVillis, J. and Brooker, G. (1974). *Science*, **186**, 1221.

Dinnendahl, V., Peters, H. D. and Schonhafer, P. S. (1973). *Naunyn-Schmiedeberg's Archives of Pharmacology*, **278**, 293.

Dismeekes, R. K. and Daly, J. W. (1976). *Journal of Cyclic Nucleotide Research*, **2**, 321.

Donnelly, Jr., T. E. (1976). *Archives of Biochemistry and Biophysics*, **173**, 375.

Dorigo, P., Visco, L., Fiandini, G. and Fassina, G. (1973). *Biochemical Pharmacology*, **22**, 1957.

Dousa, T. P., Hui, Y. F. S. and Barnes, L. D. (1975). *Endocrinology*, **97**, 802.

Ebert, R. and Schwabe, U. (1974). *Naunyn-Schmiedeberg's Archives of Pharmacology*, **286**, 297.

Evans, D. B., Parham, C. S., Schenck, M. T. and Laffan, R. J. (1976). *Journal of Cyclic Nucleotide Research*, **2**, 307.

Fallon, E. G., Agrawal, R., Furth, E., Steiner, A. L. and Cowden, R. (1974). *Science*, **184**, 1089.

Ferrendelli, J. A., Johnson, Jr., E. M., Chang, M-M. and Needleman, P. (1973). *Biochemical Pharmacology*, **22**, 3133.

Fichman, M. P. and Brooker, G. (1972). *Journal of Clinical Endocrinology and Metabolism*, **35**, 3547.

Fireman, P. (1973). *International Archives of Allergy*, **45**, 123.

Fleisch, J. H. and Tituse (1972). *Journal of Pharmacology and Experimental Therapeutics*, **181**, 425.

Flores, J. and Sharp, G. W. G. (1975). *Journal of Clinical Investigation*, **56**, 1354.

Franklin, T. J. and Twose, P. A. (1976). *FEBS Letters*, **66**, 225.

Franklin, T. J., Morris, W. P. and Twose, P. A. (1975). *Molecular Pharmacology*, **11**, 485.

Friedmann, N. and Dambach, G. (1973). *Biochimica et Biophysica Acta*, **307**, 399.

Ganguly, U. and Greenough III, W. B. (1975). *Proceedings of the National Academy of Sciences, USA*, **72**, 3561.

Gnegy, M. E., Costa, E. and Uzunov, P. (1976). *Proceedings of the National Academy of Sciences, USA*, **73**, 352.

Goldberg, N. D., O'Dea, R. F. and Haddox, M. K. (1973). *In* "Advances in Cyclic Nucleotide Research" (Eds P. Greengard and G. A. Robison), p. 155. Raven Press, New York.

Goldyne, M. E. and Winkelmann, R. K. (1973). *Journal of Investigative Dermatology*, **60**, 258.

Gorin, E. and Brenner, T. (1976). *Biochemica et Biophysica Acta*, **451**, 20.

Gorman, R. R., Hamburg, M. and Samuelsson, B. (1975). *Journal of Biological Chemistry*, **250**, 6460.

Greenberg, S., George, W. R., Kadowitz, P. J. and Wilson, W. R. (1974). *Canadian Journal of Physiology and Pharmacology*, **52**, 14.

Greengard, P. and Robison, G. A. (1971–6). *In* "Advances in Cyclic Nucleotide Research" (Eds P. Greengard and G. A. Robison), vol. 1–7. Raven Press, New York.

Grill, V. and Rosenquist, U. (1975). *Acta Endocrinologia*, **78**, 39.

Haddock, A. M., Patel, K. R., Alston, W. C. and Kerr, J. W. (1975). *British Medical Journal*, **ii**, 357.

Harwood, J. P., Löw, H. and Rodbell, M. (1973). *Journal of Biological Chemistry*, **248**, 6239.

Haslam, R. J. and Goldstein, S. (1974). *Biochemical Journal*, **144**, 253.

Hess, H. J. (1975). *Hospital Formulary*, 9.

Hess, H. J. (1975). Postgraduate Medicine Prazosin Symposium Proceedings, 9.

Ho, H. C., Wirch, E., Stevens, F. C. and Wang, J. H. (1977). *Journal of Biological Chemistry*, **252**, 43.

Ho, R. J. and Sutherland, E. W. (1975). *Proceedings of the National Academy of Sciences, USA*, **72**, 1773.

Houssay, B. A., Foglia, V. G. and Rodriquez, R. R. (1954). *Acta Endocrinologia*, **17**, 146.

Hsu, C-Y, Leighton, H. J., Westfall, T. C. and Brooker, G. (1976). *Journal of Cyclic Nucleotide Research*, **2**, 359.

Huang, Y-C, Wolff, D. J. and Brostrom, C. O. (1975). *Federation Proceedings*, **34**, 2253.

Ishikawa, Y., Ciosek, Jr., C. P., Fahey, J. V. and Newcombe, D. S. (1976). *Journal of Cyclic Nucleotide Research,* **2,** 115.

Issekutz, T. B. (1975). *American Journal of Physiology,* **229,** 291.

Iwangoff, P. and Enz, A. (1973). *Experientia,* **29,** 1067.

Izumi, H., Hideko, O. and Ozawa, H. (1975). *Japanese Journal of Pharmacology,* **25,** 375.

Johnson, G. L. and Perkins, J. P. (1976). *Federation Proceedings,* **35,** 191.

Johnson, R. A., Pilkis, S. J. and Hamet, P. (1975). *Journal of Biological Chemistry,* **250,** 6599.

Kacew, S. and Singhal, R. L. (1973). *Life Sciences,* **13,** 1363.

Kahn, R. H. and Lands, E. M. (1973). *In* "Prostaglandins and Cyclic AMP" (Eds R. H. Kahn and E. M. Lands). Academic Press, New York and London.

Kakiuchi, S., Yamazaki, R. and Teshima, Y. (1971). *Biochemical and Biophysical Research Communications,* **42,** 968.

Kalish, M. I., Pineyro, M. A., Cooper, B. and Gregerman, R. I. (1974). *Biochemical and Biophysical Research Communications,* **61,** 781.

Kanamori, T., Hayakawa, T. and Nagatsu, T. (1974). *Biochemical and Biophysical Research Communications,* **61,** 781.

Kemp, R. G., Huang, Y-C. and Duquesnoy, R. J. (1973). *Journal of Immunology,* **111,** 1855.

Kempen, H. J. M., DePont, J. J. H. H. M. and Bonting, S. L. (1974). *Biochimica et Biophysica Acta,* **370,** 573.

Khac, L. D., Harbon, S. and Clauser, H. J. (1973). *European Journal of Biochemistry,* **40,** 177.

Kimura, N., Nakane, K. and Nagata, N. (1976). *Biochemical and Biophysical Research Communications,* **70,** 1250.

Kletzien, R. F., Pariza, M. W., Becker, J. E. and Potter, V. R. (1975). *Nature,* **256,** 46.

Kuehl, Jr., F. A., Humes, J. L., Mandel, L. R., Cirillo, V. J., Zanetti, M. E. and Ham, E. A. (1971). *Biochemical and Biophysical Research Communications,* **44,** 1464.

Kuo, J. F., Davis, C. W. and Tse, J. (1976). *Nature,* **261,** 335.

Kuo, W-N., Hodgins, D. S. and Kuo, J. F. (1973). *Biological Chemistry,* **348,** 2705.

Kuo, W-N., Shoji, M. and Kuo, J. F. (1976). *Federation Proceedings,* **35,** 2093.

Kuster, J., Zapf, J. and Jakob, A. (1973). *FEBS Letters,* **32,** 73.

Lacombe, M-L. and Hanoune, J. (1974). *Biochemical and Biophysical Research Communications,* **59,** 474.

Laudat, N-H. and Pairault, J. (1975). *European Journal of Biochemistry,* **56,** 583.

Lauzon, G. J., Kulshrestha, S., Starr, L. and Bär, H-P. (1976). *Journal of Cyclic Nucleotide Research,* **2,** 99.

Lefkowitz, R. J. (1975). *Journal of Biological Chemistry,* **250,** 1006.

Lehotay, D. C. and Murphy, E. P. (1975). *Endocrinology Research Communications,* **2**(647), 431.

Levey, G. S. (1972). *Journal of Molecular and Cellular Cardiology,* **4,** 283.

Limbird, L. E. and Lefkowitz, R. J. (1976). *Molecular Pharmacology,* **12,** 559.

Lovell-Smith, C. J. and Sneyd, J. G. T. (1974). *Diabetologia,* **10,** 655.

Manganiello, V. and Vaughan, M. (1973). *Journal of Biological Chemistry,* **248,** 7164.

Manganiello, V. and Vaughan, M. (1976). *Journal of Biological Chemistry,* **251,** 6205.

Manku, M. S., Nassar, B. A. and Horrobin, D. F. (1973). *Lancet,* **i,** 991.

Martin, T. J., Hunt, N. H., Boyd, H., Ellison, M., Michelangeli, V. P. and Atkins, D. (1976). *Clinical Endocrinology,* **5,** S373.

Martres, M-P., Baudry, M. and Schwartz, J-C. (1975). *Nature,* **255,** 731.

Maugh II, T. H. (1976). *Science*, **193**, 220.

Mavier, P. and Hanoune, J. (1975). *European Journal of Biochemistry*, **59**, 593.

Mawatari, S., Takagi, A. and Rowland, L. P. (1974). *Archives de Neurologie*, **30**, 96.

Mickey, J., Tate, R. and Lefkowitz, R. J. (1975). *Journal of Biological Chemistry*, **250**, 5727.

Mickey, J. V., Tate, R., Mullikin, D. and Lefkowitz, R. J. (1976). *Molecular Pharmacology*, **12**, 409.

Mui, M. M., Hsia, S. L. and Halprin, K. M. (1975). *British Journal of Dermatology*, **92**, 225.

Muirhead, M. and Himms-Hagen, J. (1974). *Canadian Journal of Biochemistry*, **52**, 176.

Mukherjee, C., Caron, M. G. and Lefkowitz, R. J. (1975). *Proceedings of the National Academy of Sciences, USA*, **72**, 1945.

Mullin, B. R., Fishman, P. H., Lee, G., Aloj, S. M., Ledley, F. D., Winand, R. J., Kohn, L. D. and Brady, R. O. (1976). *Proceedings of the National Academy of Sciences, USA*, **73**, 842.

Murad, F. (1973). *Biochimica et Biophysica Acta*, **304**, 181.

Murphy, D. L., Donnelly, C. and Moskowitz, J. (1973). *Clinical Pharmacology and Therapeutics*, **14**, 810.

Nagasaka, A. and Hidaka, H. (1976). *Biochimica et Biophysica Acta*, **438**, 449.

Najjar, V. A. and Constantopoulos, A. (1973). *Molecular and Cellular Biochemistry*, **2**, 87.

O'Donnell, E. R. (1974). *Journal of Biological Chemistry*, **249**, 3615.

Orly, J. and Schramm, M. (1975). *Proceedings of the National Academy of Sciences, USA*, **72**, 3433.

Parker, C. W., Huber, M. G. and Baumann, M. L. (1973). *Journal of Clinical Investigation*, **52**, 1342.

Parker, C. W. and Smith, J. W. (1973). *Journal of Clinical Investigation*, **52**, 48.

Peters, H. D., Dinnendahl, V. and Schonhofer, P. S. (1975). *Naunyn-Schmiedebergs Archiv für Experimentelle Pathologie und Pharmakologie*, **289**, 29.

Pfeuffer, T. and Thomas, R. (1974). *Hoppe-Seyler's Zeitschrift für Physiologische Chemie*, **355**, 1237.

Pichard, A-L. and Cheung, W. Y. (1976). *Journal of Biological Chemistry*, **251**, 5726.

Pichard, A-L. and Kaplan, J-C. (1975). *Biochemical and Biophysical Research Communications*, **64**, 342.

Pull, I. and McIlwain, N. (1973). *Biochemical Journal*, **136**, 893.

Rajerison, R., Marchetti, J., Roy, C., Bockaert, J. and Jard, S. (1974). *Journal of Biological Chemistry*, **249**, 6390.

Rapaport, E. and Zamecnik, P. C. (1976). *Proceedings of the National Academy of Sciences, USA*, **73**, 3122.

Rodan, G. A. and Feinstein, M. B. (1976). *Proceedings of the National Academy of Sciences, USA*, **73**, 1829.

Rodbell, M. (1975). *Journal of Biological Chemistry*, **250**, 5826.

Rodbell, M., Lin, M. C., Salomon, Y., Londos, C., Harwood, J. P., Martin, B. R., Rendell, M. and Berman, M. (1974). *Acta Endocrinologia*, **77**, 11.

Roufogalis, B. D., Thornton, M. and Wade, D. N. (1976). *Life Sciences*, **19**, 927.

Roy, C., Guillon, G. and Jard, S. (1976). *Biochemical and Biophysical Research Communications*, **72**, 1265.

Rubalcava, B. and Rodbell, M. (1973). *Journal of Biological Chemistry*, **218**, 3831.

Rudman, D., Fleischer, A. and Kutner, M. H. (1976). *New England Journal of Medicine*, **295**, 635.

Ryan, W. L. and Durick, M. A. (1972). *Science*, **177**, 1002.
Sakai, T., Okano, T., Makino, H. and Tsudzuki, T. (1976). *Journal of Cyclic Nucleotide Research*, **2**, 163.
Sato, S., Yamada, T., Furihata, R. and Makiuchi, M. (1974). *Biochimica et Biophysica Acta*, **332**, 166.
Schmidt, J. J. and Najjar, V. A. (1976). *Federation Proceedings*, **35**, 1797.
Schultz, J. and Daley, J. W. (1973). *Journal of Biological Chemistry*, **248**, 843.
Schwabe, U., Ebert, R. and Erbler, H. C. (1973). *Naunyn-Schmiedeberg's Archives of Pharmacology*, **276**, 133.
Schwartz, J. P. and Passonneau, J. V. (1974). *Proceedings of the National Academy of Sciences, USA*, **71**, 3844.
Selstam, G. and Rosberg, S. (1976). *Acta Endocrinologia*, **81**, 563.
Sevilla, N., Steer, M. L. and Levitzki, A. (1976). *Biochemistry*, **15**, 3493.
Shier, W. T., Baldwin, J. H., Nilsen-Hamilton, M., Hamilton, R. T. and Thanassi, N. M. (1976). *Proceedings of the National Academy of Sciences, USA*, **73**, 1586.
Simon, L. N., Schuman, D. A. and Robins, R. K. (1973). *In* "Advances in Cyclic Nucleotide Research" (Eds P. Greengard and G. A. Robison), p. 225. Raven Press, New York.
Singer, A. L., Sherwin, R. P., Dunn, A. S. and Appleman, M. M. (1976). *Cancer Research*, **36**, 60.
Song, W. Y. and Cheung, W. Y. (1971). *Biochimica et Biophysica Acta*, **242**, 593.
Spitzer, J. A. (1974). *Proceedings of the Society for Experimental Biology and Medicine*, **145**, 186.
Sporn, J. R., Harden, T. K., Wolfe, B. B. and Malinoff, P. B. (1976). *Science*, **194**, 624.
Staniel, G. M., Leunz, K. M. T. and Gorski, J. (1973). *Biochemistry*, **12**, 2130.
Stawiski, M., Rusin, L., Schork, M. A., Burns, T., Duell, E. and Vorhees, J. (1976). *Clinical Research*, **24**, 267A.
Steer, M. L., Atlas, D. and Levitzki, A. (1974). *New England Journal of Medicine*, **292**, 409.
Steer, M. L. and Levitzki, A. (1975). *Archives Biochemistry and Biophysics*, **167**, 371.
Steer, M. L. and Levitzki, A. (1975). *Journal of Biological Chemistry*, **250**, 2080.
Stouffer, J. E., Armstrong, K. J., Inovergen, R. Van, Thompson, W. J. and Robinson, G. A. (1974). Abstracts, 2nd International Conference on Cyclic AMP **MP-2**, 32.
Su, Y. F., Cebeddu, L. and Perkins, J. P. (1976). *Journal of Cyclic Nucleotide Research*, **2**, 257.
Su, Y. F., Johnson, G. L. and Cebeddu, L. (1976). *Journal of Cyclic Nucleotide Research*, **2**, 271.
Sulakhe, P. V., Sulakhe, S. J., Leung, N. L-K., St. Louis, P. J. and Hickie, R. A. (1976). *Biochemical Journal*, **157**, 705.
Sulakhe, S. J., Leung, N. L-K. and Sulakhe, P. V. (1976a). *Biochemical Journal*, **157**, 713.
Süsskand, K., Siess, M. and Schultz, J. (1976). *Biochemical Pharmacology*, **25**, 1959.
Sweat, F. W. and Wincek, T. J. (1973). *Biochemical and Biophysical Research Communications*, **55**, 522.
Thompson, W. J., Johnson, D. G. and Williams, R. H. (1976a). *Biochemistry*, **15**, 1658.
Thompson, W. J., Ross, C. P., Pledger, W. J. and Strada, S. J. (1976b). *Journal of Biological Chemistry*, **251**, 4922.

Trembath, P. W. and Shaw, J. (1976). *British Journal of Clinical Pharmacology,* **3**, 1001.

Tria, E., Scapin, S., Cocco, C. and Luly, P. (1976). *Biochimica et Biophysica Acta,* **496**, 77.

Tsang, B. K., Kacew, S. and Singhal, R. L. (1976). *Biochemical Pharmacology,* **25**, 1985.

Uzunov, P. and Weiss, B. (1972). *Biochimica et Biophysica Acta,* **284**, 222.

Uzunov, P. and Weiss, B. (1971). *Neuropharmacology,* **10**, 697.

Uzunov, P., Shein, H. M. and Weiss, B. (1973). *Science,* **180**, 304.

Vesely, D. L. and Levey, G. S. (1977). *Biochemical and Biophysical Research Communications,* **74**, 780.

Vorhees, J. J., Colburn, N. H., Stawiski, M., Duell, E. A., Haddox, M. and Boldberg, N. D. (1974). *In* "Cold Spring Harbor Laboratory Symp. on Regulation of Proliferation in Animal Cells" (Eds B. Clarkson and R. Baserga). p. 635.

Wallach, D. and Pastan, I. (1976). *Biochemical and Biophysical Research Communications,* **72**, 859.

Wallach, D. and Pastan, I. (1976). *Journal of Biological Chemistry,* **251**, 5802.

Walton, K., Vogt, M. and Baldessarini, R. (1974). *The Pharmacologist,* **16**, 287.

Weinryb, I., Michel, I. M. and Hess, S. M. (1973). *Archives of Biochemistry and Biophysics,* **154**, 240.

Weiss, B. (1975). *In* "Cyclic Nucleotides in Disease" (Ed. B. Weiss).

Wolff, J. and Cook, G. H. (1975). *Journal of Biological Chemistry,* **250**, 6897.

Yamashita, K. and Field, J. B. (1973). *Biochimica et Biophysica Acta,* **304**, 686.

Zakarija, M. and McKenzie, J. M. (1973). *Life Sciences,* **12**, 225.

Zenser, T. V., DeRubertis, F. R., George, D. T. and Rayfield, E. J. (1974). *American Journal of Physiology,* **227**, 1299.

Zenser, T. V., DeRubertis, F. R. and Curnow, R. T. (1974). *Endocrinology,* **94**, 1404.

Cyclic Nucleotides and the Heart[1]

WINIFRED G. NAYLER, DSc

Cardiothoracic Institute, University of London, England

1 Introduction and history: cyclic AMP and the two messenger theory

In 1965, when it was already firmly established that certain hormones, including noradrenaline, stimulate the production of cyclic adenosine mono-phosphate (cyclic AMP, or $3'5'$-AMP) in a wide variety of tissues, Sutherland (Sutherland *et al.*, 1965) formulated his now famous two messenger theory of hormone action. According to this theory the primary hormone, e.g. noradrenaline in Fig. 1, interacts with specific receptors located at the surface of the effector cell. The resultant stimulation of these surface-located receptors (in Fig. 1, the hypothetical β-adrenoceptor) results, in an as yet unidentified way, in the activation of the adenyl cyclase enzyme. In the presence of Mg^{2+}, this enzyme catalyses the conversion of adenosine triphosphate (ATP) to cyclic AMP, which then acts as a *second messenger* to evoke the physiological response—in the case of the catecholamines, for example, the increase in peak developed tension or the abbreviated systole which we will be discussing in a later section of this chapter. It seems probable that the cyclic AMP that is formed as a result of the activation of the adenyl cyclase system evokes its various physiological responses by activating one of the many cyclic AMP-dependent protein kinases that are present both in the cytosol and in various intracellular organelles, including the mitochondria. These protein kinases exist as two subunits—one regulatory (R) and the other catalytic (C) (Bronstrom *et al.*, 1970). When closely complexed with one another, these two subunits are

[1] Supported in part by grants from the Medical Research Council and the British Heart Foundation.

essentially inactive. Apparently cyclic AMP interacts with the regulatory subunit R, thereby allowing the active catalytic subunit C to exert its effect, which
is the *transfer* of the terminal phosphate moiety of ATP to a specific *recipient
protein*. The rate of transfer of the terminal phosphate from ATP to the
receptor proteins, and hence the rate of formation of the active phosphorylated
sites (Fig. 2), can be monitored using ^{32}P-labelled ATP. Many protein kinases,
including those that are cyclic AMP dependent, have been isolated. Some of
them are cytosolic, others protein bound. However, it is the ensuing changes
in the properties of the membranes that contain these newly phosphorylated
proteins that is of prime interest to us here, because they involve alterations in
selective permeability to certain ions, including Ca^{2+}, and the activation of
certain enzymic pathways as described below.

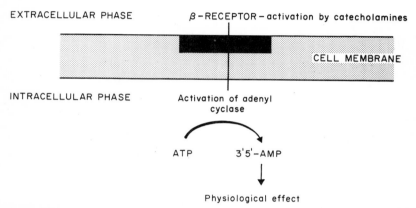

FIG. 1. Schematic representation of the two messenger theory illustrated for the
catecholamines.

For convenience, therefore, we can summarize the sequence of events that
we are interested in here, as follows: stimulation of adenyl cyclase → formation
of cyclic AMP → stimulation of cyclic AMP dependent protein kinase →
protein phosphorylation → physiological effect.

Obviously a counterbalance system must exist to regulate this cascade of
events. As currently understood, the regulatory process involves two other
classes of enzymes: (a) the *cyclic AMP phosphodiesterases*, that convert *active*
cyclic AMP to physiologically inactive 5'-AMP, and (b) *phosphoprotein
phosphatases*, that dephosphorylate the phosphorylated proteins.

In this introductory section, attention has been deliberately directed towards
the adenyl cyclase system. However, before considering in detail the
consequences of its activation, mention should be made of the guanosine-based
nucleotide system found in heart and other tissues, particularly since it is

believed that cyclic AMP and cyclic guanosine monophosphate (cyclic GMP) play opposing regulatory roles in the heart (Goldberg *et al.*, 1975). This hypothesis is based on the observation that the positive inotropic response to β-adrenoceptor stimulation is accompanied by an increase in the cyclic AMP and a concomitant decrease in the cyclic GMP content of heart muscle (George *et al.*, 1973). Despite the undoubted importance of cyclic GMP in heart muscle, our current discussion will be restricted to its counterpart—cyclic AMP.

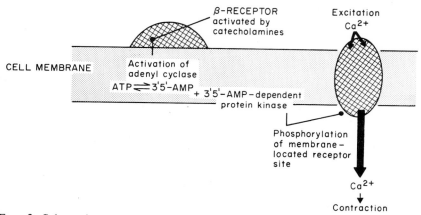

FIG. 2. Schematic representation of the 3'5'-AMP mediated phosphorylation of proteins in the cell membrane of a cardiac muscle cell and the ensuing increase in the permeability of the membrane to Ca^{2+}.

2   Cyclic AMP levels in heart muscle

Before considering the consequences that can result from changes in the tissue concentrations of cyclic AMP in heart muscle, it may be interesting to note the levels of cyclic AMP that are normally found. According to the assays performed on isolated guinea-pig hearts (Robison *et al.*, 1965, 1967; Mayer *et al.*, 1970; Kukovetz and Pöch, 1972; Gardner and Allen, 1976) the concentration ranges from 200 to 800 pmol g^{-1} wet weight. In left ventricular wall samples frozen *in situ* in open chest dogs, Wollenberger *et al.* (1969) found an average cyclic AMP concentration of 740 pmol g^{-1}. These relatively high values contrast with the lower levels found in blood plasma, 12–27 pmol ml^{-1} (Issekutz, 1975; Wehmann *et al.*, 1974). This relatively large difference between the cardiac and plasma levels of cyclic AMP is interesting, particularly when it is recalled that cyclic AMP can escape from cells (Wehmann *et al.*, 1974) and that various hormones, including the catecholamines and glucogen (Issekutz, 1975; Strange and Mjøs, 1975; Messerli *et al.*, 1976) activate the release.

3 Cyclic AMP and glycogenolysis

There is little doubt that the most prominent effect that the catecholamines exert on the metabolism of heart muscle is the accelerated breakdown of glycogen. This is mediated in the cytoplasm of cardiac muscle cells and involves Sutherland's second messenger—cyclic AMP. By activating the adenyl cyclase system, and not by activating the phosphodiesterases, the catecholamines raise the cytosolic concentration of cyclic AMP. Then, provided that the intracellular ionic environment is appropriate, this increased availability of cyclic AMP precipitates the cascade of events shown

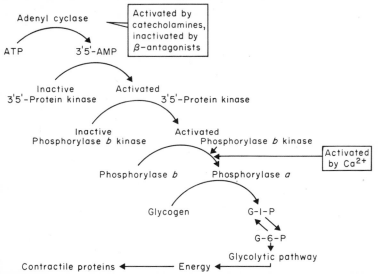

FIG. 3. Schematic representation of the cascade of events linking cyclic AMP and glycogenolysis.

schematically in Fig. 3. Thus, cyclic AMP activates a protein kinase. The activated protein kinase then activates the conversion of a relatively inactive phosphorylase kinase into an activated form. The activated phosphorylase kinase in turn catalyses the phosphorylation and hence the activation of glycogen phosphorylase, i.e. the transformation of phosphorylase b to phosphorylase a. It is perhaps worth noting here that this phosphorylase kinase is Ca^{2+} dependent and that its activation via its phosphorylation increases its sensitivity to Ca^{2+}. Activated phosphorylase a is then able to activate the breakdown of glycogen to glucose-1-phosphate (Fig. 3); at the same time glycogen synthetase is converted into its nonactive glucose-6-dependent or D form (Soderling et al., 1970). The important point to grasp here is that it is the phosphorylation of the phosphorylase kinase that confers Ca^{2+} sensitivity on the cascade. This phosphorylation, discovered by Walsh, Perkins and Krebs (1968), was the first known example of a cyclic AMP dependent phosphorylation of a protein, a process which we now know to result in an enhanced sensitivity of the complex to Ca^{2+}.

A similar cascade reaction, started by the catecholamines in adipose tissue, results in the mobilization of free fatty acids. In this case, it is the hormone sensitive lipase that is phosphorylated and activated by a cyclic AMP-dependent protein kinase. This is why heart muscle responds to catecholamines and to certain cyclic AMP derivatives with an increased triglyceride mobilization and a release of free fatty acids (Christian et al., 1969; Crass, 1973)—free fatty acids which, according to some investigators (Opie, 1968), are an important source of metabolic energy for the heart, but unfortunately (Opie and Lubbe, 1975) may be arrhythmogenic. At one time it was thought that the cyclic AMP-induced activation of the myocardial phosphorylase system and the resultant acceleration of glycogenolysis and glycolytic energy production might be either causally or directly related to the increase in contractile force brought about by the catecholamines (Haugaard and Hess, 1965). This idea we now know is untenable because (a) small doses of catecholamines that have a positive inotropic effect do so without increasing phosphorylase a activity (Mayer et al., 1963); and (b) the positive inotropic response and the activation of the phosphorylase a do not occur at the same time (Drummond et al., 1964; Robinson et al., 1965). However, despite this lack of a direct causal link between the activation of phosphorylase a and the positive inotropic response, the stimulation of glycogenolysis most probably provides the energy required for the exhibition of a sustained positive inotropic response. This raises the theoretically exciting possibility of using the cyclic AMP-induced activation of the phosphorylase system to provide the energy needed for the support of metabolically failing heart muscle. If this is to become feasible, then drugs must be designed to specifically stimulate cyclic AMP-dependent glycolytic energy production without simultaneously mobilizing the free fatty acids, which may be arrhythmogenic. In ischaemic heart muscle, this process is partly brought into play—for heart muscle responds to an ischaemic episode by releasing its endogenous stores of noradrenaline (Shahab et al., 1969), a process that must result in the activation of the phosphorylase pathway described above. Unfortunately, it is also accompanied by the mobilization of the free fatty acids.

4 Cyclic nucleotides, catecholamines and heart rate

Little information exists as yet as to the levels of cyclic AMP and adenyl cyclase activity in cardiac pacemaker cells and tissues, but the fact that spontaneously beating cultured heart cells are sensitive to added noradrenaline, dibutyryl cyclic AMP and dibutyryl cyclic GMP (Goshima, 1976), indicates that the pathways that are involved in regulating pacemaker activity are nucleotide sensitive. Krause et al. (1973) showed that both carbamylcholine (an acetylcholine derivative) and dibutyryl cyclic GMP decreases the rate of spontaneous beating in cultured rat myocytes. Conversely the catecholamine-induced stimulation of beating in cultured rat heart cells has been found to be accompanied by a stimulation of their adenylate cyclase activity (Wollenberger, 1976). Adenylate cyclase activity has also been found in the conducting Purkinje fibres of adult dog heart (Dhalla et al., 1973). Here, as in the working cells of the myocardium, the activity of the adenylate cyclase system is enhanced by concentrations of catecholamines that normally evoke an increase in heart rate. Tsien et al. (1972) have shown that the effect of the dibutyryl derivative of cyclic AMP (used because it is more lipophilic than cyclic AMP) on the configuration of the action potential closely resembles that of noradrenaline, whilst Tuganowski et al. (1973) was able to restore spontaneous electrical activity in arrested cardiac pacemaker tissue by adding either dibutyryl AMP or adrenaline. These and other data support the conclusions reached by earlier workers—that cyclic AMP is probably involved in the positive chronotropic actions of the catecholamines (Krause et al., 1970; Kukovetz and Poch, 1970). Likewise it seems probable that cyclic GMP is involved in mediating the negative chronotropic effects of acetylcholine and other cholinergic agents on heart muscle. However, we do not know whether an intermediate process of membrane phosphorylation is involved.

5   Cyclic nucleotides and the positive inotropic effect of the catecholamines

If the positive inotropic effect of the catecholamines cannot, as discussed earlier, be accounted for in terms of the catecholamine-induced activation of the phosphorylase system, then there must obviously be another system that is involved. Remembering that it was shown more than ten years ago (Grossman and Furchgott, 1964; Reuter, 1965) that the positive inotropic effect of the catecholamines is accompanied by an increased influx of Ca^{2+} into cardiac muscle cells, that it is the amount of Ca^{2+} that is available for interaction with the troponin tropomyosin complex, as shown schematically in Fig. 4, that determines the peak tension developed during contraction, and that in cardiac, but not skeletal muscle, the major part of this "activator Ca^{2+}" is derived from the extracellular phase (Fig. 5) and hence must be transported across or through the cell membrane, then it is not surprising to find that many laboratories have been searching for and have now identified phosphorylation-dependent systems for transporting Ca^{2+} across the cell membrane. Indeed in recent years, the regulation of membrane calcium transport by cyclic AMP- and Ca^{2+}-dependent phosphorylation of membrane proteins has been

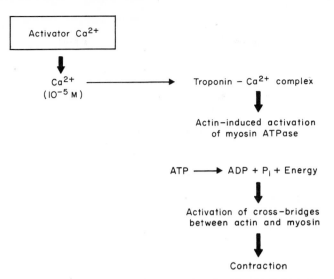

FIG. 4. Schematic representation of the events involved in the Ca^{2+}-induced activation of the interaction between actin and myosin.

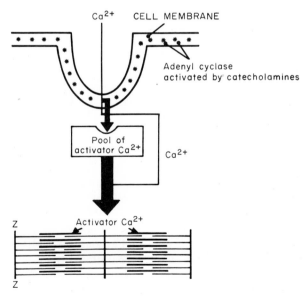

FIG. 5. Schematic representation of the displacement of Ca^{2+} needed to activate contraction.

investigated for cardiac muscle, not only at the level of the plasmalemma, but also for the sarcoplasmic reticulum (Sulakhe and St Louis, 1976; Kirchberger et al., 1972; La Raia and Morkin, 1974; Nayler and Berry, 1975).

At the level of the plasmalemma, we have the conditions shown schematically in Fig. 5. Thus, exogenous catecholamines (adrenaline, noradrenaline and isoprenaline) activate the adenylate cyclase enzyme, thereby increasing the concentration of cyclic AMP either in or in the immediate vicinity of the membrane. Under these conditions, and provided that the appropriate cofactors are present, it seems certain (Wollenberger, 1976) that some of the membrane proteins are phosphorylated. This either directly, or because it evokes a configurational change either in the membrane, or selectively in the "Ca^{2+} channels", increases the permeability of the membrane to Ca^{2+}, thereby evoking a rapid increase in the concentration of Ca^{2+} in the cytosol, and hence

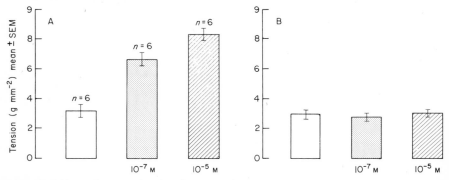

FIG. 6. Effect of adrenaline (10^{-7} and 10^{-5} M) on peak tension developed by rabbit trabecular muscle (A) immersed in normal Krebs solution and (B) after the muscles had been treated chemically (Winegrad, 1971) to render them freely permeable to Ca^{2+}. Stimulation rate, 6 per minute at 37°C. Note that after the muscles had been made freely permeable to Ca^{2+}, they no longer developed an inotropic response when adrenaline was added.

in a positive inotropic response. Hence there is little reason to doubt that there is a link between the catecholamine-induced increase in calcium influx across the cell membrane during the plateau phase of the action potential (Reuter, 1967; Shigenobu and Sperelakis, 1972) and the activation of the adenylate cyclase system. One test for this hypothesis would be to add catecholamines, or the lypophilic derivative of cyclic AMP, dibutyryl AMP, to heart muscle preparations before and after these preparations (papillary or trabeculae muscles) have been treated chemically to render them freely permeable to Ca^{2+}. If the positive inotropic effect of these drugs is due to an enhanced cytosolic Ca^{2+} dependent upon a raised Ca^{2+} influx, then the positive inotropic response should be abolished under conditions which allow Ca^{2+} to freely enter the cell. The results from a series of such experiments are summarized in Fig. 6.

They show quite clearly that adrenaline no longer exerts its normal inotropic effect if selective permeability of the membrane for Ca^{2+} has been abolished. Under these same conditions of nonselective permeability (Fig. 7) the normal positive inotropic response to dibutyry cyclic AMP is also abolished.

Other recent findings indicate a role for cyclic AMP in the regulation of calcium transport *within* myocardial cells, particularly within the sarco- plasmic reticulum where it seems likely that the cyclic AMP protein kinase

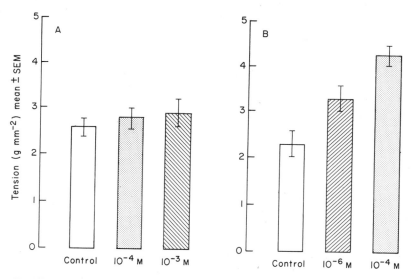

FIG. 7. Effect of dibutyryl cyclic AMP on tension development in isolated rabbit trabecular muscles before (B) and after (A) the muscles had been treated to render them freely permeable to Ca^{2+}. Stimulation rate, 6 per minute at 37°C (Winegrad, 1971).

system can control the transport of calcium into the sarcoplasmic reticulum. This cyclic AMP-induced regulation appears to be dependent upon a protein kinase phosphorylation of a specific component of the reticulum membrane (Kirchberger *et al.*, 1974; Tada *et al.*, 1974; La Raia and Morkin, 1974). The accumulation of Ca^{2+} by the sarcoplasmic reticulum involves the activation of a specific Ca^{2+}-activated ATPase enzyme, and recently Tada and Kirchberger (1975) have shown that the rate of turnover of this ATPase is stimulated through the cyclic AMP-mediated phosphorylation of a specific protein. In our laboratory, we have shown that the increase in Ca^{2+}-accumulating activity of the isolated sarcoplasmic reticulum that occurs under these conditions of enhanced phosphorylation is not blocked by the β-adrenoceptor antagonist, propranolol. The results of these experiments are summarized in Fig. 8.

In general, therefore, we can link the increase in peak tension that develops in response to added catecholamines with their ability to abbreviate systole, because both phenomenon are mediated via a common pathway—i.e. a cyclic AMP-phosphorylation-mediated change in the permeability of the cell membrane and the limiting membranes of the sarcoplasmic reticulum to Ca^{2+}. At the level of the plasmalemma, this results in a greater influx of Ca^{2+} during the excitatory phase of the action potential, and hence in an enhanced supply of activator Ca^{2+} (Nayler, 1967). The rapid removal of Ca^{2+} from the cytosol (Fig. 9) will ensure that systole is abbreviated, and probably that more Ca^{2+}

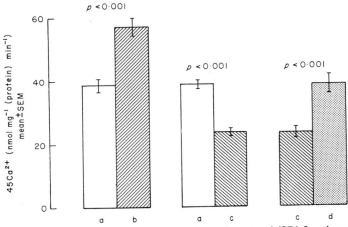

FIG. 8. Calcium-accumulating activity of cardiac microsomal (SR) fractions incubated with $^{45}Ca^{2+}$ in the presence and absence of cyclic AMP and the cyclic AMP-dependent protein kinase. a, Control; b, ($\pm$)-propanolol (10^{-4} M); c, 3'5'-AMP (5×10^{-6} M) + protein kinase (5 μg ml^{-1}); d, 3'5'-AMP (5×10^{-6} M) + protein kinase (5 μg ml^{-1}) + ($\pm$)-propanolol (10^{-4} M). For details of methods, see Nayler and Berry (1975).

will be available for release from the sarcoplasmic reticulum during the next excitation-contraction coupling event (Nayler, 1967). At the same time, of course, additional energy will be made available as a result of the enhanced glycolytic energy production discussed above.

It is also possible that the cyclic nucleotides may play an important role in phosphorylating the regulatory proteins embodied in the troponin-complex. In the case of cardiac troponin, Solaro et al. (1976) have recently reported that the cyclic AMP-mediated phosphorylation of the regulatory proteins of cardiac muscle results in a decreased sensitivity to Ca^{2+}, an observation that led these investigators to conclude that this would "smooth out" the positive inotropic response evoked by the catecholamines. Contrary findings, however, have been reported by other investigators and clearly until more data are available, the significance of this cyclic AMP-mediated phosphorylation of the regulatory proteins can only be the subject for speculation. Likewise, the significance of the cyclic AMP-phosphorylation dependent efflux of Ca^{2+} from mitochondria (Borle, 1973) awaits evaluation.

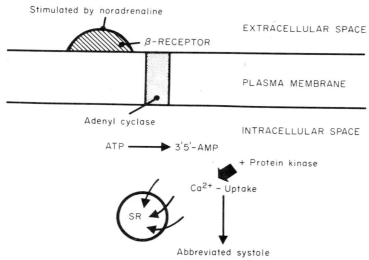

Fig. 9. Schematic representation of the basis of the catecholamine-induced reduction in the duration of systole in heart muscle. Note that the β-adrenoceptor antagonists act only at the primary level of the β-receptor.

6   Conclusion

In conclusion, therefore, there can be no doubt of the fact that the cyclic nucleotides play an important role in heart muscle. In the case of the adenyl-based nucleotides, their production via the activation of the adenyl cyclase system can be regulated by appropriate drug therapy. Likewise their rate of destruction via the phosphodiesterases can be modified, i.e. by the xanthine drugs. But, whichever mechanism is used to elevate the cardiac stores of cyclic AMP, the fact that the mobilization of free fatty acids is also enhanced in the presence of the raised cyclic AMP raises problems, because of the known arrhythmogenic properties of the free fatty acids (Cowan and Vaughan Williams, 1977).

There are many facets of nucleotides in heart muscle that have not been discussed here, particularly with respect to the role of GMP. This omission is partly deliberate, because of my own interest in the adenyl nucleotides and the multiplicity of sites within cardiac muscle, pacemaker and conducting cells (plasmalemma, myofibrils, sarcoplasmic reticulum, mitochondria and cytosol) at which cyclic AMP-dependent protein kinases act to facilitate the phosphorylation of membrane-bound proteins. When phosphorylated, the properties of these membrane-bound proteins are altered, often in such a way that their sensitivities to specific stimuli, e.g. Ca^{2+}, are enhanced.

References

Borle, A. B. (1973). *International Research Communication,* **1**, 9.

Brostrom, C. O., Hunkeler, F. L. and Krebs, E. G. (1971). *Journal of Biological Chemistry,* **246**, 1061.

Christian, D. R., Kilsheimer, G. S., Pettet, G., Paradise, R. and Ashmore, J. (1969). *Advances in Enzyme Regulation,* **7**, 71.

Cowan, J. C. and Vaughan Williams, E. M. (1977). *Journal of Molecular and Cellular Cardiology,* **9**, 527.

Crass, M. F. (1973). *Recent Advances in Cardiac Structure and Metabolism,* **3**, 275.

Dhalla, N. S., Chernecki, W., Gandhi, S. S., McNamara, D. B. and Naimark, A. (1973). *Recent Advances in Studies on Cardiac Structure and Metabolism,* **3**, 233.

Drummond, G. I., Valadares, J. R. E. and Duncan, L. (1964). *Proceedings of the Society of Experimental Biology and Medicine,* **117**, 307.

Gardner, R. M. and Allen, D. O. (1976). *Journal of Pharmacology and Experimental Therapeutics,* **198**, 412.

George, W. J., Wilkerson, R. D. and Kadowitz, P. J. (1973). *Journal of Pharmacology and Experimental Therapeutics,* **184**, 228.

Goldberg, N. D., Haddox, M. K., Nicol, S. E., Glass, D. B., Sandford, C. H., Kuehl, Jr, F. A. and Estensen, R. (1975). *In* "Advances in Cyclic Nucleotide Research" (Eds G. I. Drummond, P. Greengard and G. A. Robison), vol. 5, p. 307 Raven Press, New York.

Goshima, K. (1976). *Journal of Molecular and Cellular Cardiology,* **8**, 713.

Grossman, A. and Furchgott, T. (1964). *Journal of Pharmacology and Experimental Therapeutics,* **145**, 162.

Haugaard, N. and Hess, M. E. (1965). *Pharmacological Reviews,* **17**, 27.

Issekutz, T. B. (1975). *American Journal of Physiology,* **229**, 291.

Kirchberger, M. A., Tada, M., Repke, D. I. and Katz, A. M. (1972). *Journal of Molecular and Cellular Cardiology,* **4**, 673.

Kirchberger, M. A., Tada, M. and Katz, A. M. (1974). *Journal of Biological Chemistry,* **249**, 6166.

Krause, E. G., Will, H., Pelauch, V. and Wollenberger, A. (1973). *Acta Biologica et Medeca Germanica.* **31**, 37.

Krause, E. G., Halle, W., Kallabis, E. and Wollenberger, A. (1970). *Journal of Molecular and Cellular Cardiology,* **1**, 1.

Kukovetz, W. R. and Pöch, G. (1972). *In* "Advances in Cyclic Nucleotide Research" (Eds P. Greengard and G. A. Robison), vol. 1, p. 261. Raven Press, New York.

Kukovetz, W. R. and Pöch, G. (1970). *Archives Intérnatoinales de Pharmacodynamie et de Thérapie,* **266**, 236.

La Raia, P. J. and Morkin, E. (1974). *Circulation Research,* **35**, 298.

Mayer, S. E., Cotten, M. de V. and Moran, N. C. (1963). *Journal of Pharmacology and Experimental Therapeutics,* **139**, 275.

Mayer, S. E., Namm, D. H. and Rice, L. (1970). *Circulation Research,* **26**, 225.

Meinertz, T., Nawrath, H. and Scholz, H. (1973). *Archives of Pharmacology,* **279**, 327.

Messerli, F. H., Kuchel, O., Hamet, P., Tolis, G., Guthrie, G. P. Jr., Fraysse, J., Nowaczynski, W. and Genest, J. (1976). *Circulation Research,* **38,** Suppl II, 42.

Nayler, W. G. (1967). *American Heart Journal,* **73,** 379.

Nayler, W. G. and Berry, D. (1975). *Journal of Molecular and Cellular Cardiology,* **7,** 387.

Opie, L. H. (1968). *American Heart Journal,* **76,** 685.

Opie, L. H. and Lubbe, W. F. (1975). *Journal of Molecular and Cellular Cardiology,* **7,** 115.

Rasmussen, H. and Tennenhouse, A. (1968). *Proceedings National Academy of Sciences (Washington),* **59,** 1364.

Reuter, H. (1965). *Naunyn-Schmiedebergs Archiv für Experimentelle Pathologie und Pharmakologie,* **251,** 401.

Reuter, H. (1967). *Journal of Physiology,* **192,** 479.

Robison, G. A., Butcher, R. W., Øye, I., Morgan, H. E. and Sutherland, E. W. (1965). *Molecular Pharmacology,* **1,** 168.

Robison, G. A., Butcher, R. W. and Sutherland, E. W. (1967). *Annals of New York Academy of Sciences,* **139,** 703.

Shahab, L., Haase, M., Schiller, U. and Wollenberger, A. (1969). *Acta Biologica et Medeca Germanica,* **22,** 135.

Shigenobu, K. and Sperelakis, N. (1972). *Circulation Research,* **31,** 932.

Soderling, T. R., Hickenbottom, J. P., Reimann, E. M., Hunkeler, F. L., Walsh, D. A. and Krebs, E. G. (1970). *Journal of Biological Chemistry,* **245,** 6317.

Solaro, R. J., Moir, A. J. G. and Perry, S. V. (1976). *Nature,* **262,** 615.

Strange, R. C. and Mjøs, O. D. (1975). *European Journal of Clinical Investigation,* **5,** 147.

Sulakhe, P. V. and St Louis, P. J. (1976). *Journal of General Pharmacology,* **7,** 713.

Sutherland, E. W., Øye, I. and Butcher, R. W. (1965). *Recent Progress in Hormone Research,* **21,** 623.

Tada, M. and Kirchberger, M. A. (1975). *Acta Cardiologica,* **30,** 231.

Tsien, R. W. (1973). *Nature,* **245,** 120.

Tuganowski, W., Krause, M. and Korezak, (1973). *Archives Intérnationales de Pharmacodynamie et de Thérapie,* **280,** 63.

Walsh, D. A., Perkins, J. P. and Krebs, E. G. (1968). *Journal of Biological Chemistry,* **243,** 3763.

Wehmann, R. E., Blonde, L. and Steiner, A. L. (1974). *Journal of Clinical Investigation,* **53,** 173.

Winegrad, S. (1971). *Journal of General Physiology,* **58,** 71.

Wollenberger, A., Krause, E. G. and Heier, G. (1969). *Biochemical and Biophysical Research Communications,* **36,** 664.

Wollenberger, A. (1976). *In* "Contraction and Relaxation of the Myocardium" (Ed. W. G. Nayler), p. 113. Academic Press, London and New York.

Integrated Control of Trematode Diseases

NORMAN O. CROSSLAND, BSc, ARCS

Shell Research Ltd, Shell Toxicology Laboratory (Tunstall), Sittingbourne, Kent, England

1 Introduction

The liver flukes of grazing animals and the human blood flukes are parasites that belong to a class of flatworms known as the Trematoda. There are numerous kinds of parasitic trematodes that affect all kinds of vertebrate hosts, including fish, amphibia, birds and mammals. However, the liver flukes belonging to the genus *Fasciola* and the blood flukes belonging to the genus *Schistosoma* have a far greater impact on human health and wealth than other trematodes. Worldwide, the trematode disease problems of livestock and humans, called fascioliasis and schistosomiasis respectively, are getting worse rather than better. The diseases are more often chronic than acute and their effects on livestock productivity and human health are difficult to measure.

Their control is equally difficult because no single method can be expected to solve the problems and a combination of several control methods can be prohibitively expensive. Successful control depends on the intelligent application of a combination of methods. The rational choice of methods and the allocation of resources between them depends on an understanding of the epidemiology of the disease and its effects on the mammalian hosts. The problem of control is not the lack of effective tools but rather the rational allocation of resources to those tools that are available. Although there has been significant progress, particularly within the last two decades, this problem has not been satisfactorily resolved for either of the major trematode diseases.

The problems of control cannot be divorced from pathological, economic and epidemiological considerations. The severity of trematode diseases varies widely depending, among other factors, on the numbers of parasites acquired by the hosts. A few parasites may cause little or no disease whereas many parasites may cause severe illnesses and death. Because of the wide spectrum of pathological effects associated with varying intensities of infection the economic consequences can be equally variable.

The numbers of parasites depend on the numbers of hosts, both snails and mammals, and the ways in which these host populations are distributed to provide opportunities for transmission of the free-living larval parasites. In this paper some of the quantitative aspects of trematode diseases are reviewed, particularly those that affect control strategies. The development of control methods for fascioliasis has followed a similar pattern to that for schistosomiasis because there are basic similarities in the biology of *Schistosoma* and *Fasciola*, the epidemiology of the diseases they cause and the effects of these diseases on the mammalian hosts.

In section 2 the life-cycles of *Schistosoma* sp. and *Fasciola* sp. are described and these illustrate the basic similarity of their biology. There are, however, important differences. Whereas *Schistosoma* is bisexual, *Fasciola* is hermaphroditic; in the life-cycle of *Schistosoma* there is no metacercarial stage but this is an important feature of the *Fasciola* life-cycle.

In section 3 some pathological and economic effects of trematode diseases are discussed. Although there is an extensive literature on this subject only a few studies have concentrated on the relation between effects of disease and parasite numbers.

In section 4 the use of incidence and prevalence data is critically examined in relation to evaluating the effectiveness of control programmes.

Section 5.1 deals with parasite population dynamics and their dependence on mammalian and snail populations. It is largely based on the work of Professor Nelson G. Hairston of the University of North Carolina who was the first to understand and describe these interrelationships in a quantitative sense.

Section 5.2 deals with host population dynamics. Within the life-span of trematode parasites the population dynamics of snail hosts interact with parasite population dynamics to a greater extent than do the population dynamics of mammalian hosts.

In section 6, the role of mathematical models is reviewed. The author suggests that there is scope for the development of a systems approach to the problem.

In section 7 integrated control is defined as a combined attack on parasitic and adult larval stages. Examples of integrated control of trematode diseases are described.

2 Life-cycles

2.1 LIFE-CYCLE OF THE COMMON LIVER FLUKE

Several species of liver flukes affect sheep and cattle. The common liver fluke, *F. hepatica*, causes more economic damage and has been studied in more detail than have other species. It is infective to all kinds of wild and domesticated mammals but the disease it causes is most prevalent among sheep and cattle. Animals become infected by ingesting herbage infested with metacercariae, the encysted larval stages of the liver fluke. Inside the mammalian gut the larva escapes from its cyst and migrates via the intestinal wall and the peritoneal cavity into the parenchyma of the liver. The young liver fluke tunnels its way through its host's liver until, when it becomes adult, it settles in the bile ducts. The adult fluke is an hermaphrodite. It lays numerous eggs which are passed with the bile into the host's gut and are then voided with the faeces.

After deposition onto pastures the fluke eggs can survive from one to more than twelve months, depending on prevailing weather conditions. In warm, moist weather the fluke eggs hatch and a free-swimming, ciliated larva called a miracidium escapes from the egg. The miracidium cannot feed and can survive for only a few hours unless it is able to find a suitable host species of snail. Various species of snail may become infected but in Europe the only one of any economic significance is the mud snail, *Lymnaea truncatula*. The miracidium infects the snail by boring into the snail's tissues with the aid of glandular secretions.

Inside the snail the miracidium loses its ciliated epithelium, becomes round in shape, about half the size of the miracidium, and is then known as a sporocyst. The sporocyst grows and groups of germinal cells inside it give rise to the next larval stage, called a redia. The redia feeds and grows in the digestive gland or "liver" of the snail and gives rise to a new generation of daughter rediae. These may produce another generation of daughter rediae but eventually the rediae produce the next larval stage called the cercaria.

The cercaria is round with a long, unforked tail used for swimming and two suckers used for adhesion onto blades of grass or other surfaces. It escapes from the pulmonary cavity of the snail when conditions are suitably warm and moist and swims freely until it attaches itself to a suitable object with the aid of its suckers. It then loses its tail and forms a cyst wall around itself, when it is known as a metacercaria. The metacercaria is infective to mammals and can survive for up to twelve months. The life-cycle of the liver fluke is illustrated diagrammatically in Fig. 1.

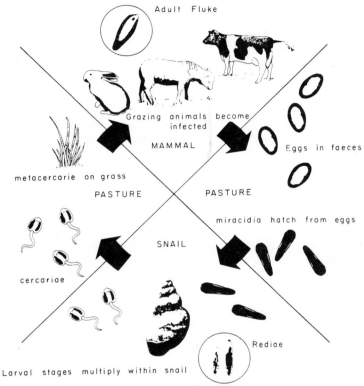

FIG. 1. The life-cycle of *Fasciola hepatica*.

2.2 LIFE-CYCLES OF THE HUMAN SCHISTOSOMES

Several species of schistosomes infect humans but the three most important species are *S. mansoni*, *S. haematobium* and *S. japonicum*. Worldwide, these three species affect about 200 million people in tropical and subtropical countries.

S. mansoni is endemic in the Middle East, most of Africa south of the Sahara and in parts of the western hemisphere. The infective larval stages, or cercariae, are relatively specific to humans, although Nelson (1960) has shown that baboons may act as reservoir hosts. People may become infected after bathing or washing in infected water. The cercaria is round with a long forked tail used for swimming and has two suckers used for adhesion to the skin of its human host. It is able to penetrate the human skin with the aid of glandular secretions emitted from around the oral sucker of a penetrating cercaria.

After penetrating the skin the cercaria loses its tail and becomes worm-like, when it is called a schistosomule. The schistosomules enter peripheral veins or lymphatic vessels within a day or two and migrate via the heart, lungs and liver to the mesenteric veins of the hepatic portal blood system where they develop into sexually mature worms. The adults are bisexual and the female is held by the male within a ventral fold of the body wall. The average life-span of an adult worm is from three to five years, although some may live for over 20 years and the average egg output is about 100–300 eggs per female per day. Some of these eggs become lodged in the tissues of the host, particularly in the liver, spleen and the walls of the lower gut but many are passed to the exterior with the host's faeces.

Eggs that are deposited in water, hatch releasing the miracidia which are unable to survive for long unless they are able to locate and penetrate an aquatic species of snail belonging to the genus *Biomphalaria*. An asexual multiplicative phase takes place inside the snail, similar to that already described for the liver fluke, and after a period of 3–4 weeks the cercariae begin to emerge. An infected snail may continue to shed cercariae every day for a period of several months. The life-cycle of *S. mansoni* is illustrated in Fig. 2.

The life-cycles of the other two species of schistosomes differ in several important respects. *S. japonicum* is endemic in China, Japan, the Philippines and Celebes. It can infect a variety of mammalian hosts, including rats, dogs and pigs. It is transmitted via amphibious species of snails belonging to the genus *Oncomelania*. *S. haematobium* is endemic in the Middle East and most of Africa south of the Sahara. It is specific to man. The adult worms live in the renal portal system of veins and the eggs are passed to the exterior with the host's urine. The parasite is transmitted via several species of freshwater snails, most of them belonging to the genus *Bulinus*. In most other respects the life-cycles of *S. haematobium* and *S. japonicum* are similar to that described for *S. mansoni*.

3 The relation between parasite numbers and effects of disease

Effects on morbidity, mortality and productivity can more easily be measured for acute than for chronic diseases. In general it is possible to assess the economic impact of acute diseases on populations even though the interpretation of epidemiological data may be problematical. It is much more difficult to assess the economic impact of chronic diseases partly because of the need for longitudinal surveys, i.e. surveys that follow the effects of disease on cohorts, or age-groups within a population, for some considerable time.

Trematode diseases can affect their hosts in either an acute or a chronic form, although the chronic form of the disease is the more important, both to livestock productivity and to human health. The acute disease occurs when a mammalian host is invaded within a short period of time by a large number of parasites. The infection takes place quickly and the host is unable to mount an effective immunological response. The chronic disease occurs when a

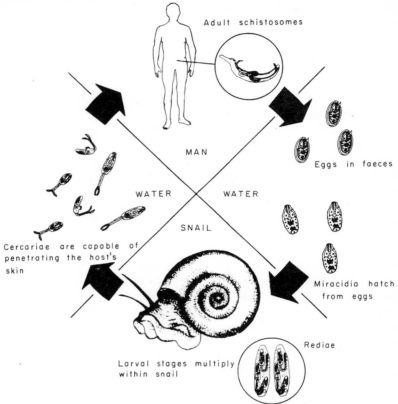

Adult schistosomes

MAN

WATER   WATER

SNAIL

Eggs in faeces

Miracidia hatch from eggs

Cercariae are capable of penetrating the host's skin

Rediae

Larval stages multiply within snail

FIG. 2. The life-cycle of *Schistosoma mansoni*.

mammalian host is invaded by a smaller number of parasites acquired over a longer period of time. Acquisition of parasites by the host may give it a certain degree of immunity to subsequent infections so that establishment of parasites in the host may become progressively more difficult.

3.1   LIVER FLUKE NUMBERS AND FASCIOLIASIS

Acute fascioliasis has a long and well-known history as a major cause of death among sheep in mild, wet climates such as in the UK. It is known to have occurred at least 1000 years ago among Welsh hill sheep and some form of flock management to control fascioliasis and other diseases was practised as long ago as the eleventh century A.D. in the time of King Howell the Good. As stocking densities increased so, too, did the incidence of disease and in the 19th century acute fascioliasis in the UK was responsible for an average annual loss of one million sheep. In the year 1879, following a succession of wet summer seasons, more than three million sheep died. The last major outbreak in the UK occurred in 1958 when over a million sheep died and in 1968 regional outbreaks were responsible for further heavy losses. The disease occurs in sheep when large numbers of invading worms cause extensive damage to the liver leading to massive internal haemorrhage and death. It is frequently associated with black disease, caused by the bacterium *Clostridium oedematiens*. Bacterial spores which are present, but dormant, in healthy sheep are activated following liver damage caused by invading liver flukes. The bacteria multiply causing further liver damage and producing toxins that are fatal to sheep.

The pathology of subacute and chronic fascioliasis has been studied by numerous workers. Development of the disease has been described recently by Dargie (1975). It is essentially a two-stage process. The first stage is associated with migration of the young flukes through the liver parenchyma. As they burrow they leave behind them long, winding tracks which become wider as they grow. The tracts become filled with debris, leucocytes and eventually with fibrous tissue. The extent of damage to the liver at this stage is proportional to the number of invading worms. If only a few worms are involved the damage to the liver may be slight and the damaged parenchyma may be regenerated. If a large number of worms are involved the damage may be severe and extensive, fibrosis may result. Monitoring of blood changes in experimentally infected sheep has shown that the invasive stage is associated with eosinophilia, elevated serum globulins and serum enzymes.

The second stage of the infection is associated with the entry of the adult flukes into the bile ducts. They are voracious blood-suckers and cause haemorrhage into the host's gastrointestinal tract via the bile. The resulting anaemia, hypoalbuminaemia and loss of appetite are associated with a decrease in weight gain of sheep and beef cattle and a decrease in the quality and quantity of milk produced by dairy cattle.

An infected animal attempts to compensate for the continual loss of red cells into its gut by increasing its rate of red cell synthesis. This leads to an increased rate of plasma-iron turnover and a greatly increased demand for iron in the diet. An infected animal may also attempt to compensate for loss of blood albumins by increasing its rate of albumin synthesis. However, it cannot increase its albumin output unless the flow of amino acids to the liver is maintained, i.e. unless it has access to a high protein diet. The extent and severity of effects of chronic fascioliasis are therefore dependent not only on the numbers of parasites present but also on the nutritional status of the host.

Among farm animals it is particularly difficult to quantify the losses attributable to chronic fascioliasis. It has already been mentioned that the diet may have a considerable influence on the animal's ability to cope with the debilitating effects of fascioliasis. Environmental stresses and other concurrent diseases may also obscure the clinical picture. Diagnosis of disease generally depends on detection of parasite eggs in faecal samples but this method is not too reliable, at least for individual animals. Furthermore, relatively small changes in productivity parameters such as weight gain can be of considerable economic importance but their reliable measurement is difficult.

Despite the difficulties of measuring the economic importance of chronic fascioliasis and the paucity of reliable data there is mounting evidence to suggest that the problem is gradually getting worse. The overall prevalence of disease can be gauged from the results of abattoir surveys. Fascioliasis is the main reason for condemnation of livers, which are routinely examined by trained meat inspectors when farm animals are slaughtered. The rate of liver condemnation reflects the prevalence of fascioliasis because only a few per cent of livers are condemned for other reasons. In a review of animal diseases encountered at meat inspection in the UK in the period 1960–8 Blamire *et al.* (1970) reported that between 600 000 and 700 000 bovine livers were condemned annually and during the latter part of this period there was an increase in the numbers of livers condemned. However, any trend in incidence of disease in cattle in the UK as revealed by abattoir statistics is obscured by the fact that large numbers of bovines are imported from Ireland where the incidence of disease is much higher than in the UK. On the other hand the trend for sheep during the same period shows a steady increase in the number of livers condemned; in 1960 about half a million ovine livers were condemned and this figure increased steadily over the period to about one million by 1968 A similar rise in the incidence of condemned livers among Dutch cattle has been reported by Donker (1971) for the period 1960–6. In 1961 about 25 per cent of all cattle livers were condemned and there was a steady increase to 50 per cent of livers condemned during the last three months of 1966. The considerable increase in the condemnations of livers in Holland was attributed to an increase in the incidence of fascioliasis among cattle because of a succession of mild, wet summers allied to intensification of farming practices. The dry summer weather of the mid-seventies has halted the trend but there is little doubt that the incidence will increase in future.

The loss of livers is of little economic significance compared with the probable losses in milk and meat production. It is generally accepted that fascioliasis has an adverse effect on milk production in dairy cattle and that its prevention and cure can lead to substantial increases in yields. Donker (1971) reported that after two years of treatment with a fasciolicide administered to farm animals only once a year, treated cattle gave on average 634 litres more milk per lactation than untreated cattle. Increased milk production was accompanied by decreased feed consumption and fewer cases of pre-natal mortality and rearing difficulties among calves.

Relatively few investigations have been concerned with the effects of light infections of liver flukes on meat production. Sewell (1966) has shown that for *F. gigantica* in zebu cattle there is a correlation between liver fluke burden and liveweight gain. In a study over a period of $8\frac{1}{2}$ months 39 zebu cattle were experimentally infected to varying degrees with *F. gigantica*. Despite considerable variation the regression of liveweight gain on initial weight and final fluke burden was very highly significant ($r = 0.55$; $t = 4.0$; $p < 0.001$) and the same regression remained significant even when the more heavily infected animals were disregarded. According to Sewell the response may have been somewhat curvilinear, smaller numbers of flukes having a proportionately greater effect.

The pathogenicity of *F. hepatica* in sheep has been described by Dargie (1975), Sinclair (1962, 1972) and Thorpe and Ford (1969). In one experiment Sinclair studied a group of six pregnant ewes each infected artificially with 1000 metacercariae and maintained under controlled laboratory conditions. The onset of a progressive anaemia was accompanied by a loss of liveweight. Abortion, still birth and lambs of low birthweight were associated with fascioliasis and there was a clear indication that lambs failed to gain weight as quickly as those from uninfected ewes.

Crossland *et al.* (1977) investigated the effect of light infections of *F. hepatica* on the productivity of sheep under field conditions. One hundred and sixty ewes were allocated at random into 10 groups of 16 ewes which were grazed on five pairs of 1.60 ha plots. Liver flukes were controlled on five of these plots while no control measures were used on the other five plots. The control methods and other details of this experiment are described in section 7. After three years the ewes were slaughtered and at postmortem examinations the liver flukes were removed and counted. There was a significant negative correlation ($r = -0.66$) between the liver fluke burden and the weight of lambs produced per ewe. Furthermore, it was shown that ewes from untreated plots gained less weight and produced fewer lambs than did those from the treated plots.

In Fig. 3 data obtained from this experiment have been plotted to illustrate the relationship between fluke numbers and productivity of sheep. The mean number of liver flukes per flock of 16 ewes has been plotted on a logarithmic scale against the mean productivity of each flock, expressed as a percentage of the productivity of control flocks. In all other respects, e.g. quality and quantity of diet, exposure to other infections, genetic variation, the control and treated groups were strictly comparable so that the depression in productivity was certainly attributable to the effects of chronic fascioliasis. This experimental work underrates the overall effect of chronic fascioliasis on productivity because no account was taken of effects on the mortality of ewes, their live-weight gain and wool production. Furthermore, most of the infection was acquired during the last 12 months of the experiment so that cumulative effects of infection on productivity were not investigated.

The relationships between liver fluke numbers, duration of infections and the pathological and economic effects of fascioliasis are complex. It is important to know the form of these relationships in order to formulate control strategies.

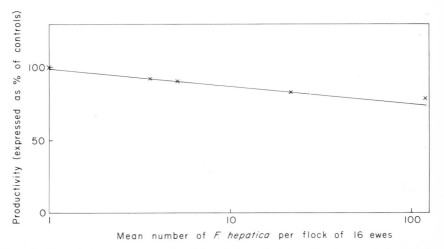

FIG. 3. The relation between productivity of sheep (weight of lambs per ewe) and liver fluke numbers.

The data presented in Fig. 3 suggest that the productivity of sheep may be related to a logarithmic rather than an arithmetic function of the liver fluke burden. Sewell's data indicate that this may also be true for *F. gigantica* in zebu cattle although the nutritional status of the animal, the duration of the infection and other factors are likely to modify this simplistic relationship.

3.2 SCHISTOSOME NUMBERS AND SCHISTOSOMIASIS

Acute schistosomiasis, sometimes known as the Katayama syndrome, has been well documented by Gelfand (1967) for expatriates in Africa but it is a rare occurrence among the indigenous people. Symptoms of disease are first observed about six weeks after exposure to infected water. A typhoid-like fever may last for several weeks accompanied by loss of appetite, lassitude, enlargement of the liver and spleen and in some cases dyspnoea and coughing. Eosinophilia is always present and is a useful diagnostic feature. Because it is relatively rare, the acute form of schistosomiasis is of no public health significance.

By contrast the chronic form of schistosomiasis is ranked by the World Health Organization as second only to malaria in its importance as a disease problem of tropical countries. In the case of *S. haematobium* infections, blood is usually passed in the urine and urination may be painful. Eggs lodging in the walls of the bladder may cause it to become thickened and calcified. The function of the kidneys may become seriously impaired and this may be associated with the formation of stones. This condition is frequently accompanied by thickening and deformation of the ureters. Cancer of the bladder occurs in some countries, e.g. in Egypt, as a late complication of urinary infection.

In the case of *S. mansoni* and *S. japonicum* infections the early phases of egg production by the parasites are associated with general symptoms of weakness, loss of appetite, weight loss and diarrhoea. The abdomen may be tender and the liver and spleen are frequently enlarged. As egg production continues, their passage through and enlodgement in the tissues may cause damage to the liver, intestine and bowel. Thickening, calcification and enlargement of the liver and spleen are frequently seen in children in areas where the disease is endemic. Severe anaemia and impairment of growth may occur. In the case of *S. japonicum* infections, there may be complications involving the lungs and the brain.

The public health and economic significance of chronic diseases is difficult to determine even in developed countries. In developing tropical countries the problem is exacerbated by lack of sufficient medical centres and trained personnel and by the presence of other parasitic diseases and malnutrition. Macdonald and Farooq (1973) have reviewed the data and conclude that, although a detailed economic analysis is scarcely feasible in most endemic areas, schistosomiasis constitutes a serious public health problem and experience in its control shows that the cost involved is generally comparable with that of other major public health programmes.

It is generally accepted that the severity of symptoms attributable to schistosomiasis is proportional to the worm burden and the duration of infection. It would be useful to know the form of this relationship but the collection of reliable data requires long-term studies by highly qualified personnel and at the present time the available resources are inadequate to cope with the problems. It is tempting to postulate that the severity of symptoms is likely to have a logarithmic rather than a linear relationship to worm burden but firm evidence is lacking.

4   The use of incidence and prevalence data to estimate the efficiency of control programmes

The importance of a trematode disease in any given area or community may be assessed by obtained data concerning (a) the number of hosts affected, i.e. the *prevalence* of infections, and (b) the rate at which uninfected hosts become infected, i.e. the *incidence* of new infections. The latter measurement is a useful indicator of the intensity of transmission of parasites and has therefore been used to evaluate the effect of snail control measures on parasite numbers.

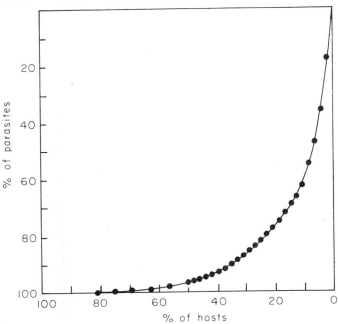

FIG. 4. Cumulative host and parasite egg frequency curve for *S. haematobium* in Tanzanian school children (after Bradley, 1972).

Assessments based on prevalence data on the other hand are insensitive to changes in parasite numbers and may lead to erroneous conclusions concerning the effect of control programmes.

In any given population of hosts a relatively large proportion of parasites may be harboured by a relatively small proportion of hosts. A control programme may therefore be very effective in reducing parasite numbers yet have no significant effect on prevalence. The significance of aggregation of helminth parasites among their hosts has been discussed by Bradley (1972) and he has illustrated their aggregation with reference to the distribution of *S. haematobium* eggs in samples of urine from Tanzanian school children (Fig. 4).

The distribution of schistosome parasites among their human hosts can only be inferred from the distribution of parasite eggs among samples of human excreta. Similar methods are generally employed to investigate the distribution of liver flukes among livestock. However, in the case of liver flukes it is possible to obtain data directly from collections of the adult parasites removed from hosts' livers at postmortem. Data of this kind were obtained by Crossland *et al.* (1977) and are presented in Fig. 5. The intensity of infection among the four groups of sheep was very different because they were maintained on different farms. The differences between rates of infection on the four different farms

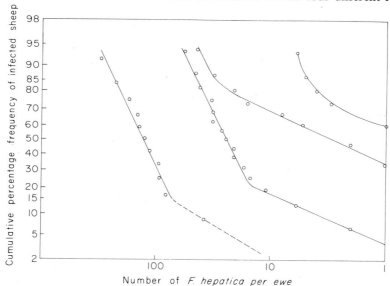

Fig. 5. The distribution of *F. hepatica* among four groups of naturally infected sheep with mean liver fluke burdens of 133, 21·8, 4·67 and 1·26 liver flukes per ewe.

were reflected in the group means of 1·26, 4·67, 21·8 and 133 liver flukes per ewe. Among the two most heavily infected groups of sheep most of the data points fit a lognormal distribution whereas among the two most lightly infected groups the distribution may more nearly approximate to a Poissonian. In the lightly infected groups a relatively small proportion of sheep carry a high proportion of the parasite population, whereas in the heavily infected groups the parasites are distributed more evenly among the hosts.

The distribution of liver flukes in experimental sheep is unlikely to parallel that of liver flukes in farm animals and it is even more unlikely that there is much similarity to the distribution of schistosomes among human beings. However, the example does illustrate that prevalence rates are not a good indicator of the abundance of trematode parasites. An important point to note is that if the mean parasite burden in either of the heavily infected groups of sheep were reduced by as much as 50 per cent the effect on prevalence might be negligible. On the other hand a reduction in mean parasite burden of the two lightly infected groups would probably be associated with a considerable reduction in prevalence.

The problems of collecting and interpreting incidence and prevalence data in relation to schistosomiasis control have been discussed by Farooq and Hairston (1966) who were concerned with measurement of the incidence of schistosomiasis in the Egypt-49 project. One of the objectives of this WHO/UNESCO-sponsored project was to demonstrate that large-scale molluscicide applications would interrupt disease transmission. An egg-counting method developed by Bell (1963) was used by Farooq *et al.* (1966) to demonstrate a significant reduction in transmission on the basis of egg-counts in urine and faecal samples collected from 0–6 year-old children. After two years of molluscicide treatments, i.e. in 1963 and 1964, the annual incidence of *S. haematobium* had been reduced from 22·8 to 8·3 per cent and the annual incidence of *S. mansoni* had been reduced from 8·5 to 1·9 per cent. These reductions in incidence compared very favourably with those in a comparable untreated area where the incidence of *S. haematobium* increased from 18·0 to 21·4 per cent and that of *S. mansoni* from 6·4 to 13·4 per cent.

Molluscicide treatments in the Egypt-49 project area continued until 1970 and Gilles *et al.* (1973) carried out a further evaluation of the effect of molluscicides on disease, this time based on prevalence data. Finding that a high proportion of the children that were negative in 1963 had become positive by 1970 Gilles *et al.* concluded: "that the *overall interruption* of transmission over the 7-year period of the project was unsatisfactory and that as a *single method* of control mollusciciding, as carried out in Project UAR 0049, is not to be recommended. Whether the intensity of infection (an important parameter in the pathogenesis of schistosomiasis) has been adversely affected or not, is not known".

It is perhaps unfortunate that the phrase "interruption of transmission" is widely used in the literature with respect to snail control. In practice control measures generally aim at reducing snail populations to a minimum at times when the snails are potentially infective. If successful, such measures may be expected to reduce the incidence of infections among mammalian hosts. However, it is not possible to assume that a reduction in snail numbers will be directly proportional to a reduction in incidence of mammalian infections.

It is difficult to obtain convincing experimental evidence of the effect of snail control measures on the incidence of mammalian infections. In this respect a basic weakness of the design of the Egypt-49 Project was that only two plots were involved, albeit very large plots, and therefore evaluation of differences between treatments depended on the comparison of human infections within only two plots, one treated with molluscicides, the other untreated. It is difficult to devise satisfactory alternatives to the unreplicated field trial in the case of schistosomiasis because of the mobility of the human host in relation to the size of the plots. In the case of fascioliasis this practical difficulty can be overcome by maintaining groups of animals entirely within the confines of a series of experimental plots.

In the field there are always considerable differences between plots, however carefully they are chosen. Variation may be attributable not only to climatic, edaphic and hydrologic factors but also to biological factors such as snail numbers, snail infection rates and rates of contamination by parasites' eggs. Variation between the infectivity of plots is therefore much greater than variation between the susceptibility of mammalian hosts, so that it is better to use a large number of plots, each with a few mammals, than to use only a few plots containing a large number of mammals.

The author (Crossland, 1976) used 17 pairs of 0·20 ha plots and seven lambs per plot to investigate the effect of a single molluscicide treatment on snail numbers and the incidence of infections among lambs. One plot in each pair was treated with a molluscicide. The numbers of snails per plot were estimated using a quadrat counting method. The lambs were grazed on the plots for varying periods before and after treatment. They were then removed from the plots and maintained on a fluke-free diet for a further six weeks before being slaughtered. The lambs' livers were examined at postmortem and liver flukes were removed and counted.

On the basis of the snail counts the overall efficiency of the molluscicide treatments was 93 per cent (85–96 per cent) and there was a highly significant reduction ($p < 0·001$) in the incidence of infections among lambs from treated plots compared with those from untreated plots. However, there was no correlation ($r = -0·03$) between snail numbers and the numbers of liver flukes acquired by tracer lambs. This finding demonstrates that, although the relation between snail numbers and incidence of infections among mammalian hosts is by no means a simple one, snail control is an effective method of controlling transmission of trematode parasites.

5 Population dynamics

5.1 PARASITE POPULATION DYNAMICS

The most detailed study of trematode population dynamics is attributable to Pesigan et al. (1958a, b, c) for S. japonicum in the Philippines. The data have been analysed by Hairston (1965, 1973) who applied the methods of classical population ecology.

Techniques for studying the population dynamics of free-living organisms are well established and if sufficient data are available changes in abundance and age structure can be predicted using the technique of matrix analysis. For trematode parasites, changes in density depend not only on the usual population parameters, i.e. age structure, birth, death, immigration and emigration rates, relating to the parasite itself but also on those parameters that describe the population dynamics of its various hosts. Hairston (1965) has described the basic technique for collating life-table data with respect to *Oncomelania quadrasi*, the amphibious snail host of *S. japonicum*. In Table 1 the probability of survival of females (l_x) and the number of female eggs produced (m_x) are listed for each of 29 different age classes. The sum of $l_x m_x$ for the 29 age classes gives the net reproductive rate per generation and in this case approximates to an expected value of 1·0 for a population whose density was neither increasing nor decreasing.

A similar technique may be used to construct a parasite's life-table but the process is more complicated because it is necessary to make separate estimates of the net reproductive rates in snails and mammals and also to estimate the death rates of the free-living larval stages. The problem may be stated as a simple equation as follows:

$$\text{net reproductive rate of schistosome} = \text{net reproductive rate in snail} \times \text{probability of infecting a mammal}$$

$$\times \text{net reproductive rate in mammal} \times \text{probability of infecting a snail}$$

If the parasite population does not change greatly with time it is legitimate to assume a stable age distribution, i.e. a net reproductive rate of 1·0. From data obtained for the village of Malirong in the Philippines, Hairston attempted to estimate the values of the parameters on the right-hand side of the above equation and assumed that the solution should approximate to a value of 1·0. Departure from this prediction was assumed to be an estimate of the total error involved in the calculations.

The net reproductive rate for the parasite in snails was estimated using life-table data in a similar way to that described for the snail host. Data for the l_x column were obtained by estimating the survival rate of infected snails in a series of laboratory and field experiments. Data for the m_x column, i.e. age-specific rates of cercarial production, were obtained from laboratory-reared infected snails. The net parasite reproductive rate had to be computed separately for male and female snails because female *O. quadrasi* live considerably longer than males. $\sum l_x m_x$ for females was 63·3 and for males 37·8. Over a two-year period the average number of infected snails in the area

TABLE 1

Life-table for *Oncomelania quadrasi* (after Hairston, 1965)

Age in days (x)	Survival of females	Female eggs produced per female (m_x)	$l_x m_x$
0	1·000		
16	0·763		
26	0·489		
46	0·240		
66	0·138		
86	0·086		
106	0·062	0·0	0·000
126	0·051	1·5	0·077
146	0·042	4·0	0·168
166	0·034	4·0	0·136
186	0·028	4·0	0·112
206	0·023	4·0	0·092
226	0·019	4·0	0·076
246	0·016	4·0	0·064
266	0·013	4·0	0·052
286	0·011	4·0	0·044
306	0·007	4·0	0·036
326	0·007	4·0	0·028
346	0·006	4·0	0·024
366	0·005	4·0	0·020
386	0·004	4·0	0·016
406	0·003	4·0	0·012
426	0·003	4·0	0·012
446	0·002	4·0	0·008
466	0·002	4·0	0·008
486	0·001	4·0	0·004
506	0·001	4·0	0·004
526	0·001	4·0	0·004
546	0·000	4·0	0·000

$\Sigma = 0\cdot997$ (= net reproductive rate per generation)

was 280 309 females and 157 674 males. The net reproductive rate for the parasite in snails was then calculated as

$$63\cdot3 \times \frac{280\ 309}{437\ 983} + 37\cdot8 \times \frac{157\ 674}{437\ 983} = 54\cdot15.$$

In order to compute the net reproductive rate in mammals it was necessary to obtain data for the age-specific survival rate of worms in mammals (the l_x

column) and the rate of production of viable eggs from these worms (the m_x column). From a consideration of age-prevalence data for the human host, together with the results of animal experiments, it was possible to estimate the death rate of adult trematodes as $0 \cdot 25$ female worms per annum. The death rate of the parasite was then combined with the death rate of its human host, $0 \cdot 012$ per annum, to obtain data for age-specific survival rates of female worms (l_x). The age-specific rate of reproduction (m_x) was estimated from the results of egg counts in urine and faecal samples obtained from people in different age groups. Multiplication of $l_x m_x$ by the proportion of 5-year-old infected children and by the average number of female worms per infected child gave $165\ 549 \times 0 \cdot 152 \times 3 \cdot 051 = 76\ 766$. Similar computations were carried out for people of all age groups, leading to a calculated net reproductive rate for the average fluke in the human population of $9 \cdot 05 \times 10^4$.

In the village of Malirong, pigs, dogs and rats are also hosts of *S. japonicum*. Life-tables and similar estimates of the parasite's net reproductive rate were obtained in these three mammals. These were much lower than in the human host; in rats, 63; in pigs, 640; in dogs, 5015.

The probability of cercariae infecting a mammal was estimated from data relating to the output of cercariae from the snail population and the infection rate of the mammalian hosts. For the waters in the vicinity of Malirong Hairston estimated that $437\ 983$ infected snails produced an average of $9 \cdot 7 \times 10^5$ cercariae per day. For field rats near the village the mean length of life was $60 \cdot 6$ days and the mean worm load $20 \cdot 4$ worms per rat. The success rate of cercariae is therefore $20 \cdot 4/60 \cdot 6 = 0 \cdot 337$ cercariae per rat per day. The number of rats was estimated to be 3075 and therefore $3075 \times 0 \cdot 337 = 1036$ successful cercariae per day. The success rate for parasites entering rats was then estimated as

$$\frac{1036}{9 \cdot 7} \times 10^{-5} = 1 \cdot 04 \times 10^{-3}.$$

The figures for cercariae infecting pigs and dogs were $9 \cdot 82 \times 10^{-6}$ and $1 \cdot 69 \times 10^{-6}$ respectively.

It is not possible to obtain direct experimental evidence concerning the rate of infection among humans. However, it is possible to deduce this rate from age-prevalence data, assuming random distribution of worms among humans. Although it is basically incorrect, this assumption may be permissible for certain kinds of data, e.g. those drawn from samples stratified between urban and rural populations. If the proportion of people acquiring female worms is p and the proportion not acquiring female worms is q, the annual incidence of disease is equal to p^2 and the mean number of worms per person may be calculated from the relationship:

$$1 - p^2 = e^{-m}$$

where m is the mean number of worms per person (this relationship is true only for a $1:1$ sex ratio and the Poisson distribution).

Using this method Hairston estimated that $4 \cdot 2$ cercariae succeeded in infecting the population of Malirong each day and therefore the probability of success of cercariae in humans was

$$\frac{4 \cdot 2}{9 \cdot 7 \times 10^5} = 4 \cdot 3 \times 10^{-6}$$

The probability of a miracidium infecting a snail was calculated using the same kind of principles as described for those in calculating the probability of success of a cercaria. The total daily output of parasite eggs from the four mammalian hosts was estimated to be 832 401 and the rate of snail infection 19 211 snails per day. The probability of success of the miracidium was therefore estimated as $19\,211 \div 832\,401 = 0 \cdot 0231$.

Hairston was now able to estimate the overall net reproductive rate of the parasite as a combination of the net reproductive rates in its various hosts multiplied by the estimated chances of success of the free-living larval stages. The solution was

$$54 \cdot 15 \times \sum \begin{Bmatrix} 4 \cdot 3 \times 10^{-6} \times 9 \cdot 05 \times 10^4 \\ 1 \cdot 04 \times 10^{-3} \times 63 \\ 1 \cdot 69 \times 10^{-6} \times 5 \cdot 02 \times 10^3 \\ 9 \cdot 82 \times 10^{-6} \times 6 \cdot 4 \times 10^2 \end{Bmatrix} \times (2 \cdot 31 \times 10^{-2}) = 0 \cdot 588$$

The result is different from the predicted value of $1 \cdot 0$, possibly because the net reproductive rate in rats has been grossly underestimated. Hairston was unable to obtain satisfactory data for this species although he suspected that the rat may play a major role in the life-cycle of *S. japonicum*.

Attempts to construct life-tables for the other species of schistosomes have yielded results which depart even more widely from predictions. It is clearly very difficult to obtain all of the necessary data required to construct a life-table for these parasites. The approach is intellectually appealing and it certainly helps to highlight weaknesses in measurements of parasite population dynamics. The resolution of life-tables in a few carefully chosen situations would be invaluable as an aid to the rational design of control programmes. However, there are very considerable technical and practical problems to be solved in order to obtain adequate data for any given area.

5.2 HOST POPULATION DYNAMICS

Estimates of the snail and mammalian populations were essential ingredients of Hairston's analysis of the population dynamics of *S. japonicum* in the

Philippines. Four mammalian populations had to be considered because of the importance of rats, dogs and pigs as reservoir hosts. In many areas the reservoir hosts carry only a small proportion of the total parasite population and may be safely ignored for practical purposes.

The population densities of human beings and their livestock have increased substantially during the last few decades, thereby increasing the chances of successful transmission of trematode parasites between their alternate hosts. Undoubtedly this has been a major factor in the spread of trematode diseases in the twentieth century. However, mammalian birth rates and death rates are low relative to those of the parasite. In considering short-term changes in parasite numbers it is therefore permissible to regard the density of the mammalian population as static, or subject only to changes arising from emigration or immigration.

On the other hand snail population densities in most areas change very rapidly and such changes have a considerable effect on the numbers of parasitic larval trematodes. In the tropics the average life-span of a snail host may be only 4–8 weeks while the average life-span of an infective snail may amount to only one or two weeks (Sturrock, 1973a, 1973b). Young snails are more susceptible to infection than old snails and development of infection within a snail reduces its chances of survival (Pan, 1965). The output of infective cercariae from any given snail population will therefore depend not only on snail density and the input of miracidia but also on the age structure of the snail population.

The key role of the snail host in regulating schistosome population densities has long been recognized by the World Health Organization, which has sponsored numerous studies. From life-tables that have been constructed for various species of host snails it is possible to calculate r, the biotic potential or intrinsic rate of natural increase, for specific environmental conditions. This parameter reflects the maximum growth rate achievable by populations in an unlimited environment for specific microclimatic conditions. Populations living in stable environments have low values for r, whereas populations living in unstable environments or subject to frequent climatic changes have high values for r. Thus Pesigan et al. (1958a, b) found that r for O. quadrasi, a snail that lives in a relatively stable environment, was 0·013 at a temperature of 27·5°C, whereas Sevilla (1965) reported a value for r of 0·123 at 25°C for B. glabrata, a snail that lives in a relatively unstable environment.

The intrinsic rate of natural increase, r, is useful for calculating the expected rate of repopulation following adverse weather conditions or molluscicide treatments. The maximum rate of population growth may be calculated from the equation:

$$N_t = N_0 e^{rt} \tag{1}$$

where N_t is the number of individuals at time t and N_0 is the number of individuals at the start.

Using this equation and the values for r given above it may be calculated that if 95 per cent of a population of B. glabrata were killed by molluscicide treatment its pretreatment population density would be restored in 25 days, given optimal environmental conditions. On the other hand it would require 235 days for a population of O. quadrasi to make a similar recovery.

The environment exerts a profound affect on the ability of organisms to achieve their biotic potential and snails are no exception to this general rule. It has been shown that temperature can have a considerable effect on the growth rate of snail populations. For some species, e.g. B. glabrata and Bulinus globosus, r varies by a factor of two or three within a 10°C range of water temperatures. For other species, i.e. those with a smaller degree of tolerance to water temperature, r varies by a factor of five or six within a 5°C range.

Values of r obtained for field populations of snails tend to be somewhat lower than those obtained for populations reared under optimal laboratory conditions. For example Dazo et al. (1966) obtained a value of 0·048 for Bulinus truncatus under field conditions in Egypt but Hairston (1973) calculated a value of 0·065 for this species reared under favourable laboratory conditions by Chu et al. (1966). Sturrock (1973a) obtained values for r in the range 0·02–0·04 for field populations of B. glabrata, whereas Sevilla (1965) obtained 0·123 under the most favourable laboratory conditions.

In all environments the growth of populations is limited by the carrying capacity of the habitat. As populations grow the individuals within it interact upon one other to a greater and greater extent and various kinds of density-dependent regulatory mechanisms become more and more important. In practice this means that the maximum growth rate defined by equation (1) is rarely achieved, even when microclimatic conditions are optimal. Recognizing the importance of environmental factors in limiting population growth Sturrock found that a logistic growth equation (2) fitted his snail population data somewhat better than equation (1).

$$N_t = \frac{K}{1 + e^{a - rt}} \qquad (2)$$

where K is a measure of the carrying capacity and a is a constant.

The role of the snail host L. truncatula in the life-cycle of F. hepatica was first described by Thomas (1883) and further studies have been carried out by Bruce et al. (1973), Kendal (1949), Ollerenshaw (1966), Morphy (1973) and Ross (1967). Under optimal conditions for snail population growth Kendal showed that one snail can give rise to 25 000 descendants in two generations in

12 weeks, from which it is possible to calculate a value for r of $0 \cdot 12$. Morphy has recently collected much of the basic data needed to construct a life-table for *L. truncatula* but the effect of temperature and other environmental factors on r have not been investigated.

The climate exerts a considerable effect on the population growth of *L. truncatula*. Popularly called the mud snail, this species lives on the margins of ponds and ditches where it feeds on blue-green algae, e.g. *Oscillatoria* sp. and possibly other algae that bloom on moist mud or in very shallow water. The extent of the available habitat and its carrying capacity are subject to unpredictable and rapid fluctuations. In warm, moist weather extensive areas of clay or peaty soil may become rapidly colonized by snails. If the weather changes the soil may dry out and the snails may crawl beneath herbage or into cracks in the soil where they aestivate by becoming immobile and applying the aperture of the shell firmly to a suitable surface. Because of their response to alternating dry and wet conditions the abundance and distribution of *L. truncatula* are constantly changing. This poses formidable sampling problems that have not been satisfactorily resolved. The rate of growth of field populations of *L. truncatula* for a range of environmental conditions is largely unknown.

6 Mathematical models

According to Walters (1971) ecological models can be evaluated in terms of three basic goals: realism, precision and generality. Realism refers to the degree with which formal mathematical statements of the model represent basic biological concepts. A mathematical model may be nothing more complicated than a simple description of a biological problem or process in mathematical terms. More frequently mathematical models of complicated biological processes are developed so that they can be used in computer programs to simulate dynamic changes in biological systems over a period of time. When used in this way the precision of a model is defined as its ability to predict change. Its generality is defined as its applicability to a range of different circumstances.

Modelling of trematode population dynamics is still in its infancy and while some valuable and instructive modelling attempts have been made, none of the modellers can claim to have developed a realistic representation of the whole of the trematode life-cycle. Cohen (1976) has critically reviewed all known mathematical models for schistosomiasis and compares the activities of himself and other modellers to those of learned blind men trying to discover the true nature of an elephant. Each one discovers a different part of the elephant's anatomy by touch and arrives at a different conclusion about the nature of the elephant.

One of the first and most interesting contributions is that of Macdonald (1965). His model followed a successful precedent set by Ross and Hudson (1931) and Macdonald (1957) with respect to the epidemiology of malaria. In his schistosomiasis model Macdonald represented transmission as occurring in four stages: an inoculation rate of snails; multiplication of parasitic larvae within infected snails; an inoculation rate of man; and the growth of infection in man.

The inoculation rate of snails was defined as $Bm\alpha$, where m is the mean number of worms per human host, α is the proportion of m which are paired (assuming random distribution of worms among hosts) and B is the probability of a snail living until cercariae develop.

If p is the probability of a snail surviving through one day, the infection rate of snails is

$$\frac{Bm\alpha}{Bm\alpha - \ln p}.$$

The inoculation rate of man, h, may be defined as a product of snail infection rate, snail density and frequency of human contact with water.

$$h = \frac{ABm\alpha}{Bm\alpha - \ln p}$$

where A = snail density $\times$ frequency of human contact with water and the rate of change of parasite numbers is defined as

$$\frac{dm}{dt} = h - rm,$$

where r is the death rate of the parasites.

In this model the infection rate of snails is therefore assumed to be a density-independent function and this is unlikely to be so.

Macdonald also assumes that there is a direct relation between worm burden in mammals and snail infection rate and this too has been challenged by Hairston (quoted by Cohen, 1976).

Macdonald used numerical values in his model to predict the outcome of various happenings, including control measures, on parasite numbers. One of his predictions was that there exists a "break-point", i.e. a critical number of parasites below which the parasite population will decline to extinction. This particular concept is based on the assumption of random distribution of worms among hosts, an assumption that cannot be true in the light of more recent work (e.g. Bradley, 1972) which shows that the distribution of adult schistosomes is highly aggregated. Another prediction of Macdonald's is that a great reduction in the number of eggs reaching water has a negligible effect on transmission, a conclusion that follows from his implicit assumption that the water in which snails live is saturated with miracidia.

Nåsell and Hirsch (1972) visualized trematode diseases as a problem in compartmental analysis, as shown in Fig. 6.

Models by Nåsell and Hirch (1972, 1973) introduce some new and better techniques for mathematical treatment of trematode population dynamics but they lack realism since they take no account of variations in the host populations and their interactions with the environment.

The relationship between incidence of acute fascioliasis in sheep and meteorological data and the use of this relationship in forecasting outbreaks of disease

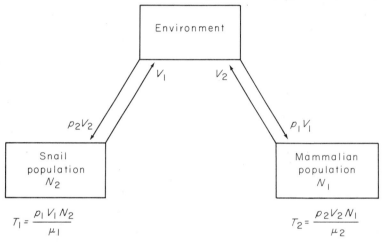

FIG. 6. Basic compartmental model (after Nåsell, 1972).

have been described by Ollerenshaw and Rowlands (1959). These workers have established that the incidence and severity of disease are dependent on both temperature and soil surface moisture. The amount and duration of rainfall during the summer months are particularly important in determining the severity of outbreaks in the UK.

Gettinby (1974a, b) and Gettinby et al. (1974) have proposed several models for predicting the prevalence of acute fascioliasis and its control from meteorological data. Building on the earlier work of Ollerenshaw and Rowlands these workers have concentrated on modelling the effect of temperature on liver fluke infection among sheep. The basic model used to relate development of eggs and parasitic stages within the snail to temperature is

$$D_T = D_0 e^{a_0 T},$$

where D_T is the development time, in days, at a constant temperature T.

$D_0 = e^a$, e is the base of natural logarithms, and a_0 and a^1 are constants derived from the regression equation $\ln D_T = a_0 T + a_1$.

The relationships between temperature and rate of development of parasitic larval stages are described in considerable detail and the models are tested by comparison with data for *F. hepatica* in sheep in the West of Ireland.

Gettinby (1974a) has proposed a matrix formulation of liver fluke population dynamics. The use of matrices is a well-established algebraic method for dealing with life-table data. If the birth rate, death rate and age distribution of a population are known the matrix technique can be used to predict how the population will change in time. Gettinby used fecundity, survival probabilities and probabilities of transition from one stage to another as elements in his matrices. From studies of disease transmission on the West coast of Ireland estimates of the fecundities, survival and transition probabilities were used in the matrices to predict the probable annual patterns of pasture infection with metacercariae. The predicted pattern of annual infection appears to fit an observed set of data reasonably well. However, Gettinby assumed that moisture conditions are not limiting, an assumption that may be justified for the high rainfall and peaty soil of the West of Ireland but is not valid for most endemic areas. One consequence of this assumption is that the model does not allow for interactions between moisture, snail population dynamics and parasite population dynamics.

Models must be used with great caution, especially as far as their predictive value is concerned. The predictions of a model can be no more reliable than the underlying biological theory on which they are based. Notwithstanding the many weaknesses and imperfections of existing models, they have made some important contributions to the understanding of trematode population dynamics and are likely to play an important role in determining future control strategies.

None of the models that have been proposed to date allows for interactions between parasite, snail and mammalian populations. The work of Hairston with respect to *S. japonicum* in the Philippines clearly demonstrates the dependence of parasite numbers on snail population dynamics and on mammalian population dynamics. Any model that aspires to realism and the possibility of development for useful predictive purposes should not ignore these essential features of the trematode life-cycle.

Perhaps there is scope for the development of a compartmental model of the kind illustrated in Fig. 7. The size of the compartments in this model are proportional to the numbers of snails, parasitic larval stages, mammals and adult parasites. The rates of change of the numbers of organisms in these four compartments are controlled by rates of birth, death, emigration and immigration and are represented by valves as shown. The numbers of mammals and the numbers of snails are controlled by their own intrinsic rates of increase and decrease and therefore they have no direct effect on the parasite system. However, as the numbers of snails and mammals change they affect the opening and closing of valves that regulate the numbers of parasitic larval and adult parasites. These interactions between the snail, mammal and parasite

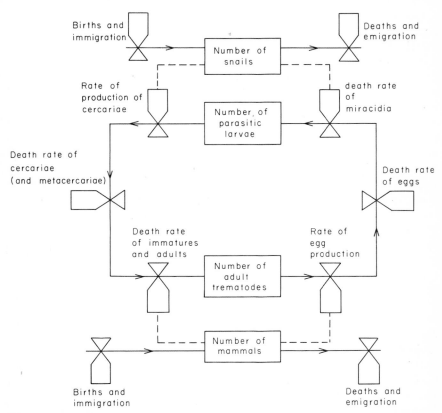

FIG. 7. Flow diagram to illustrate the interdependence of parasite, snail and mammalian populations.

populations are represented by dotted lines in the diagram. The death rates of the free-living larval stages are similarly represented by valves connected by solid lines between parasitic larvae and adult parasites. The death rates of these free-living stages are regulated by environmental influences such as temperature and moisture.

Flow diagrams of the kind illustrated in Fig. 7 do not require any mathematical skills yet allow the biologist to define his concepts in terms that can be translated into formal mathematical statements. It may then be possible to carry out meaningful computer simulations to investigate the ways in which various components of a complex biological system interact.

An important feature that needs to be considered in building a trematode model is the relative generation times of parasites, snails and mammals. Compared with the mean life-span of the adult parasites and the mammalian hosts, the life-span of the snails is relatively short.

7 Integration of control methods

In agricultural entomology "integrated control" is generally used to refer to a combination of chemical and biological control methods for control of agricultural pests. Predators and parasites of many pest species of insects play a useful role in regulating the population density of pests. If the life-cycles of pests and natural enemies are sufficiently well known the timing of insecticide treatments may be selected so as to achieve maximum reduction of the population densities of the pests but have minimum effect on populations of natural enemies. In recent years the term "pest management" has become more widely used to describe systems of pest control involving both biological and chemical control methods. Pest management systems may include the introduction of pesticide-resistant predators and often involve biological monitoring of insect populations as an aid to selection of the best time for insecticide treatments.

The concept of integrated control of trematode diseases is defined in this paper as a combination of control methods aimed at the parasitic stages of the trematode life-cycle. Only two basic control methods are required. One of these methods should aim at reducing the numbers of adult parasites in the mammalian hosts and the other should aim at reducing the numbers of parasitic larvae in the snail hosts. Control of the free-living parasitic larval stages will be an indirect consequence of the application of these two basic methods. In Fig. 7 the parasite system consists of two compartments containing parasitic adult and larval stages and six rate processes, or valves, that control the flow of parasites through the compartments. A coordinated effort to reduce the level of parasites in the compartments will have an effect on the levels in these compartments and also have a direct effect on four of the six rate processes, or valves, in the cycle.

The concept of using more than one control method is nothing new. Perhaps the first advocate of a multipronged approach was Thomas. In his classic description of the "Natural History of the Liver-fluke and the Prevention of Rot" (1883) he suggested that farmers should use a combination of control measures including drainage, grazing management and molluscicides. Early workers in the field of schistosomiasis came to similar conclusions. For example, Leiper

(1915) recommended various measures to control the free-swimming infective larval stages or the snail hosts. His proposals included the replacement of open drainage channels by pipes and mole drains, improved management of canals to discourage snail breeding and the use of molluscicides. The multipronged approach to control, using all of the available techniques, has obvious merit if the objective is to control disease at whatever cost. It has been demonstrably successful in controlling schistosomiasis in countries such as Japan, Israel, Venezuela and Puerto Rico, where economic considerations have been relatively unimportant. It has also been successful in controlling fascioliasis on farms that have been able to afford relatively expensive land improvements and farm management techniques. However, in the majority of endemic areas there are many other important demands on the available public and private funds and it is necessary for public health workers and farmers to operate within considerable financial constraints. A multipronged approach to trematode disease control while possibly offering the best chance of success is beyond the financial and technical resources available to many people.

Faced with the economic imperatives there has been a tendency for research to seek a simple panacea, a new wonder drug, vaccine, biological control agent or molluscicide that will somehow solve the problems. In fact chemical industry aided by universities, governments and international agencies has been remarkably successful in producing effective drugs and molluscicides. The available chemicals have their limitations but other pests and diseases have been successfully controlled with less perfect weaponry. There is now a basic need to develop ways of using the available chemicals and applying technology more efficiently, i.e. to increase the benefits obtainable from control programmes while minimizing their costs.

Theoretical and experimental evidence reviewed in previous sections indicates that effective control of trematode parasites requires a two-pronged attack, i.e. control of adult parasite numbers allied with control of parasitic larval stages. The only method of reducing the numbers of parasites in the mammalian hosts, other than by natural mortality, is chemotherapy. This method should be combined with one or more of the available methods of snail control. Unlike the multipronged approach this two pronged method seeks to achieve maximum effectiveness at minimum cost. Attempts to control the free-living larval stages are likely to be relatively expensive because the larval stages are widely dispersed in the environment compared with the parasitic stages.

A permanent solution to the problem of snail control, e.g. by drainage of snail habitats, may be preferable to the use of molluscicides. However, eradication of snail habitats is often impossible or expensive. When using molluscicides the timing of treatments is at least as important as the effect on snail densities. Actively growing snail populations are more important in the transmission of disease than senescent populations, because conditions that favour snail breeding also favour development of parasitic larval stages. A correctly timed molluscicide treatment may prevent a seasonal increase in the density of the snail population and at the same time prevent the development of parasitic larvae within a new generation of snails.

The following examples have been chosen to illustrate the effectiveness of integrated control programmes. They have all been based on the use of relatively new synthetic drugs and molluscicides.

The control of *S. mansoni* on a sugar estate in Tanzania has been described in papers by Crossland (1967), Foster (1967), Fenwick (1970) and Fenwick and Jorgensen (1972). The estate is situated in a low-rainfall area in the Kilimanjaro region of Tanzania at an altitude of 610 m. About 25 000 tons of sugar are produced annually. The cultivation of sugar is entirely dependent on the irrigation. For water management purposes the estate is divided into two areas, called the Old Area and the New Area. Water is supplied from the Weru Weru River via two main canals. One of these canals supplies water to the Old Area and has a discharge of 1100 litres per second, while the other one supplies water to the New Area and has a discharge of 1700 litres per second. To make the best use of available water the company has built a series of reservoirs that function as night storage dams. From the reservoirs secondary canals carry water to an extensive system of tertiary canals that run alongside the fields of sugar cane. Plastic siphons are used to feed water from the tertiary canals to the rows of sugar cane. A separate drainage system, much less extensive than the canal system, collects excess irrigation water or water that collects after rain.

During the period of the studies described by the above-mentioned authors, i.e. from 1960 to 1970, the company employed a resident labour force of 2250 workers. Together with wives and families the total resident population was about 5000. Some of the labourers were from the Kilimanjaro region but the majority were migrants from a much wider geographical area.

The estate's hospital has 75 beds, a doctor, medical assistant and two nurses. All patients at the hospital were routinely examined and infected persons were treated. All new employees were examined for infection with *S. mansoni* and periodic surveys were carried out on all of the workers and their families. All those found to be infected were given an antimonial preparation during the early years of the investigation but hycanthone was introduced when this was shown to be more effective and produced fewer side effects.

The irrigation system was treated with molluscicide (trifenmorph, triphenylmethylmorpholine, Frescon) using a simple, automatic dispenser to apply a prolonged low dosage of molluscicide from the headwaters. The drainage system was treated with niclosamide using knapsack sprayers. Two snail searchers were employed to monitor the effectiveness of molluscicide treatments. These measures were successful in keeping the snail population at a permanently low density in an area where breeding and disease transmission can occur all year round.

Before control measures started the prevalence of *S. mansoni* in adults was greater than 50 per cent and in school children up to 75–100 per cent as revealed by surveys carried out in 1961–5. The overall prevalence was reduced to about 20 per cent in 1970 and new cases among young children were reduced to zero. The cost of the control programme was virtually covered by savings in the cost of treating hospitalized patients.

The control of *S. haematobium* in the lower Mangoky region of Madagascar has been described in considerable detail by Degrémont (1973). The project area was situated in the delta of the river Mangoky in Southwest Madagascar. The flood plain of the delta has a rich alluvial soil and therefore has considerable potential for agricultural development. The mean monthly air temperature varies from 20 to 28°C. The average annual rainfall is 60 cm. About 90 per cent of this rainfall occurs in the rainy season, from December until March. Cyclonic tropical storms sometimes occur at this time and may cause flooding of the river, considerable damage to property and disruption of communications. It was a noteworthy achievement that the project was carried through to a satisfactory conclusion despite catastrophic flooding of the region in 1969 and 1970 and many other practical difficulties associated with the remoteness of the area and poor communications.

In an introduction to Degrémont's report Professor Geigy of the Swiss Tropical Institute describes the objectives of the project as follows:

Knowing that schistosomiasis considerably slows down economic development in endemic regions, particularly in irrigated areas, we considered that it would be preferable to prevent introduction of the disease to the area rather than to control an already established and perfectly adapted infestation. The irrigated area, already partly developed, provided an excellent example in which to confirm this idea and to demonstrate its profitability. By examining all inhabitants of the region and all immigrant workers before they settled in the area, and then treating all infected people we intended to prevent the occurrence of a human reservoir. Similarly, by rigorously controlling the irrigation system and by applying molluscicide where necessary, we intended to remove all intermediate hosts and reduce the chances that a transmission cycle could be set up. These two lines of attack must be consolidated by a continued effort to provide health education for the people.

The project was carried out over a five-year period from 1966 to 1971 during the development phase of an irrigated area. About 3000 ha of land were irrigated from a main canal discharging 10 000 litres per second into secondary, tertiary and quaternary canals. For cotton cultivation 600 000 litres of water per ha are used every 10 days and for rice the fields are flooded for a period of three months at a time. There are some 30 reservoirs varying in size from about $\frac{1}{20}$ to 1 ha in surface area. There are also numerous "borrow pits", i.e. excavations resulting from road, canal and drain construction, that become filled with water during the rainy season. The drainage system is of variable quality and the principal, secondary and tertiary drains are frequently choked with aquatic weeds.

About 10 000 inhabitants were living in the area, including 2000 to 3000 annual migrants. All of these people were required to submit to a compulsory medical examination at a Health Centre and to hold a health card. Samples of urine from all inhabitants were examined at least twice. At 30th June, 1969 it was estimated that 1335 people were infected with S. haematobium. There was a sudden appearance of transmission foci in two villages resulting in a very rapid increase in infections among the people living there. For example at the village school of Ambahikily it was found that 154 out of 155 pupils were positive in June, 1969.

Soon after this situation was discovered an integrated control programme was launched. Most of the snail habitats were treated with molluscicide (trifenmorph) on two separate occasions between November and February, which are the most important months for snail breeding. All infected people were treated with niridazole (Ambilhar), which was given as a 7-day course at 25 mg kg^{-1} d^{-1}. A daily dose was given in two parts, one in the morning, the other in the afternoon. All tablets were swallowed in the presence of the person distributing them. Treatment was generally well tolerated although there were some transient effects of minor importance such as dizziness, headache and abdominal pains.

As a result of these measures transmission of disease in the two foci was stopped. Habitats of the snail hosts elsewhere in the project area were similarly treated with molluscicide and infected people were treated with niridazole. As a result of these measures the overall level of infection was reduced to around 4 per cent, which corresponds approximately to the level of infections outside the project area.

The cost of the project was about 23 Swiss francs per person protected per year and this figure includes the cost of equipment, buildings and vehicles. Bearing in mind the extremely difficult conditions in which the project was undertaken it is highly probable that with the experience gained a similar result could be achieved at a greatly reduced cost if such a project were undertaken elsewhere.

These notable but somewhat limited successes in schistosomiasis control were possible because the administration of drugs and the control of snails were under the control of a single management, thereby permitting the proper integration of control techniques.

The control of chronic fascioliasis in sheep using a combination of drugs and molluscicides has been reported by Crossland et al. (1977). An experiment was carried out during a period of three years on five pairs of 1·60 ha plots located in Shropshire, UK. Each of these plots was divided into four paddocks and the paddocks were grazed in rotation by 16 ewes plus their lambs. The fence lines were arranged such that each paddock included an area of snail habitat, generally about 25 per cent of the total grazing area.

One hundred and sixty Welsh Half Bred yearling ewes, each with a single lamb, were allocated at random into 10 groups of 16 ewes plus their lambs. They were introduced onto the experimental plots in spring, 1970. In summer the original crop of single lambs was weaned and in autumn the ewes were mated with Suffolk Down rams. After mating the ewes were kept on the plots until late December when they were removed and managed as a single flock in preparation for lambing. In February and March, 1971 the new born lambs were weighed and tagged and in spring each group of ewes plus their lambs were returned to their original plots. This second crop of lambs, containing single births, twins and triplets, was weaned in summer and the schedule of mating, lambing and producing fat lambs was repeated in 1971–2. The productivity of each group of 16 ewes was measured in terms of the weight of lambs produced at weaning in 1971 and 1972. The performance of the ewes was also monitored by weighing them at intervals during the experiment.

Within each pair of five 1·60 ha plots fascioliasis was controlled on one plot only using chemotherapy plus molluscicide treatments. The basic strategy of the control programme was to use a single molluscicide treatment plus a single dose of a fasciolicide whenever weather conditions were unfavourable for snail breeding and development of larval parasites. When weather conditions were favourable two molluscicide plus two fasciolicide treatments were used. In practice the ewes were dosed routinely with oxyclozanide (Zanil) in the winter of 1970, 1971 and 1972. They were given one additional dose in November, 1971, following warm, moist summer weather. The snail habitats were treated routinely with molluscicide (trifenmorph) in the spring of 1970, 1971 and 1972. They were also treated in August, 1971, i.e. when conditions were favourable for snail breeding.

Lambs' livers were removed when successive lamb crops were slaughtered in 1970, 1971 and 1972. Very few liver flukes were found among the lambs and there was no significant difference between the numbers found in treated and untreated groups. This was not surprising because the lambs were grazed on the plots for only a few months in each year, i.e. from April to July. Ewes' livers were removed when the ewes were slaughtered in 1972, at the end of the experiment. By this time they had been grazing the plots continuously for two and a half years except for two winter breaks for lambing. A total of 2640 liver flukes were recovered from 72 ewes grazed on untreated plots, compared with only 17 liver flukes from 74 ewes grazed on treated plots.

The weight gain of ewes from untreated plots was significantly less ($p < 0.05$) than that of ewes from treated plots. The relatively poor health of infected ewes was reflected in a reduced output of lambs from the untreated groups compared with that from the treated groups. The relationship between numbers of *F. hepatica* and weight of lambs produced per ewe is shown in Fig. 3.

8 Conclusions

The trematode parasites discussed in this chapter have two parasitic stages that are associated with high rates of multiplication at the expense of the alternate hosts. They also have two or three free-living stages that are associated with high death rates. Attempts to control the parasitic stages are likely to be more effective than attempts to control the free-living stages. The latter are more widely dispersed in the environment, they are more numerous and are subject to relatively high mortality rates compared with the parasitic stages. Attempts to control only one of the parasitic stages, e.g. by chemotherapy or snail control, have not been successful in reducing the prevalence of disease on a large scale or for a sufficiently long period of time. It seems clear that successful control depends on a two-pronged attack on both adult and larval parasitic stages. Examples of this approach to control have been discussed and its success has been demonstrated for both schistosomiasis and fascioliasis. However, these statements do not imply that measures such as environmental sanitation, health and farmer education are unimportant. On the contrary they may be essential in order to gain the cooperation of people in pursuing the successful implementation of integrated control programmes and they may contribute to the control of other kinds of diseases.

Mathematical models may have a valuable role to play in understanding complex interactions between parasite numbers, their host populations and environmental factors. They have potential value as tools for predicting the outcome of alternative control strategies. However, mathematical models must be based on sound biological concepts and they must be validated by comparison with data collected in the field. The classical methods of studying population dynamics, as described by Hairston, seem to be the best starting point for the development of life-cycle models.

A relatively large reduction in the mean parasite burden of mammalian populations needs to be achieved in order to have an effect on prevalence rates in the majority of endemic areas. The severity of pathological and economic effects is related to the duration of infections and to a logarithmic rather than an arithmetic function of parasite burden. For these reasons it is suggested that, in order to achieve a worthwhile, measurable effect on chronic trematode diseases, control programmes must aim at reducing parasite numbers by an order of magnitude. The best hope of realizing such an objective is through the use of an integrated control programme, as defined in this paper.

Implementation of nation-wide control programmes depends not only on successful control technology but also on measurement of the pathological and economic effects of disease as a basis for the rational allocation of resources to control programmes. Expenditure on control tends to receive a low priority because trematode diseases are mostly chronic and their effects on mammals are difficult to measure. The few studies that have been carried out indicate that even light infections can have significant effects on productivity and health. It is probable that trematode diseases deserve a higher priority than they currently receive.

Acknowledgements

I am grateful to my colleagues Mr M. H. Breese and Dr E. Thorpe for helpful comments on the manuscript and to Mr P. F. Hunt for discussions concerning systems analysis.

References

Bell, D. R. (1963). *Bulletin of the World Health Organization,* **29**, 525.

Blamire, R. V., Crowley, A. J. and Goodhand, R. H. (1970). *Veterinary Record,* **87**, 234.

Bradley, D. J. (1972). *Transactions of the Royal Society of Tropical Medicine and Hygiene,* **66**, 697.

Bruce, R. G., Armour, J. and Corba, J. (1973). *Veterinary Record,* **92**, 518.

Chu, K. Y., Sabbaghian, H. and Massoud, J. (1966). *Bulletin of the World Health Organization,* **34**, 121.

Cohen, J. E. (1976). *In* "Theoretical Ecology: Principles and Applications" (Ed. Robert M. May), Blackwell Scientific, Oxford.

Crossland, N. O. (1967). *Bulletin of the World Health Organization,* **37**, 23.

Crossland, N. O. (1976). *Veterinary Record,* **98**, 45.

Crossland, N. O., Johnstone, A., Beaumont, G. and Bennett, M. S. (1977). *British Veterinary Journal,* **133**, no. 5, in press.

Dargie, J. D. (1975). *In* "Facts and Reflections", p. 43. Publ. CDI Lelystad, The Netherlands.

Dazo, B. C., Hairston, N. G. and Dawood, I. K. (1966). *Bulletin of the World Health Organization,* **35**, 339.

Degrémont, A. A. (1973). "Mangoky Project: Campaign against Schistosomiasis in the Lower-Mangoky (Madagascar)." Swiss Tropical Institute, Basle.

Donker, K. (1971). Proceedings of the Second International Liverfluke Colloquium, Wageningen, The Netherlands, p. 36. Publ. Merck International, Rahway, New Jersey.

Farooq, M. and Hairston, N. G. (1966). *Bulletin of the World Health Organization,* **35**, 331.

Farooq, M., Hairston, N. G. and Samaan, S. A. (1966). *Bulletin of the World Health Organization,* **35**, 369.

Fenwick, A. (1970). *Bulletin of the World Health Organization,* **42,** 589.
Fenwick, A. and Jorgensen, T. A. (1972). *Bulletin of the World Health Organization,* **47,** 579.
Foster, R. (1967). *Journal of Tropical Medicine and Hygiene,* **70,** 185.
Gelfand, M. (1967). *In* "A Clinical Study of Intestinal Bilharziasis in Africa". Edward Arnold, London.
Gettinby, G. (1974a). Mathematical models for the control of liverfluke infection. PhD Thesis. New University of Ulster.
Gettinby, G. (1974b). *In* "Ecological stability" (Eds M. B. Usher and M. H. Williamson). Chapman and Hall, London.
Gettinby, G. Hope-Cawdery, M. J. and Grainger, J. N. R. (1974). *International Journal of Biometeorology,* **18,** 319.
Gilles, H. M., Abdel-Aziz Zaki, A., Soussa, M. H., Samaan, S. A., Soliman Soliman, S., Hassan, A. and Barbosa, F. (1973). *Annals of Tropical Medicine and Parasitology,* **67,** 45.
Hairston, N. G. (1965). *Bulletin of the World Health Organization,* **33,** 45.
Hairston, N. G. (1973). *In* "Epidemiology and Control of Schistosomiasis (Bilharziasis)" (Ed. N. Ansari), p. 250. S. Karger, Basel.
Kendal, S. B. (1949). *Journal of Helminthology,* **23,** 57.
Leiper, R. T. (1915). Quoted by Farooq, M. (1973). *In* "Epidemiology and Control of Schistosomiasis (Bilharziasis)" (Ed. N. Ansari), p. 1. S. Karger, Basel.
Macdonald, G. (1957). "The Epidemiology and Control of Malaria". Oxford University Press, London.
Macdonald, G. (1965). *Transactions of the Royal Society of Tropical Medicine and Hygiene,* **59,** 489.
Macdonald, G. and Farooq, M. (1973). *In* "Epidemiology and Control of Schistosomiasis (Bilharziasis)" (Ed. N. Ansari), p. 337. S. Karger, Basel.
Morphy, M. J. (1973). A study of the ecology of the snail *Lymnaea truncatula* Müller. PhD Thesis, Queen's University, Belfast.
Nåsell, I. (1972). "Mathematical Models of Some Parasitic Diseases Involving an Intermediate Host", PhD Thesis, New York University.
Nåsell, I. and Hirsch, W. M. (1972). *Communications on Pure and Applied Mathematics,* **25,** 459.
Nåsell, I. and Hirsch, W. M. (1973). *Communications on Pure and Applied Mathematics,* **26,** 395.
Nelson, G. S. (1960). *Transactions of the Royal Society of Tropical Medicine and Hygiene,* **54,** 301.
Ollerenshaw, C. B. and Rowlands, W. T. (1959). *Veterinary Record,* **17,** 591.
Ollerenshaw, C. B. (1966). *Agricultural Meteorology,* **3,** 35.
Pan, C. T. (1965). *American Journal of Tropical Medicine and Hygiene,* **14,** 931.
Pesigan, T. P., Farooq, M., Hairston, N. G., Jauregui, J. J., Garcia, E. G., Santos, A. T., Santos, B. C. and Besa, A. A. (1958a). *Bulletin of the World Health Organization,* **18,** 345.
Pesigan, T. P., Farooq, M., Hairston, N. G., Jauregui, J. J., Garcia, E. G., Santos, A. T., Santos, B. C. and Besa, A. A. (1958b). *Bulletin of the World Health Organization,* **18,** 481.
Pesigan, T. P., Farooq, M., Hairston, N. G., Jauregui, J. J., Garcia, E. G., Santos, A. T., Santos, B. C. and Besa, A. A. (1958c). *Bulletin of the World Health Organization,* **19,** 223.
Ross, J. G. (1967). *Veterinary Record,* **80,** 214.

Ross, R. and Hudson, H. P. (1931). "*A priori* Pathometry". Harrison and Sons, London.

Sevilla, J. Z. (1965). PhD Thesis, University of Michigan, Ann Arbor, Michigan. Quoted by Hairston (1973).

Sewell, M. M. H. (1966). *Veterinary Record,* **78**, 98.

Sinclair, K. B. (1962). *British Veterinary Journal,* **118**, 37.

Sinclair, K. B. (1972). *British Veterinary Journal,* **128**, 249.

Sturrock, R. F. (1973a). *International Journal of Parasitology,* **3**, 165.

Sturrock, R. F. (1973b). *International Journal of Parasitology,* **3**, 175.

Thomas, A. P. (1883). *Journal of the Royal Agricultural Society of England,* 2nd series, **19**, 276.

Thorpe, E. and Ford, E. J. H. (1969). *Journal of Pathology,* **97**, 619.

Walters, C. J. (1971). *In* "Fundamentals of Ecology" (2nd Edition), p. 276. W. B. Saunders, Philadelphia.

Chemical and Biological Studies on Indomethacin, Sulindac and their Analogs

TSUNG-YING SHEN, PhD

Merck Sharp and Dohme Research Laboratories,
Rahway, New Jersey, USA

and

CHARLES A. WINTER, PhD

8540 S.E. 78th Street,
Mercer Island, Washington, USA

1   Introduction

The introduction of indomethacin (**1**) as a new antiarthritic agent more than a decade ago marked the beginning of a new direction of antiinflammatory research. Salicylates had been in use since the end of the nineteenth century, and research interest in the pyrazolones during the 1940s culminated in the discovery of the antiinflammatory properties of phenylbutazone (Domenjoz, 1952). Following the epoch-making report by Hench *et al.* (1949) of the antirheumatic activity of cortisone, corticosteroids held the center of research attention during the 1950s, while the 1960s witnessed major advances in the aryl acids. In the 1970s a new generation of aryl acids has become available, including such compounds as ibuprofen, naproxen, and many others. Among these new compounds is sulindac (**2**). These efforts followed the announcement of the properties of indomethacin (Shen *et al.*, 1963; Winter *et al.*, 1963).

At present, research is moving forward in several directions. Immuno-pharmacological approaches may permit new kinds of antirheumatic therapy, while at the same time new light is being shed on the physiological and biochemical aspects of inflammation, often with indomethacin as a tool (Sherrer and Whitehouse, 1974; Robinson and Vane, 1974). It therefore seems timely for us to present a perspective review of the chemical and biological efforts involved in the discovery and development of indomethacin (**1**) and of sulindac (**2**) in our laboratories.

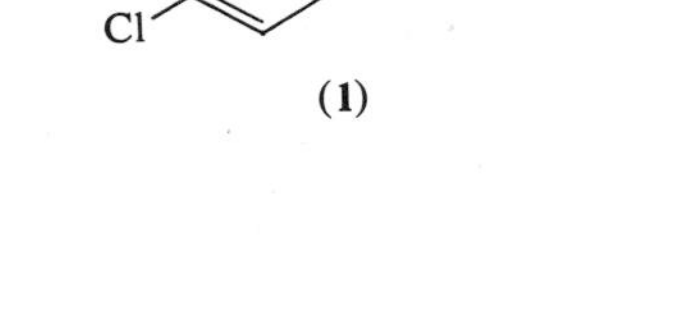

(1) 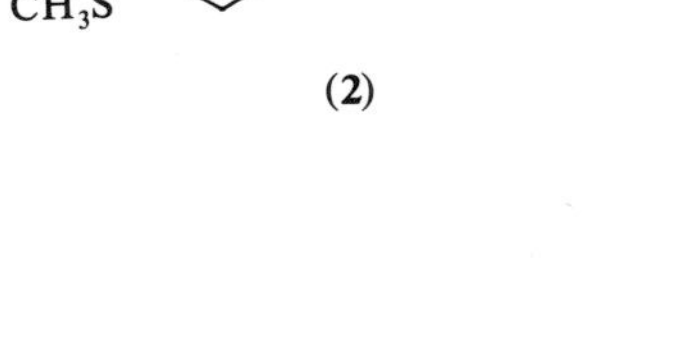   (2)

2   Discovery and early development of the indole lead

2.1   RATIONALE

Antiinflammatory activity has been found in a wide variety of structures. However, at the beginning of our work, only salicylates and phenylbutazone were typical nonsteroidal antiinflammatory drugs. As grams of sample were needed for a limited "random screening" assay some thought had to be given to the types of structures that might be especially rewarding.

As candidates for such a study, indole derivatives had an especial appeal. There has been much discussion of 5-hydroxytryptamine (serotonin) as a possible mediator of inflammation (for reviews see Erspamer, 1961; Spector, 1964), and Shaw and Wooley (1954) demonstrated that some indole derivatives possessed antiserotonin activity. While our study of indole compounds was in progress, evidence of abnormalities of tryptophan metabolism in some rheumatic patients was obtained (McMillan, 1960; Bett, 1962a; Spiera, 1963). The antiinflammatory activity of indole derivatives may seem to confirm this simple rationale but it must be admitted that the finding of such activity may be largely fortuitous.

Indeed, subsequent studies in inflammation have modified the views concerning the role of serotonin in inflammation, and there is no parallelism between antiserotonin activity and antiinflammatory activity in general (Winter, 1966a). Furthermore, abnormalities in tryptophan metabolism in rheumatic patients are not necessarily related to their disease, and may be corrected by pyridoxine (Bett, 1962b). As it turned out, indomethacin lacks specific antiserotonin activity, and there is no evidence that it may correct errors in tryptophan metabolism.

In the laboratory, the speculation that certain indole compounds might have antiinflammatory activity, was quickly tested and bore fruit from the beginning. It was fortunate that a group of indole derivatives, including their intermediates, were available for selection from a serotonin antagonist program which had been actively pursued in our laboratories (Clark et al., 1957).

At the time of this development, the test employed in our laboratories for antiinflammatory screening was based on the demonstration by Meier et al. (1950) that the response of tissue to the inflammatory stimulus of a subcutaneous implant of cotton wool was reduced by treating the animal with cortisone. This method was widely adopted for screening steroids for antiinflammatory activity, and several modifications were devised (Winter, 1966a, b). When we undertook to test non-steroids, we performed the assay as described by Winter and Porter (1957).

2.2 DEVELOPMENT OF THE LEAD

The first compound with an indole nucleus to be tested was 1-benzyl-5-methoxy-2-methylindole-3-acetamide (3). Some of the structural features of indomethacin were foreshadowed by this compound, including the substituents at C-2 and C-5, and a benzyl group at N-1, later replaced by a more effective 1-benzoyl group.

In a three-level direct comparison with phenylbutazone, the new compound was found to share with phenylbutazone the property of inhibiting granuloma formation, yielding responses related to log dose. Of particular interest, this activity was exhibited at dose levels which did not significantly inhibit body weight gain, or weights of adrenals or thymus. Hence, the antiinflammatory activity could reasonably be presumed not to be due to corticoadrenal stimulation or to any extraordinary toxic effects. It was estimated that the compound was nearly half as potent as phenylbutazone. There was no assurance that this potency ratio would hold for man—and, indeed, it later turned out that the granuloma inhibition test in rats exaggerated the potency of these compounds relative to phenylbutazone in man.

The result with compound 3 was considered to be of sufficient interest to justify the initiation of a synthetic program. In spite of the relatively good activity of compound 3, more than three and a half years were to elapse before the first sample of indomethacin was available for testing in the biological laboratory. During this time, more than two thousand other compounds, including over 350 indoles, were tested for granuloma inhibiting properties.

After the activity of the lead compound had been established, there was need for further delineation of the essential features for chemical modification. Attention was first given to the amide function at C-3 and a number of compounds were prepared with modifications of the side chain at C-3. Compounds 4–8 (Table 1) are illustrative of the changes made and the activities encountered. Compound 8, the acetic acid, represented a clear advance in antigranuloma activity over that seen in the lead compound without exhibiting the side effects on body weight and thymus weight encountered with the amine 4 and the chloro derivative 6.

From these and similar tests, it became clear that the lead should be designated as an indole-3-alkyl carboxylic acid. The amine (4), though active, in addition to its CNS activities produced unfavorable effects upon body and thymus weights, and similar actions were seen with other amines. Compounds 5 and 7 were judged to be nearly inactive at the 100 mg kg^{-1} level.

Several retests of compound 8, including formal assays with phenylbutazone as a standard, indicated a potency ratio of about 1·3 for the new compound. Several homologs of compound 8 were evaluated. Testing data as

TABLE 1

Steps toward establishing the indole-3-acetic acid lead: granuloma inhibition assay of compounds **4–8**

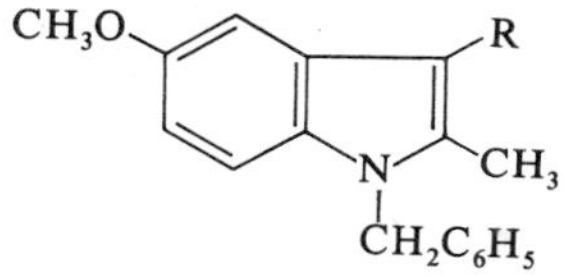

Compound R	Daily dose po $mg\ kg^{-1}$	Body weight gain g	Adrenals mg	Thymus mg	Granuloma inhibition %
Saline controls		46	34·0	543	—
4 $CH_2CH_2NH_2 \cdot HCl$	100	14^a	39·6	365^a	22
5 CH_2CH_2OH	100	40	37·8	526	14
6 CH_2CH_2Cl	100	-5^a	34·3	333^a	30
7 H	100	40	40·5	549	14
8 CH_2COOH	18·75	41	34·2	515	15
	37·5	43	34·7	513	20
	75	43	34·5	511	33

^{a} Body weight gain and thymus weight significantly lower than controls.

TABLE 2

Granuloma inhibition activity of homologs of compound **8**

Compound	C-3 Chain	Dose $mg\ kg^{-1}$	Granuloma inhibition %
(**8**)	$-CH_2COOH$	75	33^a
(**9**)	$-CH(CH_3)COOH$	75	33^a
(**10**)	$-COOH$	100	8
(**11**)	$-CH_2CH_2COOH$	100	5
(**12**)	$-C(CH_3)_2COOH$	100	6

^{a} Statistically significant, $p < 0.05$.

exemplified in Table 2 clearly indicated that the acetic acid side chain at C-3 was optimal in length.

As a consequence of experiments such as these, the lead could now be described as a substituted 1-aralkyl indole-3-acetic acid (**13**) with many positions available for systematic structural modifications. Such modifications yielded data on structure-activity relationships, as discussed in section 4.

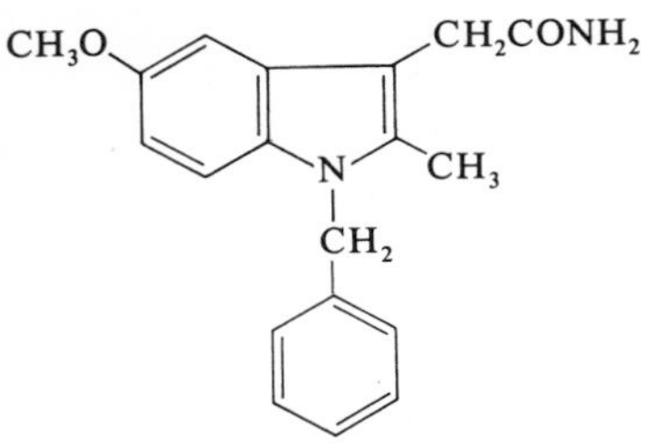

(3)

The lead compound

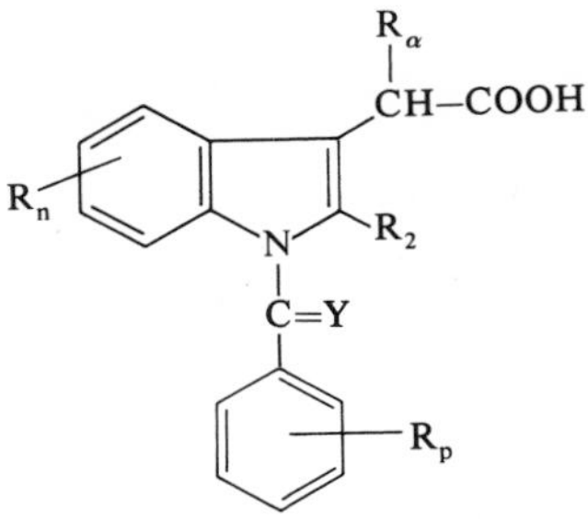

(13)

The basic structure for study of
structure–activity relationships
of indomethacin analogs

3   Pharmacodynamic properties of indomethacin and its analogs

The pharmacodynamic actions of indomethacin and its congeners are rather
limited. Antiinflammatory, antipyretic and analgesic activities can be detected
at rather low doses of the more active compounds, but many tests for
pharmacodynamic activity yield negative results. The varieties of adverse
effects are also limited. Virtually all the toxic manifestations in animals can be
accounted for on the basis of the induction of gastrointestinal lesions, and even
then, the doses required are significantly higher than those needed to
demonstrate antiinflammatory activity.

3.1   ANTIINFLAMMATORY TESTS

Since rheumatic disorders seem to be characterized by chronic inflammation, it
is a common practice to test compounds for antiinflammatory activity, then
hopefully predict that active ones should be useful antirheumatic drugs.
Although the methods are nonspecific, the correlation between test results and
therapeutic activity seems to be fairly good. In the case of indomethacin and its
congeners, six of the compounds to be discussed in the review have received
clinical trial. The rank order of effectiveness, as evidenced by the dose required
to show an effect, and insofar as incomplete data enable one to judge, appears
to be the same as that obtained in the laboratory (see Table 3).

3.1.1   *Methods*

The "cardinal signs" of inflammation most frequently employed for antiinflammatory testing are those relating to: (1) the edema produced by loss of
fluid through the small vessels in an inflamed tissue, (2) the reddening

(erythema) seen when the small vessels dilate, and (3) the proliferation of tissue with granuloma formation which occurs when a foreign body continues to irritate the tissue for some time.

During the early stages of our program, we adopted as a primary screen the granuloma inhibition test mentioned in section 2. This test had been in use in our laboratories for several years in testing steroids. Later, an acute test based on inhibition of foot edema in rats was developed which met our requirements

TABLE 3

Correlation of analgesic, antipyretic and antiinflammatory potencies of several indomethacin analogs which have been submitted to clinical trial

Compound[a]	Granuloma inhibition	Carrageenan edema	Antipyretic (rats)	Analgesia (inflamed foot assay)
MK-615 (1) (Indomethacin)	1	1	1	1
MK-825 (46)	0·5	0·7	0·2	0·4
MK-231 (2)	0·5	0·5	0·5	1·3
MK-715 (97)	0·2	1·0	2·0	0·3
MK-409 (33)	0·03	0·14	0·1	0·07
MK-555 (32)	0·01	0·1	<0·1	<0·01

[a] For structures, see section 4.

(Winter et al., 1962). Of the compounds exhibiting activity in these assays, those of particular interest were then submitted to secondary tests, including analgesia, antipyresis, inhibition of adjuvant arthritis, gastrointestinal effects, and others, as described below.

As pointed out by Swingle (1974) granuloma formation may also be inhibited by compounds which stimulate the adrenal cortex, either directly or by an indirect toxic effect. This possible source of error was controlled in our experiments by monitoring adrenal, thymus and body weights. Some investigators have determined cotton pellet weight only 24 hours after insertion. Although this modification is time saving, the results are more closely related to vascular events than to granuloma formation.

The foot edema inhibition test, requiring only a single dose of compound, is more economical than the granuloma inhibition procedure, and permits a more prompt decision as to the activity of a given compound. In addition, the relatively small sample of material required makes available a large number of compounds which might not be obtainable in sufficient supply for a test requiring repetitive administration. The acute tests for antiinflammatory activity have been reviewed elsewhere (Winter, 1965, 1966a, b; Swingle, 1974).

The original description of the carrageenan edema procedure (Winter et al., 1962) showed that the edema responded to antiinflammatory drugs with single oral doses within a nontoxic range. Several other laboratories confirmed and extended these observations (Arrigoni-Martelli and Conti, 1964a, b; Niemegeers et al., 1964; Fontaine et al., 1965). Several authors have pointed out that the carrageenan edema assay became the most frequently used method to support claims of antiinflammatory activity. A fair correlation exists between this assay and therapeutic activity, though false positive findings may occur (Sofia et al., 1975) and the procedure exaggerates somewhat the potency of the more active compounds. These discrepancies may be clarified from the current quantitative studies of the pathways involved in this acute model (Vinegar et al., 1976) as well as other inflammatory systems.

The activity of indomethacin in assays for antigranuloma and anti-carrageenan edema has been discussed in previous publications from this laboratory (Winter et al., 1963; Winter, 1965; Winter and Risley, 1965). These findings—which have been confirmed in other laboratories—may be summarized as follows:

i. In both tests, indomethacin was more potent than most of the known antiinflammatory drugs, including aspirin, phenylbutazone, the fenamates, and hydrocortisone, but less potent than dexamethasone.

ii. It inhibited granuloma formation when locally applied directly to the cotton pellet. It was also fully active in the absence of the adrenal gland.

iii. The inhibition of carrageenan-induced edema is somewhat specific; that is, the compound is not a general antiedema agent and it fails to inhibit several types of foot edema in the rat (Winter, 1965).

Other antiinflammatory procedures in which indomethacin was said to be highly active include: reduction in the accumulation of dye in skin exposed to ultraviolet light (Sim, 1965), suppression of the lymph node permeability factor (Walters and Willoughby, 1965) inhibition of crystal-induced synovitis in dogs (Phelps and McCarty, 1966; Van Arman and Carlson, 1970; Van Arman et al., 1970a), diminution of the Schwartzman reaction in rabbits (Van Arman et al., 1970b), reduction of acute ocular inflammation in sensitized rabbits challenged by intracameral injection of specific antigen (Hanna and Keatts, 1967), and modification of adjuvant arthritis in rats (Winter and Nuss, 1966; Ward and Cloud, 1966; Piliero et al., 1966; Bogden et al., 1967; Glenn et al., 1967). The suspension of Mycobacterium tuberculosis in mineral oil commonly used to induce adjuvant arthritis also produces an acute development of localized edema at the injection site, which can be inhibited by anti-inflammatory drugs. Sofia et al., (1975) viewed this action as a more specific test than the carrageenan edema assay; indomethacin was about equally active in both procedures.

3.1.2 *Topical activity*

Most of the antiinflammatory activities mentioned above were seen after oral or parenteral administration, but indomethacin has also been described as being active when topically applied. Hanna and Keatts (1967) and Hanna and Sharp (1972) reported topical activity in experimental uveitis, while Podos *et al.* (1963) and Conquet *et al.* (1975) found that topical indomethacin prevented the rise in intraocular pressure after application of arachidonic acid. Van Arman (1974) described the antiinflammatory activity of indomethacin when applied topically to the ear of the mouse. Topical indomethacin has also been reported to relieve inflammation in human skin after exposure to ultraviolet rays; one group of investigators characterized it as superior to a potent steroid cream (Snyder and Eaglstein, 1974a, b).

3.2 ANTIPYRETIC ACTIVITY

In previous publications, we have shown that indomethacin was effective in rats against fever induced by injections of yeast or bacterial pyrogen, and in rabbits with pyrogen fever (Winter *et al.*, 1963; Winter, 1965). The compound was effective at lower dose levels than those required for any previously known antipyretic agent. Similar data were obtained by others (Benzi and Frigo, 1964).

For routine assay of antipyretic activity, 2 ml of 7·5 per cent suspension of brewers' yeast was injected under the skin in the back of the neck on the afternoon before a test, using Sprague–Dawley rats of either sex. A fever of about 2·5°C above normal temperature was well maintained throughout the test day. An electrical thermometer activated by a thermocouple inserted rectally to a uniform depth of 3 cm enabled a reading to be made within a few seconds. In some experiments, an "antipyretic index" was calculated by recording temperatures at 30-minute intervals for 2 hours after drug administration; the sum of the differences between these temperatures and the pre-drug temperature was the "antipyretic index".

The example in Table 4 shows how this method works in practice, when several compounds are examined simultaneously. Such data readily lend themselves to statistical manipulation and calculation of relative potencies. In the experiment shown, the approximate ratios of the compounds were: aspirin 1, phenylbutazone 1·9, aminopyrine 4·8, indomethacin 38. These ratios are based on data for only the first 2 hours after administration of drug, and might be different if the experiment had continued for the full time of drug action. Winder (1966) found a slightly higher activity of indomethacin relative to phenylbutazone, but more recent work from the same laboratory reported a potency ratio of 6·1 for indomethacin to phenylbutazone (Wax *et al.*, 1975). Investigators commenting upon the high antipyretic effectiveness of indomethacin include Benzi and Frigo (1964), Bianchi et al. (1967), Cashin and Heading (1968), Lange (1966), and Kobayashi and Takagi (1968). According to Ramunni (1966) indomethacin in relatively small doses—25 to 50 mg daily—in tubercular patients with fever, produced a defervescence unobtainable with other antipyretic agents.

TABLE 4

Example of an assay for antipyretic activity of indomethacin in comparison with other known antipyretic agents in groups of 6 yeast-fevered rats receiving single oral doses of drugs

Compound	Dose mg kg^{-1}	Initial temperature °C	Change in temperature °C Time after drug (min)				Antipyretic index
			30	60	90	120	
Normal controls	—	36·9	+0·3	+0·2	+0·2	+0·2	−0·9
Fevered controls	—	39·5	+0·3	+0·1	+0·1	+0·1	−0·6
Indomethacin	0·78	39·4	−0·7	−1·0	−0·9	−0·9	3·5
	1·56	39·3	−0·9	−1·4	−1·3	−1·3	4·9
	3·12	39·5	−1·2	−1·6	−2·1	−2·2	7·1
Phenylbutazone	25	39·6	−1·4	−1·3	−1·2	−0·9	4·8
	50	39·5	−1·3	−1·7	−1·7	−1·6	6·3
	100	39·4	−1·1	−1·8	−1·9	−2·0	6·8
Aspirin	25	39·5	−0·9	−0·7	−0·6	−0·5	2·7
	50	39·4	−1·2	−1·3	−1·1	−1·1	4·7
	100	39·4	−1·4	−1·6	−1·7	−1·8	6·5
Aminopyrine	6·25	39·3	−0·9	−0·8	−0·7	−0·5	2·9
	12·5	39·5	−1·1	−1·5	−1·4	−1·3	5·3
	25	39·4	−1·4	−1·8	−1·9	−2·0	7·1

3.2.1 Antipyretic mechanisms

Gander and Goodale (1969) considered the antipyretic effect to be exerted at the level of the leucocytes, since leucocytes are known to release a centrally acting pyrogenic substance (leucocytic pyrogen) when stimulated by bacterial endotoxin. Observations in our laboratory (unpublished) indicate that yeast-induced fever in rats may also be related to release of leucocytic pyrogen. There is no direct evidence, however, that indomethacin prevents formation or release of pyrogen from leucocytes. There is evidence, summarized by Milton (1973) and Feldberg (1974) that the central action of leucocytic pyrogen is mediated by a release of prostaglandins (probably PGE_2). According to this view, antipyretic activity is related to inhibition of the release of PGs, rather than to a direct action on the fever induced by PGs after their release. Feldberg also described a fever produced in cats by perfusion of the cerebral ventricles with calcium-free sodium solution which was not mediated by PGs. Such fever was not prevented by antipyretic agents.

The data in Table 5 show that indomethacin has a rather wide spectrum of antipyretic action, but not all types of experimental fever are equally well controlled. Hyperthermia induced by bacterial pyrogen in rabbits or rats, or by yeast in rats, responded especially well. Fever induced by LSD in rabbits, on the other hand, was only slightly affected; morphine-induced fever in rats also proved to be resistant. The brief and rather low-grade fever after LSD in rats was rather well controlled, though only by a rather high dose.

Body temperatures of normal rats and rabbits were not affected by indomethacin. The distinction between hypothermia in normal animals and antipyresis in fevered animals is an important one (Swingle, 1974). Vane (1973) observed some hypothermia in afebrile cats receiving indomethacin directly into the cannulated third ventricle. Such an effect has not to our knowledge been observed in afebrile animals receiving indomethacin by any other route.

The experiments in Table 5 were performed before the relationship between antipyresis and prostaglandin synthetase activity had been described, but some of the data may be of some theoretical interest in this connection. There is a widespread belief that bacterial pyrogens and morphine produce only hypothermia in rats, rather than the hyperthermia observed in most species. With respect to morphine, this impression has been obtained by observations on rats injected with sufficient opiate to render the animal depressed and quiescent. Temperatures of rats are rather labile, and drop when animals become exceptionally relaxed. The data in Table 5 show that a *small* dose of morphine results in a fever of 2 to 3 hours duration; the effect was easily reproducible in our hands. We have summarized elsewhere the background for the common belief that bacterial pyrogen does not produce fever in rats, but we demonstrated that under proper conditions bacterial pyrogen in appropriate doses produces fever in rats which responds to antipyretic drugs as in other species of animals (Winter and Nuss, 1963; Winter et al., 1963). Similar results were reported recently by Sharkawi (1972).

If we accept the hypothesis that fever which responds to antipyretic agents is mediated by prostaglandins, while fever unresponsive to the drugs is produced by some other mechanism, pyrogen fever in both rats and rabbits must be mediated by PGs. Likewise, yeast-induced fever in rats and LSD fever in rabbits must be related to release of PGs. LSD fever in rabbits and morphine fever in rats responded poorly to indomethacin, so perhaps such fever may be only partly mediated by PGs. There remains the possibility, of course, that inhibition of PG synthetase is a mechanism of antipyresis but not the only one.

3.2.2 Congeners of indomethacin

We conducted assays of antipyretic activity of a large number of analogs of indomethacin and of sulindac. Most of the compounds were not investigated as

TABLE 5

Antipyretic actions of indomethacin in fevers of diverse origins

Species	Type of fever	Dose $mg\,kg^{-1}$ po	Initial	Time after drug (h) Body temperature (°C)					
				0·5	1	1·5	2	3	4
Rabbits	Controls—no fever	0	38·3	38·4	38·3	38·3	38·3	38·6	38·5
		9	38·4	38·3	38·3	38·2	38·2	38·3	38·3
Rats	Controls—no fever	0	37·0	37·0	36·9	36·9	36·9	37·1	37·1
		6·25	36·9	36·9	37·0	37·0	36·8	36·8	36·9
Rabbits	E. coli pyrogen 10 µg iv, 30 min after drug	0	38·3	38·9	39·6	39·7	40·0	40·5	40·5
		9	38·3	38·4	38·9	38·7	38·7	38·9	38·9
Rats	E. coli pyrogen 0·5 $mg\,kg^{-1}$ ip, 1 h after drug	0	37·3		37·8		38·6	39·0	39·2
		3·12	37·1		36·8		37·8	37·9	38·3
Rabbits	LSD 50 µg kg^{-1}, 30 min after drug	0	39·3	40·2	40·9	41·1	41·1	40·9	40·5
		9	39·2	40·3	40·8	40·5	40·6	40·3	40·0
Rats	LSD 100 µg kg^{-1} ip, 30 min after drug	0	36·9	38·1	38·0	37·8	37·2		
		12·5	37·0	37·7	37·2	37·0	36·6		
Rats	Morphine 1 $mg\,kg^{-1}$ sc, 30 min after drug	0	36·8	39·0	39·0	38·6	37·9	37·5	
		12·5	36·8	38·2	38·4	38·0	37·5	36·9	
Rats	Brewers yeast 7·5% 2 ml sc, 17 h before drug	0	40·0	40·0	40·0	39·9	39·8		
		3·12	40·0	39·0	38·2	37·8	37·8		

thoroughly as those of major interest, but several were tested against pyresis induced by pyrogen in both rats and rabbits and by yeast in rats. In general, antipyretic activity paralleled antiinflammatory potency, and there were no findings that merit detailed discussion. It may be noted that data on the indene isosteres (Table 3) demonstrated that antipyretic activity is fully retained in this series.

3.3 ANALGESIC STUDIES

Antiinflammatory-antipyretic drugs as a class possess mild analgesic properties. The analgesia can sometimes be demonstrated by testing the reaction to pressure on a rat's tail as described by Green et al. (1951) but more readily by measuring the response to pressure on a foot inflamed by local injection of yeast (Randall and Selitto, 1957). Such procedures as the hot plate and thermal stimuli to the tail do not elicit an easily detected response to these compounds.

Our adaptation of the Randall–Selitto procedure has been described elsewhere (Winter and Flataker, 1965a, b). A non-narcotic analgesic (peripherally acting) could readily be distinguished from a narcotic (centrally acting) analgesic, both by the differential response of the yeast-inflamed foot compared to the normal foot, and by the slope of the dose–response curves. Indomethacin gave responses like aspirin or other non-narcotic analgesics or narcotic antagonists, but unlike morphine. In potency, indomethacin exceeded aspirin, as noted by Swingle et al. (1971a, b).

Since our testing of analogs of indomethacin was primarily directed toward antiinflammatory potentialities, and only secondarily to analgesia, relatively few of the analogs listed in section 4 were tested in the inflamed foot assay. In those which were examined, analgesic potencies usually followed rather well the results of the antiinflammatory assays, but it is of interest that sulindac (MK-231) exhibited analgesic potency in the inflamed foot assay in rats two to four times greater than might be expected on the basis of its antiinflammatory activity (Table 3).

The data in Table 6 agree with previous reports of the effectiveness of indomethacin on the threshold of the inflamed foot, and demonstrates that this action is not antagonized by nalorphine. The table also shows the inactivity of the compound in the D'Amour–Smith (1941) tail-flick procedure which is widely used for testing potent narcotic analgesics.

3.3.1 *Evidence of a central component in the analgesic action*

Since the work of Lim and coworkers (Lim, 1960, 1967; Guzman et al., 1964; Lim et al., 1967) the analgesic action of antiinflammatory drugs has generally been regarded as due primarily if not entirely to peripheral action. More recent investigators have emphasized the probable role of prostaglandins in the genesis of pain, and of PG synthetase inhibition in the peripheral inhibition of pain (Vane, 1973; Collier *et al.*, 1973). Vane (1973) and Ferreira *et al.* (1973) suggested that PGs may have only a facilitatory role, and they may act by sensitizing the sensory nerves to other mediators. Some of our data support (but do not prove) the idea that at least a small degree of central action may also be involved, as suggested some years ago by Winder (1959).

TABLE 6

Analgesic activity of indomethacin as determined in the rat by pressure on the yeast-inflamed foot and the normal foot, and by the tail-flick test

A. Foot pressure test (modified Randall–Selitto)

| | Threshold 1 hour after drug | |
| | Inflamed foot | Normal foot |
Treatment	mmHg $\pm$ SE	mmHg $\pm$ SE
Saline controls	$8 \cdot 7 \pm 0 \cdot 5$	$28 \cdot 2 \pm 0 \cdot 5$
Indomethacin 3 mg kg^{-1} po	$34 \cdot 0 \pm 1 \cdot 6$	$30 \cdot 2 \pm 0 \cdot 5$
Indomethacin 3 mg kg^{-1} po + nalorphine 1 mg kg^{-1} sc	$34 \cdot 8 \pm 1 \cdot 9$	$33 \cdot 0 \pm 1 \cdot 7$
Nalorphine 1 mg kg^{-1} sc	$14 \cdot 8 \pm 1 \cdot 4$	$29 \cdot 0 \pm 0 \cdot 9$

B. Tail-flick test—D'Amour–Smith

| | Reaction time, s $\pm$ S.E. | | |
Treatment	Before drug	15 min	30 min
Saline controls	$4 \cdot 3 \pm 0 \cdot 1$	$3 \cdot 9 \pm 0 \cdot 1$	$3 \cdot 9 \pm 0 \cdot 1$
Indomethacin 3 mg kg^{-1} po	$3 \cdot 8 \pm 0 \cdot 2$	$4 \cdot 2 \pm 0 \cdot 1$	$4 \cdot 0 \pm 0 \cdot 1$

In previous papers (Winter and Flataker, 1965a, b) the relative ineffectiveness of indomethacin on the threshold of the non-inflamed foot was pointed out. However, the ineffectiveness is not absolute. Not only in the present Table 6 but also in Table 6 of the 1965a paper and Table 1 of the 1965b paper, the threshold of the normal foot was slightly higher in the rats receiving indomethacin than in saline treated controls, though the difference did not reach statistical significance. This slight effect has prompted us to review the data, with the result shown in Table 7. In this instance, the change in threshold induced by the drug was taken as a measure of the effect, rather than merely a comparison in final threshold level attained. Data from three experiments are shown, and in all of them the action of indomethacin, though small, was highly significant. Data for only one dose level are shown, but in experiment 3, three dose levels were used. Mean changes in threshold for controls, and for indomethacin 1, 3, and 9 mg kg^{-1} were, respectively, $0 \cdot 3$, $0 \cdot 7$, $2 \cdot 2$ and $6 \cdot 0$ mmHg. The small effect was, therefore, related to log dose.

In Table 6 it appears that the action of indomethacin-nalorphine combination was slightly, though not significantly, higher than that of either compound alone. With this observation as a cue, the experiment in Table 8 was performed. In this case, a significant degree of synergism between the two drugs was apparent, with indomethacin administered orally and nalorphine subcutaneously.

TABLE 7

Analgesic effect of indomethacin upon the noninflamed foot; thresholds taken 2 hours after oral ingestion of drug, 3 mg kg^{-1}, 6 rats per group

Experiment	Drug	Threshold (mmHg) Before drug	After drug	Change in threshold
1.	Saline	29·3	28·7	−0·6
	Indomethacin	28·8	31·5	2·7
2.	Saline	29·2	28·7	−0·5
	Indomethacin	29·0	31·3	2·3
3.	Saline	29·0	29·3	0·3
	Indomethacin	28·5	30·7	2·2

Analysis of variance, change in threshold (post-drug − pre-drug)

Source of variation	Degrees of freedom	Sums of squares	Mean square	F
Among groups of rats	5	68·22		
1. days	2	0·72	0·36	<1
2. saline versus indomethacin	1	64·00	64·00	26·0[a]
1. × (2)	2	3·50	1·75	<1
Animals within groups (error)	30	73·67	2·46	
Total	35	141·89		

[a] $p < 0.001$.

Mattila and Saarnivaara (1967a, b) obtained evidence that indomethacin also potentiated the analgesic action of morphine in mice (hot plate test) and rabbits (electrical stimulation of tooth pulp). Serotonin was also said to potentiate morphine, but indomethacin did not further potentiate the morphine-serotonin combination, not did indomethacin potentiate morphine in reserpinized animals. The authors interpreted these results as indicating that biogenic amines mediate the analgesic action of indomethacin.

3.3.2 Analgesia in man

Indomethacin is usually compared with aspirin; however, some recent clinical reports suggest the possibility that in certain types of pain in humans, indomethacin may give relief quite beyond anything that one usually expects from compounds of this category. The reports include bone pain, pleurisy and pericarditis, and even some instances of headache (Baron, 1968; Sacks and Kanarek, 1973; Asp, 1974; Brodie, 1974; Minuth *et al.*, 1975; Sjaastad, 1975). In some applications wherein pain relief is related to antiinflammatory action as shown by reduction of swelling, a distinction between antiinflammatory action and analgesia *per se* cannot readily be determined (Fitch and Gray, 1974).

TABLE 8

Effect of nalorphine in varying proportions upon the analgesic effect of indomethacin as determined by threshold of pressure response on the inflamed foot of the rat

Indomethacin (oral) mg kg^{-1}	Nalorphine (sc 30 min after indomethacin) mg kg^{-1}	Response threshold after indomethacin 60 min mmHg $\pm$ SE	90 min mmHg $\pm$ SE
None	none	8·5 $\pm$ 0·3	9·2 $\pm$ 0·5
1·0	none	22·2 $\pm$ 1·0	27·5 $\pm$ 1·3
0·75	0·25	36·0 $\pm$ 2·4[b]	36·8 $\pm$ 3·1[a]
0·5	0·5	37·3 $\pm$ 1·9[b]	31·5 $\pm$ 1·7
0·25	0·75	24·3 $\pm$ 1·7	24·7 $\pm$ 3·5
None	1·0	18·3 $\pm$ 1·1	18·3 $\pm$ 1·8

[a] Combination superior to either drug alone $p < 0.05$.
[b] Combination superior to either drug alone $p < 0.01$.

3.4   SECONDARY PHARMACOLOGICAL PROPERTIES

The therapeutic benefits of nonsteroid antiinflammatory drugs are denied to a significant number of people because of side effects. Much time and effort would be saved if laboratory tests were available which would predict the type, incidence and severity of side effects. Available animal models are imperfect in this respect, but an approach can be made by subjecting a new compound to a wide variety of pharmacological challenges.

3.4.1   *Miscellaneous pharmacodynamic tests*

Indomethacin is frequently referred to as an "aspirin-like" drug (Ferreira and Vane, 1974) but it differs from aspirin in several respects. Aspirin has long been regarded as remarkable for its pharmacological versatility. Indomethacin, on the other hand, has failed to demonstrate pharmacologic activity in many systems as shown in Table 9.

    The procedures listed in Table 9 are designed to demonstrate activity of such drugs as diuretics, antihistaminics, hypotensive agents, tranquilizers, local anesthetics, and a variety of agents possessing depressant or stimulant actions in the central or autonomic nervous system. Compounds known to have effects upon the sympathetic or central nervous systems exhibit activity in some of these tests, and hence the results with indomethacin suggest the prediction that whatever side effects the new agent might have, they would not be related to

TABLE 9

Miscellaneous pharmacodynamic tests in which indomethacin was inactive

Species	Indomethacin dose schedule	Criterion of effect
Dog, unanesthetized	2·5 mg kg^{-1} iv prime + 3 mg kg^{-1} per h infusion	Urine volume Glomerular filtration Sodium excretion Potassium excretion
Rhesus monkey, trained	0·3 to 5 mg kg^{-1} po single dose, and 3 mg kg^{-1} day^{-1} for 5 days po	Discriminated avoidance behavior
Rhesus monkey, implanted epidural electrodes	10 mg kg^{-1}, 5 days per week for 3 weeks po	Electroencephalographic recording
Dog, anesthetized, vagotomized	10 mg kg^{-1} iv	Blood pressure responses to carotid occlusion, vagus stimulation (central, peripheral), injection of methacholine, epinephrine, norepinephrine, phenethylamine, angiotensin II
Mouse	4 to 324 mg kg^{-1} ip	Observations on behavior, pupillary diameter, anti-convulsant properties (electroshock), corneal and pinnal reflexes
Guinea pig	0·5 to 12·5 mg kg^{-1} ip	Protection from histamine aerosol

CNS or sympathetic actions. Also, apart from the relevance of such tests in predicting side effects, an examination of the pharmacological potential of any new compound is an important part of the safety assessment. In addition to indomethacin, all the compounds listed in Table 3 were subjected to the same tests, and all yielded negative results.

The results indicated that these compounds do not possess central nervous system properties commonly associated with some indole derivatives. Nucifora and Malone (1971) also noted in animals an absence of CNS effects with indomethacin. On the other hand, several clinical investigators have noted transient side effects suggestive of CNS action in a significant proportion of patients treated with indomethacin (Boardman and Hart, 1967; Mills, 1974). Indeed, headache and vague affective symptoms are more frequently encountered than any other side effects with the possible exception of gastrointestinal intolerance. Tests such as those in Table 9 fail to predict such observations in the human.

Sulindac (MK-231) was subjected to a considerably expanded battery of tests. For example, in addition to the investigation of cardiovascular actions in anesthetized dogs (with intravenous doses up to 10 mg kg^{-1}) the compound was administered to rats with spontaneous hypertension. Effects on behavioral performance were examined in squirrel monkeys after oral doses up to 30 mg kg^{-1}, and a large battery of behavioral and CNS tests was performed in mice. Possible diuretic actions were tested, including effects on excretion of electrolytes and modification of the action of known diuretics. The compound was also tested for uricosuric activity. In all these tests, doses of sulindac considerably higher than those found to have antiinflammatory or analgesic action in rats or dogs yielded negative results.

3.4.2   Gastrointestinal actions

Gastrointestinal effect of indomethacin have received considerable attention; hence, the pharmacological background becomes of some importance. Such effects also need to be put in perspective relative to the therapeutic actions of the drug and to comparable properties of other antiinflammatory agents. Subjective symptoms of epigastric distress have been noted with therapeutic doses of all antiinflammatory drugs, but not all observers have agreed on actual ulcerogenicity. Several investigators have thought that the problem of g.i. toxicity has sometimes been exaggerated; peptic ulcer is not uncommon in rheumatoid arthritis. Atwater *et al.* (1965) expressed the view that incidence of ulcers is a function of the severity of the disease rather than of the therapy. Some authors—for example, Anderson (1965)—have commented upon the frequent association of antiinflammatory and gastrointestinal effects.

With specific reference to indomethacin, reports range all the way from "no ulcerogenic activity" (Casolo *et al.*, 1965) or even "improvement in previous symptoms" (Berman, 1965) to reports indicating high incidence of peptic ulcers (Lövgren and Allander, 1965). A more moderate opinion is exemplified by Ballabio's view (1965) that indomethacin causes gastric distress in a significant proportion of cases, but the distress does not necessarily have an ulcerative basis, and that drug-induced ulcers, though undoubtedly occurring, are uncommon. This view is consistent with that of Rothermich (1966).

In spite of these differences of opinion, there remains a core of evidence that indomethacin, in common with other antiinflammatory drugs, has adverse effects upon the gastrointestinal mucosa in some individuals, and the results with animal experiments demonstrate that a potential for mucosal damage exists. It is pertinent to inquire whether such experiments demonstrate a margin of safety as shown by the ratio of antiinflammatory doses to those inducing g.i. toxicity. Other questions include a comparison among various antiinflammatory agents, inquiries into the mechanism of gastrointestinal actions, and progress toward separating antiinflammatory and g.i. properties with a view toward designing useful drugs as free as possible from this type of toxicity.

The tendency of aspirin to induce bleeding from the g.i. tract is well known and has frequently been commented upon; such bleeding is often symptom-free, and is not necessarily related to ulcerogenicity. According to Wanka *et al.* (1964), in studies involving fecal excretion of red cells labelled with ^{51}Cr in human subjects, indomethacin has less tendency than aspirin to induce occult bleeding. On the other hand, Brodie *et al.* (1970) produced ulcers in the small intestine of rats with indomethacin but not with aspirin.

Levy (1974) stated that there appears to be no species difference in susceptibility—rats, dogs, guinea pigs, cats and humans all suffer g.i. disturbances. The statement needs to be qualified; although there is some susceptibility in all the species mentioned (and in others) there are differences in the doses required to produce ulcers, in the portions of the g.i. tract which are most susceptible, and in the ratio between antiinflammatory and ulcerogenic doses. Wilhelmi (1974), for example, determined the "median ulcerogenic dose" of indomethacin to be 4 mg kg^{-1} in mice, and 150 mg kg^{-1} in guinea pigs, administered orally in two consecutive doses 15 hours apart. Peck (1968) reported that in animals receiving indomethacin subacutely or chronically, minimal doses producing g.i. lesions ranged from 0·5 mg kg^{-1} day^{-1} in dogs to 20 mg kg^{-1} day^{-1} in rabbits. Susceptibility is increased if additional stress is present; thus, the incidence of ulcer is increased in rats with adjuvant arthritis (DiPasquale and Welaj, 1973).

There is not full agreement on which portion of the g.i. tract is involved in the ulcerogenic action of indomethacin. Lee *et al.* (1971), Wilhelmi (1974) and Lippmann (1974) mentioned only "gastric ulceration", though they did not agree on the dose requirements. On the other hand, several authors have emphasized a relative or absolute absence of gastric ulcers in rats receiving indomethacin. According to Somogyi *et al.* (1969) ulcers were never seen in the stomach, ileum or colon, but only in the jejunum of rats receiving up to 8 mg kg^{-1} of the drug. Kent *et al.* (1969) said, "surprisingly, the drug did not produce upper gastrointestinal ulcers"; the ulcers appeared only in the mesenteric side of the distal jejunum and ileum. Brodie *et al.* (1970) observed no ulcers in the stomach, cecum or colon, and found them only in the "mid-portion" of the small intestine, even after the massive dose of 64 mg kg^{-1} day^{-1} for 3 days. Intestinal rather than gastric lesions were also emphasized by Vecchio *et al.* (1964), Drees *et al.* (1974) and Volterra *et al.* (1974).

Although it is possible that these discrepancies may be due in some degree to differences in strains of animals, it seems likely that differences in criteria for rating an animal as a "responder" or a "nonresponder" may account for major divergencies. Brodie considered an animal positive only if at least one perforation was present, and in general those observers emphasizing intestinal effects considered anything less to be negative. Those workers reporting on "gastric ulceration" apparently considered any erosion a positive finding, and generally did not mention examining the intestines. Wong *et al.* (1973) and Wax *et al.* (1975) devised scores taking both gastric and intestinal damage into account (see section 3.4.4).

Route of administration seems not to be a critical factor in the production of gastrointestinal lesions. Brodie *et al.* (1970) obtained similar results with either the oral or subcutaneous route. Somogyi *et al.* (1969) employed intravenous injection.

3.4.3   *Mechanisms of gastrointestinal actions*

From such reports, one must conclude that antiinflammatory compounds in general, including indomethacin, produce erosions in the gastric mucosa; some of them, including indomethacin (but not aspirin according to Brodie *et al.*, 1970) may also produce intestinal perforations at appropriate doses. Gastric erosion seems not to be due to increase in acid secretion. Direct measurement of gastric acid secretion in human subjects receiving indomethacin either in basal conditions or during histamine stimulation failed to reveal any effect of the drug (Winship and Bernard, 1970). Indomethacin also failed to affect gastric juice volume or acidity in pylorus-ligated rats (Lee *et al.*, 1971) even in a dose which others have shown to be sufficient to produce perforating lesions in the small intestine. Still higher doses, according to Main and Whittle (1973), though not stimulating acid secretion in rats during basal conditions, do increase acid secretion during maximal secretory response to pentagastrin. The practical significance of results with such large doses is questionable.

Even in the absence of acid secretory effects, the gastric mucous barrier may be affected. Menguy and Desbaillets (1967) found a reduction in the rate of mucous secretion in antral pouches of dogs receiving ulcerogenic doses of indomethacin by mouth. The same authors in a subsequent paper (1968) related the effect to a decrease in the amount of carbohydrate bound to the protein of the mucous, rendering the mucous more easily degradable by proteolytic enzymes. Defects in the mucosal barrier were also described by Chivasta and Cooke (1972), who determined movement of electrolytes across the mucosa, and transmucosal potential differences. Protection against indomethacin-induced gastric lesions by 2,3-dihydro-1*H*-pyridino-(2,3-b)-(1,4)-thiazine-2-one (Abbott-2950) was described by Dodge *et al.* (1974) and was said to be related to a "tightening" of the mucosal barrier, a condition not further defined.

Brodie *et al.* (1970) were unable to prevent indomethacin-induced erosions of the small intestine by a variety of drugs, including anticholinergic agents and antacids, but Lee *et al.* (1971) claimed complete protection against gastric lesions by the anticholinergic drug propantheline. Selye (1970a, b, 1971) coined the term "catatoxic steroids" to describe substances which reportedly protect rats from lethal doses of indomethacin and certain other compounds. The most active of these steroids were said to be virtually devoid of hormonal properties. Rats pretreated with such substances did not develop jejunal ulcers. The mechanism by which this was accomplished and the effect upon anti-inflammatory activity was not established, but Aspinall (1970) found spirono-lactone to be more effective in antagonizing the ulcerogenic actions than the antiinflammatory effect. He suggested that spironolactone might be clinically useful in reducing g.i. irritation during antiinflammatory therapy.

The effect of such compounds upon the antiinflammatory action of indo-methacin might be worth more thorough evaluation, in view of the report by Solymoss et al. (1971) that spironolactone owes its ability to prevent jejunal ulcers by hastening the metabolism of indomethacin and increasing its rate of disappearance from the blood. The dose of indomethacin employed in these studies was higher than that needed to demonstrate antiinflammatory activity, and if the blood level effects were comparable at the lower doses, an unfavorable effect upon antiinflammatory action—especially in long term tests—would be anticipated.

More recently low doses of sodium salicylate were reported to exert a pro-tective action in rats versus indomethacin and other nonsteroidal anti-inflammatory drugs (Ezer al al., 1976). Any clinical significance of this laboratory observation remains to be clarified.

Roberts (1974a) pointed out that the reason for the localization of the lesions in the small intestine is unknown. Much of the injury to the wall after the initial lesion may be due to bacterial invasion, according to the results of Kent et al. (1969). Reducing the intestinal bacteria by oral administration of neomycin, polymycin B or bacitracin gave 100 per cent protection from lethal effects of indomethacin in doses as high as 40 mg kg^{-1} in rats.

Although starvation increases the ulcerogenicity of certain procedures, such as physical restraint (Brodie and Hanson, 1960), it offers protection against indomethacin-induced ulcers. The protective effect of fasting was studied in detail by Brodie et al. (1970), who found that it was necessary to withhold food only on the day the drug was given to afford complete protection. Food deprivation before and after that day had no effect. The effect of food appeared to be related to bile flow, since ligation of the bile duct prevented the appearance of ulcers, even in fed animals. Furthermore, ulcers did not appear in an isolated segment of intestine (Thiry-Vella loop) without access to bile.

Further evidence on this point was the finding by Volterra et al. (1974) that ulcerogenicity was considerably reduced by feeding a fat-free diet, and that fasting further reduced the incidence of ulcers. An effect identical with that of fasting was obtained by the use of a low residue diet described by Drees et al. (1974). Volterra argued that his results could not be entirely explained on the basis of enhanced bile flow by the regular diet, since a choleretic agent failed to increase ulcerogenicity unless solubilized in sesame oil, and the oil alone increased ulcer formation.

Walter and Diener (1971) confirmed Brodie's observation on the protective effect of bile duct ligation in rats, and extended it to dogs. They further found that in dogs given ulcerogenic doses of indomethacin, collection of the bile by catheter protected the animals but such bile intubated into other dogs induced ulcers in the recipients. They interpreted these results as evidence for biliary excretion of an ulcerogenic hepatic metabolite rather than ulcerogenicity of the parent drug in direct contact with the mucosa.

The most thorough study of the relation of bile flow to intestinal lesions is that of Duggan et al. (1975). They studied total biliary clearance, and both peripheral and portal plasma values to obtain the total exposure of the intestinal mucosa to indomethacin and also to its desbenzoyl and desmethyl metabolites, and to their respective conjugates. These studies were made in five species of animals with widely varying susceptibility to the gastrointestinal effects of the compound, and estimates were made for man. The total exposure of the intestinal mucosa to the drug depended to a large degree upon the importance of the enterohepatic circulation of indomethacin (see also Hucker et al., 1966; Yesair et al., 1970, and section 6 below).

The total recirculation of indomethacin through the bile was calculated as a single parameter, and ranged from 13 per cent of the administered dose in the rabbit to 362 per cent in the dog. An estimate of 9·5 per cent was made for man. The value for the rat, 134 per cent, was the highest for any species except the dog. In the five laboratory species studied, the figure was inversely proportional to the minimal toxic dose of the compound. These workers also reported that the desmethyl and desbenzoyl metabolites of indomethacin did not produce intestinal lesions.

The concensus of all these studies is that the antiinflammatory compound can cause lesions in the mucosa of either the stomach or the intestine. In the intestine, these lesions can perforate the wall and produce fatal peritonitis. It is not clear that gastric perforations can occur in man although they can occur in animals, but in view of the relationship between total exposure and ulcerogenic potential in the intestine and its dependence upon enterohepatic circulation, it is doubtful if the exposure of the gastric mucosa would ordinarily be sufficient to induce perforations. The facts known at this time do not exclude the possibility that gastric erosions and intestinal perforations may be related to a similar causal mechanism.

The mechanism by which gastrointestinal lesions are produced is unknown. It is tempting to speculate that prostaglandins play an important role in the maintenance of the integrity of the mucosa, and that interfering with the synthesis of PGs, as indomethacin is known to do, might lead to tissue breakdown. Evidence along this line is far from complete. Guinea-pig ileum apparently releases PGE_2 during contraction (Botting and Salzmann, 1974), and indomethacin is said to antagonize this release as well as the contraction resulting from field stimulation. Both PGE_1 (Robert, 1974a) and PGE_2 (Bennett et al., 1973) are said to have a vasodilating effect on the gastric mucosa, while indomethacin was reported to reduce gastric mucosal blood flow (Main and Whittle, 1973). Such considerations prompted Bennett (loc. cit.) to speculate that prostaglandin synthetase inhibitors might produce vasoconstriction, leading to ischemia, tissue death, and bleeding.

As a correlate to such views, one would expect that treatment with a prostaglandin or prostaglandin analog would prevent the ulcerogenic effect of indomethacin, and indeed there are several reports that it does, for both gastric (Lippmann, 1974) and intestinal (Robert, 1974a, b) lesions. Brodie et al. (1970) observed a marked difference among indomethacin, aspirin and phenylbutazone in producing lesions in the small intestine during dosage regimens fully adequate to demonstrate PG-synthesis inhibition. Such differences further indicate the complexity of relating in vitro PG-synthetase inhibitory activities to a myriad of in vivo effects.

3.4.4   Separation of gastrointestinal and antiinflammatory actions

If both antiinflammatory activity and ulcer-producing potential are explicable solely on the basis of PG-synthetase inhibition, it might be futile to attempt a separation of the two activities and find a potent antiinflammatory compound with little or no ulcerogenic action. There is evidence, however, that considerable separation can be achieved; Dodge et al. (1974) described an antiinflammatory compound said not to damage the gastric mucosa. Wax et al. (1975) judged the potential of compounds for producing g.i. lesions by observing both gastric and intestinal effects, and antiinflammatory potency by a combined score incorporating results of several antiinflammatory tests. Their "relative ulcerogenicity" scores (ratio of antiinflammatory potency to ulcerogenicity) as well as "relative lethality" scores varied about 24-fold among 14 antiinflammatory compounds examined.

Various authors have disagreed on the safety factor of indomethacin as determined by the anti-inflammatory ulcerogenic ratio. In the original report on the pharmacology of indomethacin (Winter et al., 1963) the lowest dose used for demonstration of inhibition of granuloma formation was 0.1 mg kg^{-1} day^{-1}. Subsequently, an extended study of a wide range of doses indicated a threshold of activity as low as 0.015 mg kg^{-1} d^{-1} (Phelps et al., 1968). The latter study also reported the "no effect" dose in a 6-month chronic toxicity study to be between 1 and 2 mg kg^{-1} d^{-1}, yielding a safety ratio of 83 to 166, compared to a ratio of 22 to 43 for phenylbutazone.

Acute tests also show a safety factor for indomethacin. In the carrageenan edema assay, a single dose of 1 mg kg^{-1} was effective; lower doses were not reported (Winter et al., 1963; Winter, 1965), while the LD_{50} in the rat is about 12 mg kg^{-1} (Peck, 1968). Some authors have found a more favorable safety ratio for indomethacin than for phenylbutazone or aspirin (Hitchens et al., 1967; Lorenzetti, 1970). In contrast, Menasse-Gdynia and Krupp (1974) and Wilhelmi (1974) found little difference between the antiinflammatory dose and the dose affecting the g.i. tract for either indomethacin, phenylbutazone or aspirin.

During the course of our investigation of structure–activity relationships (see section 5) we studied a number of indene isosteres of the indole acetic acid derivatives. One of these, compound 97 (MK-715), was the indene analog of indomethacin. Its profile of antiinflammatory-antipyretic-analgesic activities (Table 3) suggested that it would be worthy of a more complete study of its pharmacological properties. The most interesting finding in these experiments related to the gastrointestinal activities. When it was found that no g.i. lesions appeared in rats after 4 months on a diet containing the equivalent of 10 mg kg^{-1} day^{-1} or in dogs after daily doses of 20 mg kg^{-1} for 20 weeks, it was clear that a considerable degree of separation of antiinflammatory activity from ulcerogenic potential had been achieved. Higher doses did produce g.i. damage, but the data indicated a ten-fold greater margin of safety for the new compound than for indomethacin. The only adverse sign seen at low or moderate dose level was occasional hematuria in a few animals.

Based on these encouraging findings, a cautious trial in human subjects was begun, but had to be stopped because of occasional crystalluria at higher doses. This proved to be related to relative insolubility in urine of the glucuronide conjugate. Further exploration of the indene-3-acetic acid series has led to a compound which does not have that disadvantage. This compound (2) has received the designation of MK-231 and the name sulindac (Shen et al., 1972). The properties of this compound have been described by Van Arman et al. (1972), Hucker et al. (1972, 1973) and Hare et al. (1974). It was also the subject of a recent symposium (Huskisson and Franchimont, 1976).

Sulindac has antiinflammatory-antipyretic-analgesic potencies ranging from 0·5 to 1·3 times that of indomethacin (Table 3). When it was found that oral doses of 10 mg kg^{-1} d^{-1} for periods up to 3 months in monkeys or 6 months in dogs or rats did not produce gastrointestinal lesions, it was clear that the separation of antiinflammatory from g.i. toxicity observed in MK-715 was retained in the new indene derivative, sulindac.

3.4.5   Comparative studies with sulindac and other compounds

A comparison between indomethacin and sulindac (Table 10) confirms the improved safety ratio for the new compound. It is especially interesting that the

TABLE 10

Comparison of antiinflammatory and gastrointestinal effects of indomethacin and MK-231 (sulindac) in rats[a]

A Short-term effects

Drug	Carrageenan edema inhibition ED_{50}, mg kg^{-1}	Gastric hemorrhage ED_{50}, mg kg^{-1}	Ratio of ED_{50}s
Indomethacin	2·72	6·2	2·3
MK-231	5·39	27·4	5·1

B Long-term effects

Drug	Adjuvant arthritis ED_{50}, mg kg^{-1}	Intestinal perforation ED_{50}, mg kg^{-1}	Ratio of ED_{50}s
Indomethacin	0·24	5	21
MK-231	0·42	71	169

[a] C. G. Van Arman, M. L. Torchiana and co-workers, personal communication. ED_{50} for antiinflammatory tests, dose for 50 per cent inhibition of swelling. ED_{50} for gastrointestinal tests, dose producing effect in 50 per cent of animals.

improvement is greater for the subacute effects than in the acute tests. The metabolism of sulindac will be discussed in a later section (section 6), but it is pertinent to mention here that the active form of the drug is the sulfide metabolite which has a relatively long half-life. On this basis, a clinical schedule of administration twice daily was adopted (see section 9).

Table 11 shows that sulindac, its sulfone metabolite, and the glucuronide conjugate of both compounds are much more freely soluble in urine than is MK-715 or its conjugate. It was therefore possible to predict that sulindac would retain the advantage of MK-715 in being relatively free from gastrointestinal toxicity at therapeutic doses, and would not induce crystalluria. All of these findings have been confirmed in human subjects.

TABLE 11

Solubilities of indene compounds in human urine at 37°C mg ml^{-1} at pH 5·3

Compound	Free acid	Glucuronide conjugate
MK-715 (**97**)	0·004	0·06
MK-231 (**2**)	0·12	1·4
Sulfone metabolite of MK-231 (**108**)	0·025	1·2
Sulfide metabolite of MK-231 (**102**)	none found	

Data by E. M. Cohen, Laboratory of Pharmaceutical Chemistry, Merck Sharp & Dohme.

Additional comparisons of sulindac with other compounds are shown in Table 12. There are minor differences in ED_{50} values in Tables 10 and 12 although all the experiments were done in the same laboratory. The data in Table 12 (supplied by Dr C. G. Van Arman and Dr M. L. Torchiana) are average figures accumulated over several months. Sulindac performed well in all the antiinflammatory tests except the assay involving reduction of synovitis

TABLE 12

Comparative activities of sulindac, indomethacin and other compounds ED_{50} mg kg^{-1}, oral administration, except as noted

Test	Indo-methacin	Sulindac	Aspirin	Phenyl-butazone	Naproxen	Profenid	Ibuprofen
Carrageenan edema, rat[a]	2·6	4·9	84	27·7	1·7	1·4	23·4
Adjuvant arthritis, rat[a]	0·27	0·55	67	14	0·37	0·22	27·6
Antipyresis, yeast, rat[b]	1·55	3·25	45	24	1·7	2·6	5·9
Synovitis, crystal, dog[a]	1·7	45	72	12	nd	0·3	nd
Topical, mouse ear[c]	2·17	6·2	5·5	4·3	1·9	6·0	5·4
Intestinal ulcer, rat[d]	5	48	ne	ne	ne	6·8	128–256
Gastric hemorrhage, rat[d]	5·4	17	81·3	60	2·8	128	8–16

[a] Dose for 50 per cent inhibition; [b] dose to reduce fever 1°C; [c] dose for 50 per cent inhibition, mg per ear; [d] dose effective in 50 per cent of animals; nd, no data; ne, no effect at highest dose tested.

in the dog induced by injection of uric acid crystals into the stifle joint. This is readily explainable on the basis of the relatively poor absorption of the compound from the g.i. tract of the dog (see section 6). In the antiinflammatory tests in rodents, sulindac is seen to be only slightly less potent than the most active compounds, indomethacin, naproxen and profenid, and significantly more effective than ibuprofen, phenylbutazone or aspirin.

3.5   SAFETY ASSESSMENT OF INDOMETHACIN AND ITS ANALOGS

Although virtually all pharmacological and biochemical investigations of a compound intended for human or animal use may have some relevance to a judgment of its safety, the term "Safety Assessment" may be taken to refer particularly to those studies specifically undertaken to study the adverse actions of a substance at whatever dose and by whatever route it takes to demonstrate such effects. Since these studies are not the field of special expertise of the present authors, we shall borrow freely from the report supplied to us for our present purpose by the Department of Safety Assessment of the Merck Institute for Therapeutic Research.

Many authors have written about the general principles guiding safety assessment; a recent discussion referring especially to antiinflammatory drugs is that of Levy (1974). Publications from the Merck laboratories include those by Beyer (1960), Peck (1964a, b, 1966, 1968), Peck *et al.* (1967) and Stone *et al.* (1974). Some of the toxicologic actions of indomethacin were described in papers by Peck (1968) and Stone *et al.* (1974).

TABLE 13

Acute toxicity values for several indomethacin analogs in female mice Carworth Farms CF$_1$ strain

Compound[a]	LD_{50} mg kg^{-1} [b]		
	Oral	Intraperitoneal	Intravenous
Indomethacin	50	28	40
Sulindac (MK-231)	567	347	
Compound (**97**) (MK-715)	348	180	
Compound (**33**) sodium salt, MK-410	925		331
Compound (**46**) (MK-825)	158	64	157
Compound (**32**) (MK-555)	809		279

[a] For structures, see section 4.
[b] Data courtesy S. E. McKinney; 7 day mortality, Weil (1952).

3.5.1   Acute toxicity

Acute toxicity values for six compounds of special interest as obtained in mice are shown in Table 13. It is at once apparent that there is a very large range of LD_{50} values, even though all the compounds were selected for relatively good activity in antiinflammatory tests. Only minor variations are seen with the same compound by different routes of administration. For example, the oral and intravenous LD_{50}s for MK-825 were nearly identical, and the same could be said for indomethacin. It may be concluded that all the compounds were relatively well absorbed by each route. Death did not occur immediately, and most animals receiving up to several times the LD_{50} showed no immediate toxic signs. A few animals receiving a lethal dose died after an hour or so, but the majority of deaths were delayed for one to seven days, and occasionally longer.

Few behavioral signs were immediately apparent, though animals receiving lethal doses exhibited decreased activity and ptosis before death. Postmortem examinations suggested that gastrointestinal lesions probably accounted for virtually all the deaths. Animals which survived the test generally recovered normal rates of growth after the first week or so.

Of the six compounds shown in Table 13, the two least active, MK-555 and MK-409 (see Table 3) were also the least toxic, while the most potent compound, indomethacin, had the lowest LD_{50}. Of special interest is the relatively low toxicity of sulindac. The data in Table 14 emphasize the low acute toxicity of sulindac in three species of animals. The Table also shows that in mice and rats the LD_{50} is essentially independent of the route of

TABLE 14

Comparative acute toxicity values for indomethacin and sulindac in several species

Species and Strain	Sex	Route	LD_{50} (95% fiducial limits) mg kg^{-1}[a] Indomethacin	Sulindac
Mice, Carworth Farms CF$_1$	females	oral	50 (29, 89)	567 (511, 630)
	females	intraperitoneal	28 (21, 37)	347 (318, 379)
	females	intravenous	40 (19, 85)	
Rats, Charles River CD	males	oral	12 (10, 14)	296 (236, 372)
	males	intraperitoneal	15 (12, 19)	265 (226, 311)
	males	subcutaneous	13 (11, 15)	
Guinea-pigs	females	oral	543 (385, 764)	
	both sexes	intraperitoneal	40 (30, 54)	
Rabbits	both sexes	oral	130 (94, 181)	413 (358, 475)

[a] See footnote to Table 13.

administration. Indomethacin in the guinea-pig is an exception, a result probably indicating relatively poor absorption from the gastrointestinal tract in this species, in contrast to other species. Comparable data for sulindac in the guinea-pig are not available.

Comparative figures for antiinflammatory potency in the granuloma inhibition test in rats and the acute LD_{50} in mice are shown in Table 15. The ratio between these two figures (shown in the last column) has been used by some authors to indicate comparative safety of compounds. The ratio should not be regarded as a "therapeutic index" since activity and toxicity are determined in different species, and the ratio does not take into account the errors involved in the determinations. The ED_{50} for granuloma inhibition with indomethacin, for example, is attainable only with doses within the range inducing gastrointestinal lesions. The ED_{50} shown is therefore an extrapolation; in several experiments ED_{50} ranged from 4 to 11 mg g^{-1} d^{-1}. This range is small compared to the large differences among compounds, so the high value of the ratio for sulindac compared to the other compounds is especially impressive.

Further details of acute toxicity studies of sulindac in various species are shown in Table 16. No deaths occurred in dogs with oral doses up to 1600 mg kg^{-1}, but emesis interfered with interpretation of the data, and it was not practicable to attempt higher doses. The highest dose not producing emesis was on the order of 400 mg kg^{-1}. Indomethacin also produced emesis at 160 mg kg^{-1}. It may be noted that dogs survived very large single doses of indomethacin, although it has been established that much smaller doses repeated

TABLE 15

Relative antiinflammatory activity and acute toxicity of several analogs of indomethacin

Compound	A[a] Granuloma inhibition ED$_{50}$ mg kg^{-1}	B[b] Oral LD$_{50}$ mice mg kg^{-1}	Ratio B/A
Indomethacin	9	50	5·5
Sulindac (MK-231)	30	567	18·9
Compound (**97**) (MK-715)	45	348	7·7
Compound (**33**), sodium salt, MK-410	450	925	2·1
Compound (**46**) (MK-825)	18	158	8·8
Compound (**32**) (MK-555)	900	809	0·9

[a] Daily oral dose (extrapolated) required to produce 50 per cent inhibition of granuloma formation; the figure for indomethacin is derived from the average of three determinations: Tables 3 and 6, Winter et al., 1963, and Table I, Winter, 1965. Figures for the other compounds are obtained by dividing 9 mg kg^{-1} by "Relative Potency for Granuloma Inhibition" in Table 3.
   [b] See Table 3.

daily induce fatal gastrointestinal lesions (Menguy and Desbaillets, 1967). Relatively small single oral doses produce antiinflammatory effects in dogs receiving intrasynovial injections of sodium urate crystals. Van Arman and co-workers have reported ED$_{50}$ values in this test of 1·73 mg kg^{-1} for indomethacin (1970a). Sulindac, being a prodrug, is active only at the high dose of 45 mg kg^{-1} by this local application.

In the acute toxicity tests of indomethacin in dogs, a wide range of doses was used (20, 40, 60, 80, 160 mg kg^{-1}). Although no deaths occurred, evidence of gastrointestinal effects was seen at all dose levels. These included blanching of the gums, diarrhea or soft stools, infrequent emesis, and occasionally fecal occult blood. Some of the dogs showed a slight initial weight loss from which they soon recovered. As there were no further signs of toxicity, one animal from each group was given a repeat dose after 3 weeks. The results of the second dose were the same as those of the first, so 19 weeks after the beginning of the test five dogs were sacrificed and examined at autopsy. There was no gross evidence of gastrointestinal lesions.

These results emphasize again the absence of toxic effects of indomethacin except for the production of gastrointestinal lesions. It also appears that if the initial lesion is not fatal, full recovery can occur.

TABLE 16

Acute toxicity of sulindac (MK-231) in several species

Species and strain	Age and sex	Weight range, g	LD$_{50}$ (95% fiducial limits)		Time of death
			Oral, mg kg^{-1}	Intraperitoneal, mg kg^{-1}	
Mice, CF$_1$S					
Carworth Farms	6 wk, F	19–21	567 (511, 630)	347 (318, 379)	1 h–7 days
Rats, Charles River CD					
Young adults	5 wk, F	100–155	365 (325, 411)	261 (234, 292)	1 h–7 days
	5 wk, M	100–155	296 (236, 372)	265 (226, 311)	1·5 h–7 days[a]
Weanlings	3 wk, F	40–55	201 (158, 254)	328 (269, 399)	2 h–7 days[a]
	3 wk, M	40–55	246 (151, 403)	244 (179, 331)	1 h–5 days[a]
Infants	24 h, M, F	6–7·3	196 (153, 251)	—	1–7 days
Rabbits, New Zealand	16–18 wk, M, F	2·4–3·1 kg	413 (358, 475)	—	1–5 days
Dogs, beagle	20–40 wk, M, F	6·5–10·2 kg 10·2 kg	>1600[b]	—	no deaths

[a] Deaths rarely occurred between days 7 and 14; such deaths are included in the calculations of LD$_{50}$.

[b] Doses employed in dogs, 400–1600 mg kg^{-1}; lethal dose could not be determined because of emesis at higher doses.

3.5.2 Subacute and chronic toxicity

Peck (1968) pointed out that repeated administration over a period up to several months is a more reliable indicator of safety of a drug than is an acute study, no matter how carefully the latter is carried out. The doses used for the subacute and chronic tests range all the way from an approximation of the pharmacological dose in the animal being employed to a dose expected to be toxic.

Tables 17 and 18 list most of the subacute and chronic tests employed in the safety assessment of indomethacin and sulindac. The tables do not include some of the "range finding" tests, that is, studies intended primarily to establish the range of doses to be used in long-term studies. The tables also do not include some tests that were essentially duplicates of those shown. With these exceptions, the tables are nearly complete. They show the impressively large numbers and varieties of experiments used to determine the safety of a compound intended for human or animal therapeutic use.

Antiinflammatory drugs are intended for long-term use in human subjects, so several of the tests of chronic toxicity in animals are of long duration—for

TABLE 17

Subacute and chronic toxicity tests of indomethacin in animals

Test number	Species and sex	Route of administration	Daily dose mg kg^{-1}	Duration weeks
1	Rats, M, F	oral, by gavage	0·1, 0·25, 0·5, 0·75, 1·6, 5·0	35
2	Rats, M, F	oral, in the diet	0·5, 1·0, 2·5, 5[a]	52
3	Rats, M, F	oral, in the diet	0·5, 1·0, 2·0[a]	81
4	Dogs, M, F	oral, capsules	2, 5, 10, 20	7
5	Dogs, M, F	oral, capsules	6 (2 mg kg^{-1}, three times daily)	6
6	Dogs, M, F	oral, capsules	3 (1 mg kg^{-1}, three times daily)	57
7	Dogs, M, F	oral, capsules	0·25, 0·5, 1·0	129
8	Dogs, M, F	intravenous	5	4
9	Dogs, M, F	rectal suppositories	c. 10	1
10	Monkeys, M, F	oral, by gavage	2, 5, 10	8
11	Monkeys, M, F	oral, by gavage	1, 5, 10	18
12	Rabbits, M, F	oral, capsules	1, 5, 10, 20	22
13	Guinea-pigs, M, F	oral, in the diet	6, 11·4, 24[a]	27
14	Guinea-pigs, M	oral, by gavage	10, 20, 100, 200	21
15	Guinea-pigs, M	intraperitoneal	10, 20, 100, 200	5
16	Mice, F	oral, by gavage	2, 5, 10	16
17	Cats, M, F	oral, by gavage	10, 20	4
18	Pigs, M, F	oral, in the diet	0·7, 2, 7, 15, 33[a]	6

[a] In tests involving drug in the diet, the doses shown are based on estimates of food consumption.

example, tests 2, 3, 6, 7, 20, 22, 24 in the tables. In the case of indomethacin, Peck (1968) has pointed out that no more than 1 month is required to define the toxicity as seen in animals; nevertheless, one would not know that until the tests had been completed for a much longer time. And no matter how long the study is, symptoms of adverse effects that are uniquely human cannot be predicted from animal studies, as several authors have pointed out (for references, see Peck, 1968, and Levy, 1974).

Each of the studies listed in Tables 17 and 18 must be accompanied by observations on the clinical state of the animals, together with periodic examinations of hematological parameters, liver and renal function tests, and

TABLE 18

Subacute and chronic toxicity tests of sulindac in animals

Test number	Species and sex	Oral administration	Daily dose mg kg^{-1}	Duration
19	Rats, M, F	by gavage	10, 20, 40	13 weeks
20	Rats, M, F	by gavage	5, 10, 20	53 weeks
20a	Rats, M, F	in diet	5, 10, 20	105 weeks
21	Mice, M, F	by gavage	20, 40, 80, 100	36 days
22	Mice, M, F	in the diet	5, 10, 20[a]	81 weeks
23	Dogs, M, F	capsules	5, 10, 20, 40	14 weeks
24	Dogs, M, F	capsules	5, 10, 20	53 weeks
25	Monkeys, M, F	by gavage	5, 10, 20, 40, 80	13 weeks
26	Mice, F (teratogenic study)	by gavage	10, 20, 40, 60	gestation days 6–15
27	Rabbits, F (teratogenic study)	by gavage	20, 40, 60	gestation days 7–15
28	Rabbits, F (teratogenic study)	by gavage	30, 60, 90	gestation days 7–15
29	Rats, F (teratogenic study)	by gavage	10, 20, 40	gestation days 6–15
30	Rats, M (fertility study)	by gavage	10, 20, 40	70 days prior to mating; mated females sacrificed day 14 of gestation
31	Rats, F (fertility study)	by gavage	10, 20, 40	14 days prior to mating[b]
32	Rats, F (late gestation and lactation)	by gavage	10, 20, 40	day 15 of gestation to day 21 postpartum
33	Mice, F (parturition study)	by gavage	10, 20, 40	day 16 of gestation to parturition[c]

[a] In Test 22, daily doses estimated on basis of food consumption.

[b] In Test 31, half were sacrificed on day 14 of gestation; the remainder were maintained with their litters until 21 days postpartum.

[c] In Test 33, parallel groups received aspirin 100, 200, 400 mg kg^{-1} day^{-1} or phenylbutazone 10, 30, 90 mg kg^{-1} day^{-1}.

biochemical analyses of body fluids. Animals dying during the test must be submitted to autopsy, as must the survivors at the end of the test. The postmortem examination includes both gross and microscopic studies. A detailed discussion of all these findings would be out of place in the present paper, since the compounds described herein are quite limited in the variety of toxic manifestations which they induce in animals. All of the compounds shown in Table 3 were subjected to several of the tests listed in Table 17 and 18, but since none of them exhibited any effects which were uniquely different, and also since current therapeutic interest centers on indomethacin and sulindac, the other compounds will be omitted from the present discussion. Several of the tests listed involved large numbers of animals—in some cases, up to 100 for each dose level. This permitted a variety of observations, including autopsy studies, to be made at intervals during the study.

Toxic signs produced by both compounds were related to the gastro-intestinal tract. Typically, these consisted of anorexia, body weight depression, general weakness, accompanied by soft stools and sometimes diarrhea, and in more severe cases, blood in the stools. Hematological changes secondary to g.i. effects were seen in those with the most marked g.i. toxicity; they consisted of decreased hemoglobin, lower hematocrit, leucocytosis and neutrophilia. Gastrointestinal lesions found at autopsy varied somewhat with different species, but they were dose related in incidence and severity.

3.5.3 Chronic toxicity of indomethacin

In rats, in Test 1, the signs just described were not seen in any of the first four groups; that is, up to and including 0.75 mg kg^{-1} d^{-1}. They appeared within 4 weeks with 1.6 mg kg^{-1} d^{-1}, and in 1 week with 5 mg kg^{-1} d^{-1}. The tests had to be terminated in both these groups. In contrast, when similar amounts of drug were administered by mixing in the diet (Tests 2 and 3) the compound was much better tolerated. Those receiving 5 mg kg^{-1} d^{-1} in the diet survived until the 34th week while those on 2.5 mg kg^{-1} d^{-1} continued for the entire 52-week period. In Test 3, survival at all dose levels was equal to that of the control animals during the 81-week period.

In these two tests, gastrointestinal lesions were confined to the small intestine and did not involve the stomach or colon, except in a few severe cases of perforating ulcer of the small intestine producing peritonitis which sometimes induced a secondary effect on the stomach. The lesions of the small intestine were especially along the mesenteric attachment of the jejunum and ileum, as has been described by others (see section 3.4.2 above).

Results in dogs were similar to those in rats, and may be summarized as follows: single oral doses of 10 or 20 mg kg^{-1} d^{-1} produced perforating ulcers within 3 weeks; the dogs survived the 7-week test at 2 or 5 mg kg^{-1} d^{-1} without perforations, though ulceration was found at autopsy. On the other hand, there were no ulcers in dogs receiving 3 mg kg^{-1} d^{-1} divided into three doses of 1 mg kg^{-1} each (Test 6). These animals survived the entire 57 weeks in good health, and no lesions were found at autopsy. However, occasional fecal blood had been observed during the year, so possibly there could have been superficial lesions which healed on continued drug administration. These results were similar to those of Test 7, in which single doses up to 1 mg kg^{-1} d^{-1} were given for about 2$\frac{1}{2}$ years. The dose of 2 mg kg^{-1} produced ulcers whether given once a day (Test 4) or three times a day for a total of 6 mg kg^{-1} d^{-1} (Test 5). Intravenous or rectal administration (Tests 8 and 9) produced results comparable to the same doses given orally. Rectal administration did not produce local ulceration.

The location of lesions in the dog were similar to that in the rat; that is, the jejunum and ileum, but with the additional factor of lesions sometimes occurring in the pyloric region of the stomach, a condition never observed in the rat.

Responses of the monkeys were more variable than those of rats or dogs, and some of the monkeys showed no signs of drug effect even at the highest dose, 10 mg kg^{-1} d^{-1} for 18 weeks, while others showed body weight loss, anorexia, emesis and diarrhea at all doses except the lowest. In contrast to findings in rats and dogs, small intestinal lesions were not found in any of the monkeys. Ulcers of the colon were found in about half the animals at the two highest doses and in two of six at the lowest dose, but also in one of the controls. These lesions were small. Perhaps the drug exacerbated a tendency already present to some degree in the colony.

It is difficult to set a figure for the maximum tolerated dose of indomethacin in rabbits or guinea pigs. The rabbits which survived the test period of 22 weeks on daily doses of 1 or 5 mg kg^{-1} maintained normal appearance and body weight throughout. However, only about half of them survived. In those which died, death was usually rather sudden, with no obvious signs of toxicity until shortly before death. These signs consisted of weight loss, weakness, soft stools and diarrhea. Although these signs resemble those described above for rats and dogs receiving doses sufficient to produce intestinal lesions, such lesions were not found in the rabbits. The only gastrointestinal lesions found in any of the rabbits were ulcers in the pyloric mucosa of two animals which died during treatment with the highest dose level, 20 mg kg^{-1} d^{-1}. All of the rabbits on the two highest dose levels were sacrificed in the 10th week, but with the two exceptions noted, there were no gastrointestinal lesions.

An unusual finding in the rabbits was an increased incidence of certain infectious processes—subcutaneous abscesses, pneumonia and pericarditis. This probably accounts for the deaths observed. The relationship of this finding to drug therapy is uncertain; in extensive studies of rats and mice, no evidence of drug-induced increase in infectious disease was seen. Robinson *et al.* (1974) have also described experiments leading to the conclusion that indomethacin does not affect resistance to infection in rats or mice, nor in rabbits except at doses which were also otherwise toxic; their results with aspirin and phenylbutazone were comparable.

Interpretation of results in Tests 13 and 14 was complicated by the relatively high mortality in all groups, including the controls, and by the tendency of the guinea-pigs to regurgitate substances given by stomach tube. However, mortality was especially high in those receiving 100 or 200 mg $kg^{-1} d^{-1}$ orally or intraperitoneally, or 24 mg $kg^{-1} d^{-1}$ in the diet. Gastrointestinal lesions were found rather irregularly, but those animals found dead exhibited peritoneal adhesions.

Responses of mice were similar to those of rats; toxic signs were evident within a few days at 5 or 10 mg $kg^{-1} d^{-1}$, and foci of necrosis were found in the wall of the small intestine. The smaller dose, 2 mg $kg^{-1} d^{-1}$ was well tolerated, with body weight gain equal to that of controls receiving the vehicle alone; after 16 weeks, no gastrointestinal lesions were found in this group except some small nodules along the mesenteric attachment of the small intestine in one of 20 animals.

The doses given to the cats, 10 and 20 mg $kg^{-1} d^{-1}$ proved to be above the tolerated levels, and although there were no deaths in the 4-week period of observation, the animals lost weight and suffered from diarrhea or blood in the stools. At autopsy, ulcers were found in the stomach, duodenum and ileum, and in the gall bladder of two cats. Hence, the safe dose for this species was not established.

Responses of the swine differed from those of any other species. The two highest doses, 15 and 33 mg $kg^{-1} d^{-1}$, were above the tolerated levels, and all those on these doses died within 4 weeks. Unlike other species, gastrointestinal ulcers were confined to the colon. All other dose levels, including 7 mg $kg^{-1} d^{-1}$, an amount which would be toxic for some species, were not only well tolerated but the animals actually gained weight better and utilized food more efficiently than did the controls. The explanation for this unsuspected finding is not immediately apparent. If the animals were suffering from some inflammatory condition which was relieved by the medication, it was not detected at autopsy.

Additional chronic studies in rats included a test in which indomethacin was started at the safe dose of 0.5 mg $kg^{-1} d^{-1}$ then increased stepwise over a 10-week period to 4 mg $kg^{-1} d^{-1}$. This experiment proved that tolerance to the gastrointestinal action of indomethacin could not be established in this way. Toxic signs were apparent only 4 days after reaching the top dose, and autopsy revealed the usual gastrointestinal lesions seen in rats repeatedly receiving such doses. Other experiments established that the 1-deschlorobenzoyl and the *O*-

desmethyl metabolites, designated by Harman *et al.* (1964) as Metabolites II and III, respectively, were entirely nontoxic in rats at doses as high as 20 mg $kg^{-1} d^{-1}$.

Altogether, the chronic studies on indomethacin can be summarized as demonstrating that:

  i. Indomethacin toxicity is limited to ulcerative actions on the gastro-intestinal tract (with the possible exception of some equivocal findings in rabbits).

  ii. The doses required to demonstrate toxicity vary among species, although dogs, rats and mice are similar.

  iii. The site of action of toxic doses also differs among species, but is most commonly the ileum or jejunum.

  iv. In those species which have been used for study of antiinflammatory activity, the toxic dose is higher than the antiinflammatory dose.

  v. Animals which survive a toxic dose recover fully (except for some residual epithelial atrophy in continued treatment) if the compound is withdrawn.

  vi. The maximum tolerated daily dose increases if it is given in several divided doses or incorporated in the diet—the size of the dose tolerated seems to depend upon the amount of drug given at one time, rather than the total for the 24-hour period.

3.5.4   *Chronic toxicity of sulindac*

The most noticeable difference in the chronic studies with indomethacin (Table 17) and sulindac (Table 18) is the contrast in the doses used. In rats, for example, gastrointestinal toxicity forced discontinuance of chronic administration of indomethacin before the end of the experiment at doses of 1·6 to 5 mg $kg^{-1} d^{-1}$ (Tests 1, 2, 3). With sulindac, on the other hand (Test 19) even at the highest dose, 40 mg $kg^{-1} d^{-1}$, there was only one death related to ulcer in 30 animals; otherwise, there was not even any occult blood detected in the feces at any dose level. At autopsy on termination of the experiment, however, ulcerative enteritis could be detected in about a third of the rats on the highest dose. The occurrence of gastrointestinal lesions in a minority of animals was confirmed by the longer term study (Test 20).

Comparable results were obtained in mice in doses up to 20 mg $kg^{-1} d^{-1}$ (Tests 21, 22), but the potentiality of the compound to induce gastrointestinal lesions at high doses was shown in mice receiving 40, 80, or 100 mg $kg^{-1} d^{-1}$.

Even more impressive evidence of the gastrointestinal safety of sulindac was the absence of gastrointestinal ulceration in dogs or monkeys at any dose level Tests 23, 24, 25). The only evidence of possible gastrointestinal effects was the appearance of soft stools, diarrhea and emesis in some animals in Test 23, but when the entire test was repeated in another group of dogs in a different laboratory, even these signs were absent. When these results are considered in comparison with the antiinflammatory-antipyretic-analgesic potency of the compound (Tables 3 and 10; also Van Arman *et al.*, 1972) it is clear that a very considerable separation of potency and toxicity has been achieved.

In the absence of deaths from ulcerative changes in the gastrointestinal tract, relatively large doses of sulindac could be administered chronically, and other types of toxicity could be investigated. In Test 19, for example, there was a slight increase in weights of kidney and liver in rats receiving 40 mg kg^{-1} d^{-1}, but no microscopic changes could be found to account for the increased weight. A similar weight increase in kidney, liver and spleen was seen also in the longer-term study (Test 20) and in this instance, microscopic changes were seen in the kidney (papillary necrosis) of one animal receiving the highest dose. One dog also had a slightly enlarged liver, and two had slightly enlarged kidneys, among those receiving the two highest doses in Test 23, but this finding could not be confirmed when the test was repeated, nor in Test 24. No enlarged organs were found in the monkeys (Test 25).

Some minor histological changes possibly related to drug administration were seen in some of the dogs and monkeys. For example, there was some focal interstitial nephritis in some monkeys on the two highest doses, but this finding is complicated by the fact that similar changes were also seen in some of the untreated control animals. More definite, perhaps, was the presence of hepatic changes in both the dogs and monkeys on the higher doses, such as slight portal fibrosis, proliferation of the bile duct, and periportal inflammatory cell infiltration. Correlated with this were changes in some biochemical tests in some monkeys receiving the higher doses. These included increased serum glutamic oxalacetic transaminase (SGOT), serum alkaline phosphatase, serum creatinine concentration and blood urea nitrogen. These were not regular nor progressive, and indeed were within the normal range near the end of the test (Week 12) in the monkeys at all dosage levels (except for serum bilirubin in one monkey on 80 mg kg^{-1} d^{-1}). Such changes in the dogs were not consistently found, nor were they ever beyond the range of normal variability for this species. Yellow crystals identified as sulindac and its metabolites were seen in the gall bladder of one dog, but there were no accompanying histological changes.

The studies designed to test the teratogenicity of sulindac or the effects of the compound upon reproductive performance (Tests 26–31, inclusive) further established the safety of the compound at doses considerably higher than those required to demonstrate antiinflammatory activity, since no teratogenicity was found, nor were there any effects upon mating performance, fertility, or growth and survival of the young. When the drug was given late in the gestation period (Test 32) there was a decrease in body weight gain in the females receiving 40 mg kg^{-1} d^{-1}. Gastrointestinal ulcers were found in a few of these animals. This finding may indicate a slightly greater sensitivity to gastrointestinal effects under the stress of late pregnancy. Accompanying this effect was a small but significant decrease in average weight of newborn pups from females receiving the highest dose (40 mg kg^{-1} d^{-1} and an increase in the number of pups dying during the first postpartum day.

The final test (33) revealed the expected increase in average duration of parturition and delay in its onset by both sulindac and aspirin. This finding confirms reports in the literature; it is presumably related to the inhibition of the synthesis of prostaglandins which are important during the process of parturition. Further discussion will be deferred until a later section (section 9). Phenylbutazone did not influence duration of gestation in the doses used.

The above discussion of the tests involved in safety assessment in animals is a general summary only, and omits many details which a trained pathologist would regard as necessary to include in a technical report. However, it may be regarded as sufficiently detailed to show the kinds of toxicity encountered, the range of doses required to demonstrate toxicity, and the margin of safety possessed by these compounds. Safety assessment, of course, requires more than studies in experimental animals, but the results outlined above give the background for the next step in assessment of safety; namely, trial in human subjects. The results further show that some separation of antiinflammatory and toxic properties can be achieved, and seem to justify the expectation that sulindac may fulfil to an important degree the hope for an antiinflammatory compound of therapeutic usefullness and reduced adverse activities.

4   Synthetic chemistry

4.1   SYNTHETIC CHEMISTRY OF INDOMETHACIN AND RELATED COMPOUNDS

4.1.1   *Synthesis of indomethacin*

To illustrate the general nature of the synthetic chemistry involved in the study of indomethacin and analogs, a brief discussion of the original synthesis is summarized below (Shen *et al.,* 1963).

(1)

Indomethacin, 1-p-chlorobenzoyl-5-methoxy-2-methylindole-3-acetic acid (1), is a substituted 3-indolylacetic acid. The key steps involved in the original synthesis were the formation of the indole ring system (a + b in 1) followed by the attachment of the p-chlorobenzoyl group c at the N-position. The entire sequence is depicted as:

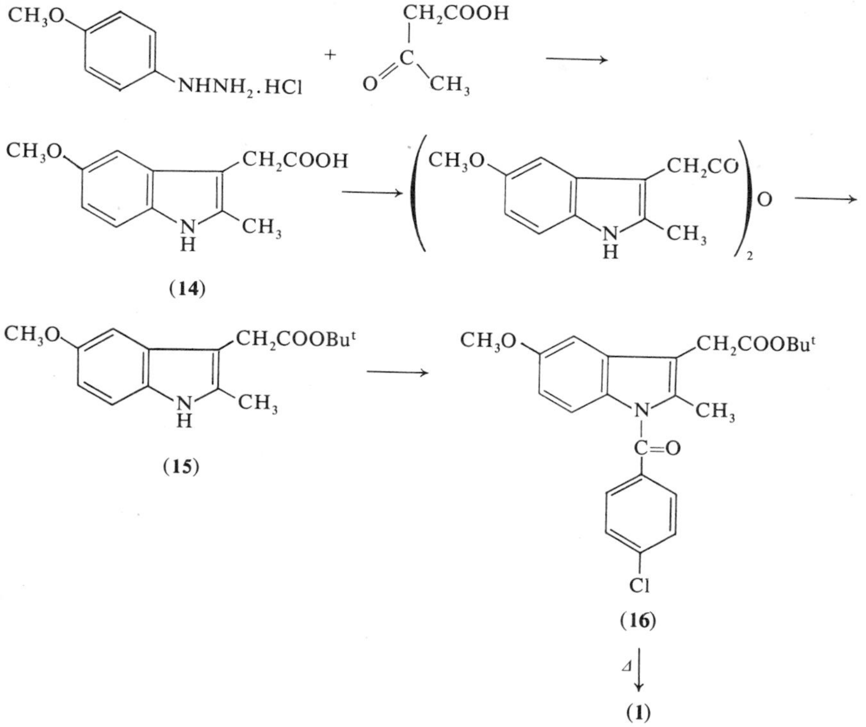

(14)

(15)

(16)

Δ

(1)

The first step (a + b) is the well-known Fischer indole synthesis which gives 14 (Shaw, 1955). However, before the next step of N-acylation the free carboxyl group in 14 had to be protected. Since acyl groups attached to the indole nitrogen are generally more sensitive than ordinary amides to cleavage under alkaline or acidic conditions, the thermal-labile t-butyl ester was chosen as the protecting group. The acid 14 was first converted to the anhydride with dicyclohexyl carbodiimide in tetrahydrofuran. The anhydride was then treated with t-butanol and zinc chloride to form the ester 15.

As described in 4.1.3 below, N-acylation with p-chlorobenzoyl chloride was achieved by first converting 15 to its sodio derivative with sodium hydride in dimethylformamide at 0°. Pyrolysis of 16, preferably in the presence of a catalytic amount of p-toluenesulfonic acid, yielded indomethacin as the final product.

An elegant variation of this basic process was developed by Sumitomo researchers (Yamamoto *et al.*, 1968). A nonhydrolytic condition was devised to couple an *N*-benzoylated phenylhydrazine (**17**) with levulinic acid to give indomethacin directly in an overall yield of about 90 per cent. It offered a significant economic advantage in the manufacture of indomethacin.

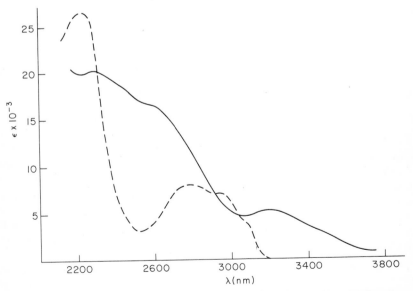

(**17**)

Indomethacin is a stable white crystalline compound, m.p. 155–156°C with an ultraviolet absorption spectrum of λ_{max} 2290, 2600 (inflection) and 3175 nm, ε 20 300, 16 700 and 5240. A comparison of its spectrum with that of the unacylated precursor is shown in Fig. 1. It is a very weak organic acid with pK_a ~5·25 (determined in 50 per cent methylcellusolve-H_2O). In phosphate buffer, solubility is about 0·3 mg ml^{-1} at pH 6·5, and 4·3 mg ml^{-1} at pH 7·2.

FIG. 1. Ultraviolet spectra of indomethacin, ————; methyl ester of **14** (in ethanol), ————.

The aqueous solution is relatively stable at pH 6–8, but prolonged standing and exposure to oxygen leads to decomposition, possibly through deacylation and ring oxidation. Additional solubility and stability data as well as aqueous formulations for biological experiments are described in section 8.

The acid chlorides of indole-3-acetic acids are generally not very stable. The acid chloride of 5-methoxy-2-methyl-3-indolylacetic acid (14) has been obtained but only under carefully controlled conditions (Shaw, 1955). From indomethacin, it was more convenient to prepare the ester and amide derivatives by direct condensation with an alcohol or amine in the presence of a carbodiimide at room temperature.

In some cases, e.g. when an unreactive alcohol was used, the acyl urea 18 was obtained as a by-product.

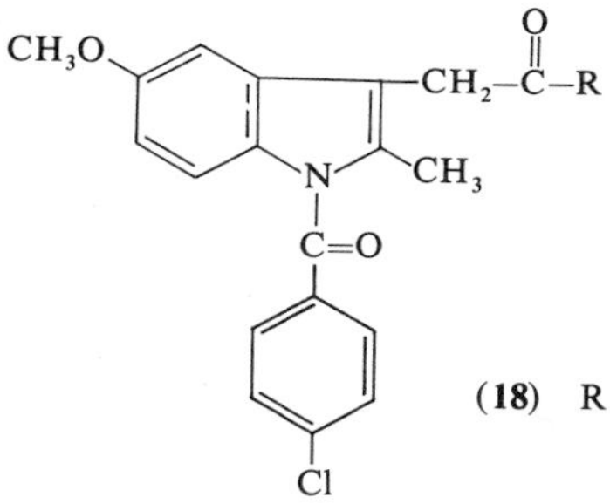

(18)   R = NCONHC$_6$H$_{11}$
                    |
                    C$_6$H$_{11}$

(20)   R = O.CO.R   (19)

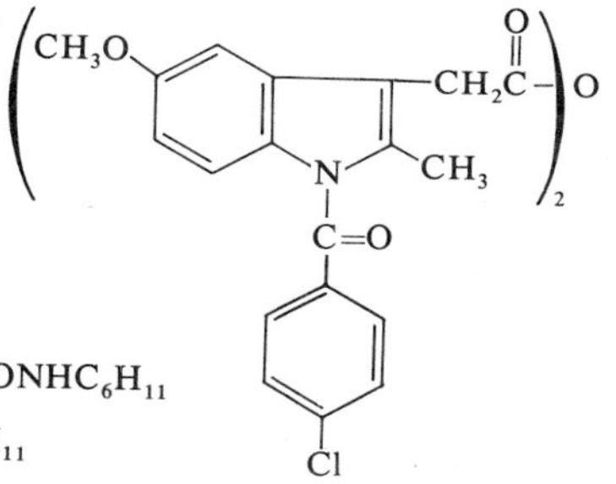

Alternatively, the anhydride 19 or a mixed anhydride of indomethacin (20) could be used as an intermediate for ester or amide formation.

As discussed below, the ester and amide derivatives of indomethacin were generally less active in the antiinflammatory assays than the free acid. The relatively good activity observed with some of them is probably attributable to in vivo cleavage to indomethacin. A number of these derivatives have been investigated for formulation or other purposes. For example, the β-diethyl-aminoethyl ester, as its hydrochloride, proved to be water-soluble and its activity was greater than that of most of the esters tested. The β-acetamido-ethyl (21) and 3-hydroxypropyl (22) esters are almost as active as the free acid in the carrageenan edema assay and are slightly less irritating to the gastro-intestinal tract in vivo. A group of substituted phenyl esters were prepared from the acid chloride of indomethacin (Dorrego et al., 1976). All are less active than the free acid. Their relative antiinflammatory potency is correlated with the lipophilicity of the phenolic moiety. An acetylated D-glucosaminide (23) and several amino acid conjugates, such as the glycyl (24), L-tyrosyl (25) and L-lysyl (26) derivatives, were found to be much less active, presumably not readily cleaved in vivo.

The amide derived from D-glucosamine, glucametacin (27), was reported to be effective in the clinic (Giordano *et al.*, 1975), but no pharmacological or metabolic details have been reported. It is not clear whether the amide linkage is cleaved before or after absorption after a daily oral dose of 420 mg.

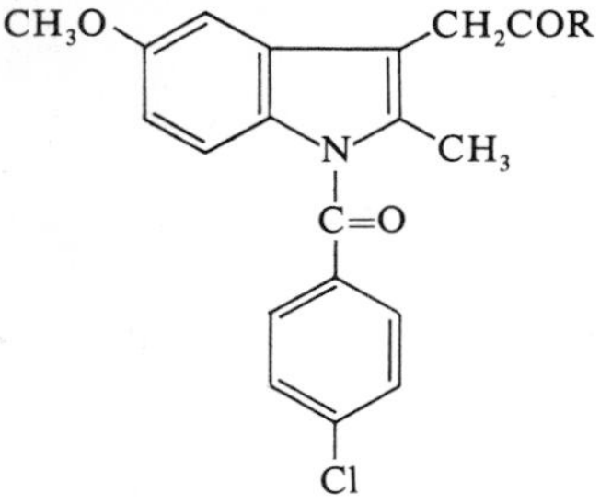

(21)   R = OCH₂CH₂NHCOCH₃

(22)   OCH₂CH₂CH₂OH

(23)   CH₂OAc

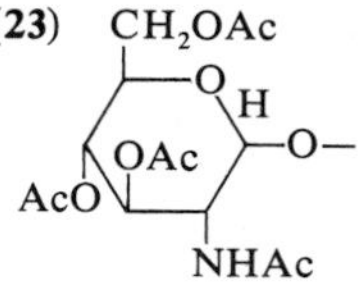

(24)   NHCH₂CO₂H

(25)   NHCHCO₂H (L)
              C₆H₄OH(p)

(26)   NHCHCO₂H (L)
              (CH₂)₄NH₂

(27)   CH₂OH ... H, OH (glucametacin)

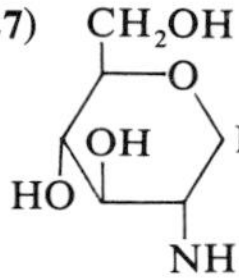

Indomethacin readily forms salts with inorganic and organic bases, e.g., Na^+, Cu^{++}, Mg^{++}, amines, etc. In our laboratory, no significant difference in biological activities was observed when these salts were administered orally in standard antiinflammatory and g.i. irritation assays.

4.1.2   *N-Alkylated analogs*

In a systematic study of indomethacin analogs one may consider the basic structure as a 3-indolyl acetic acid with substituents at the N, C-2, and C-n which are amenable to modifications of a steric or electronic nature (28).

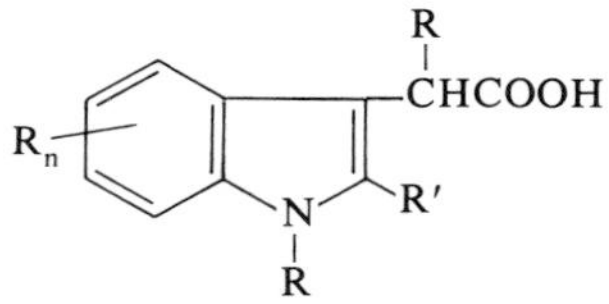

(28)

Following the characterization of **3** as a lead, our initial synthetic effort was concentrated on *N*-alkylated, particularly *N*-benzyl, indole-3-acetic acids.

Alkylation of the sodium derivative **29** with alkyl halides, benzyl halides, cinnamyl chloride, etc. proceeded smoothly in dimethylformamide at room temperature. Saponification of the *N*-alkylated methyl ester with dilute sodium hydroxide under mild conditions readily afforded the corresponding indole acetic acid for testing.

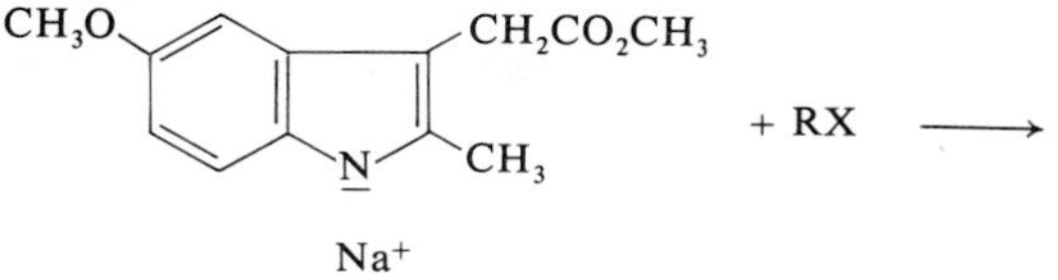

CH_3O — indole — $CH_2CO_2CH_3$, N — CH_3, Na^+ + RX $\longrightarrow$

(29)

CH_3O — indole — CH_2COOCH_3, N—R, CH_3 $\xrightarrow{OH^-}$ CH_3O — indole — CH_2CO_2H, N—R, CH_3

R = Cl—⟨⟩—CH_2—; CH_3S—⟨⟩—CH_2—; CH_3O—⟨⟩—CH_2—;

$\begin{matrix} CH_3 \\ CH_3 \end{matrix}$ NSO_2—⟨⟩—CH_2—; ⟨⟩—CH—thiophene—CH_2—, CH_3 ;

pyridine—CH_2—; ⟨⟩—$CH=CHCH_2$—; CH_3—$\overset{CH_3}{CH}$—CH_2—; cyclohexyl—CH_2—.

Cl—⟨⟩—OCH_2CH_2; ⟨⟩—$\overset{CH_3}{N}CH_2CH_2$—; $(CH_3)_2N\ CH_2CH_2CH_2$—

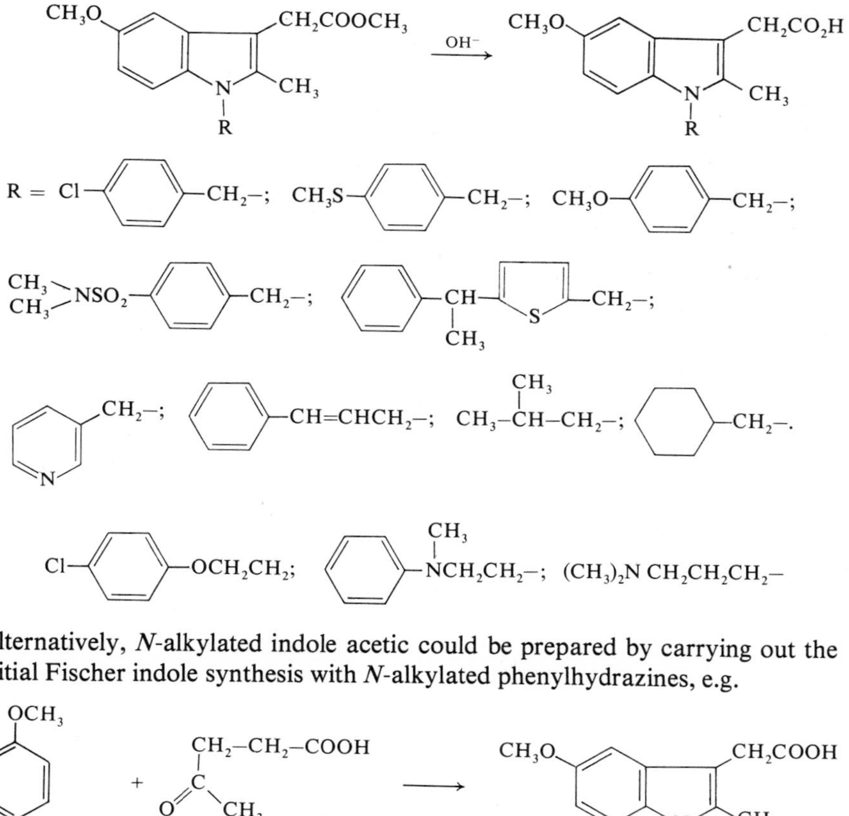

Alternatively, N-alkylated indole acetic could be prepared by carrying out the initial Fischer indole synthesis with N-alkylated phenylhydrazines, e.g.

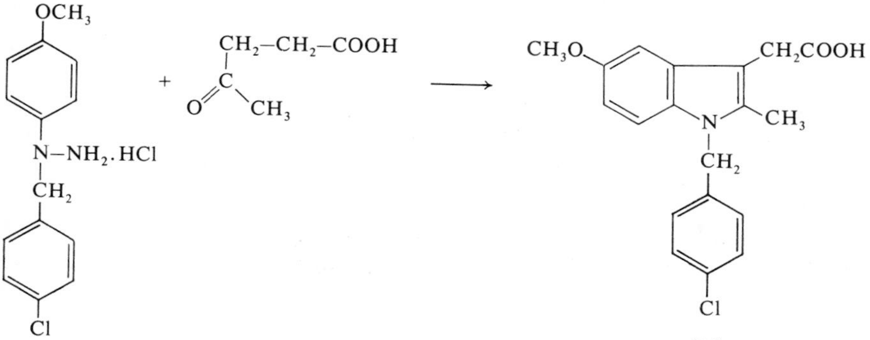

OCH_3 — ⟨⟩ — N—NH_2·HCl, CH_2 — ⟨⟩ — Cl + $\overset{O}{\underset{}{C}}\begin{matrix} CH_2-CH_2-COOH \\ CH_3 \end{matrix}$ $\longrightarrow$ CH_3O — indole — CH_2COOH, N—CH_2—⟨⟩—Cl, CH_3

(30)

The α-methyl homologs (**31**) were prepared from α-methyllevulinic acid in a similar manner. Optical resolution of several racemic mixtures showed that only the dextrorotatory enantiomers are biologically active. The absolute configuration of the dextro isomers were assigned as the sinister (*S*) form on the basis of circular dichroism studies (Shen, 1967).

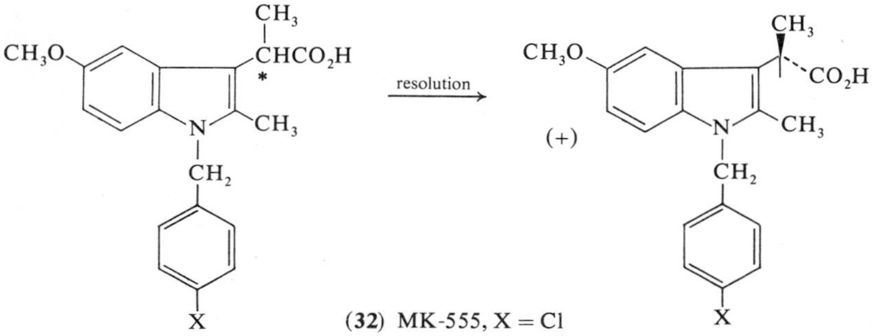

(**32**) MK-555, X = Cl
(**33**) MK-410, X = CH$_3$S

Among a number of *N*-benzyl-5-methoxy-2-methyl-indole-3-α-propionic acids investigated the (+)-*p*-chloro and (+)-*p*-methylthio analogs were chosen for clinical trials as MK-555 (**32**) and MK-410 (**33**) respectively. A modified Fischer reaction was applicable to the synthesis of *N*-arylindoles (**34**) not readily accessible by other methods.

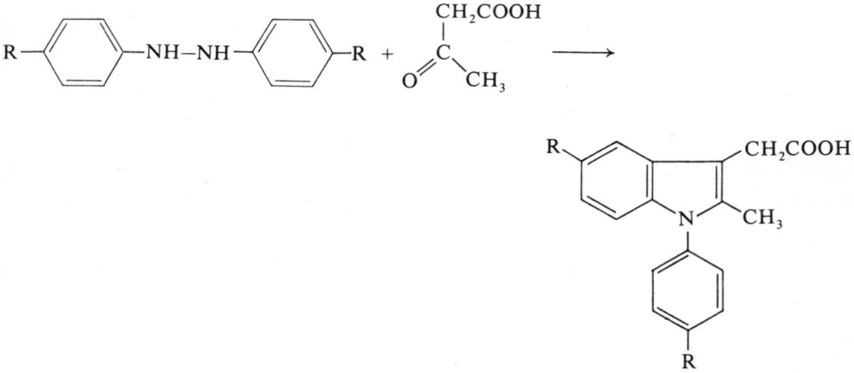

(**34**) R = H; OCH$_3$

This type of *N*-phenylindoleacetic acid with unsymmetrical substituents (**35**) was later investigated by the Sumitomo group using substituted diphenylamine as the starting material (Yamamoto, 1971).

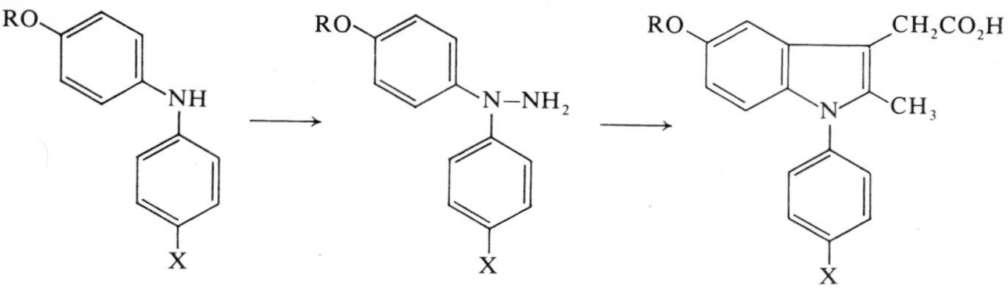

(35)

4.1.3 N-Acylated analogs

At the time of our chemical study only a few N-acylated indoles were known. For the synthesis of N-acylindoleacetic acids, optimal conditions for N-acylation were investigated extensively (T. B. Windholz, unpublished). Heating with acetic anhydride or with benzoyl chloride in pyrimidine have been effective in acylating certain indoles particularly those with a more acidic NH group (Reeve et al., 1963), but the reactivity of the nitrogen is much influenced by the nature of the ring-substituents at C-2, C-3 and by substituents on the benzenoid ring. For 2,3-dialkylated indoles like **15** and many analogs, it was found desirable to prepare the anion first with sodium hydride in dimethylformamide followed by treatment with the corresponding acid chloride at a low temperature. Other acylating agents such as anhydrides and active esters have also been used effectively in some cases.

As indicated above (4.1.1), acylation on the nitrogen of the indole was also facilitated by the formation of a sodio derivative (**29**) with sodium hydride. The p-nitrophenyl esters were particularly advantageous when a heteroaroyl acid was used, e.g.,

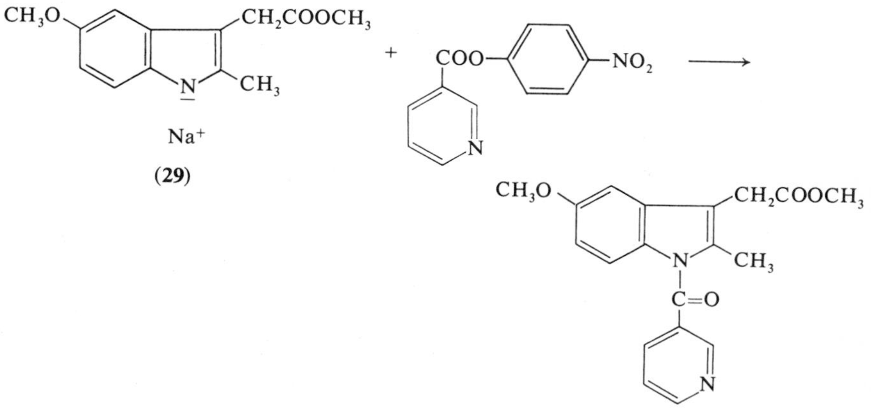

(29)

(36)

Various acyl groups evaluated in structure–activity relationship studies are exemplified by

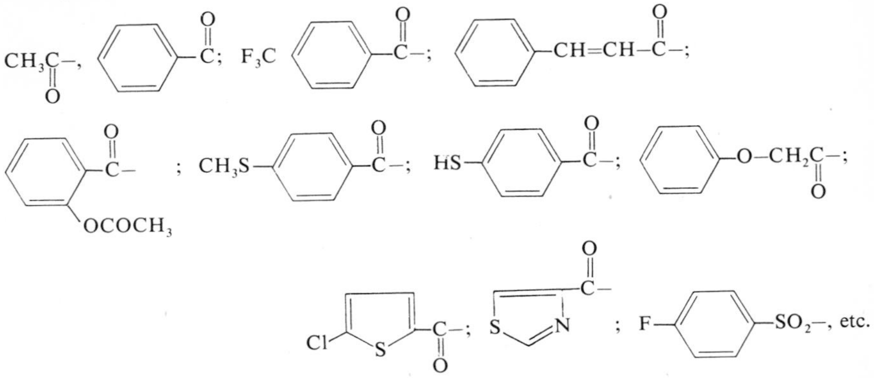

Later, three *N*-acyl analogs, Cinmetacin (Indolacin **37**), ID-133 (**38**) and ID-955 (**39**), prepared by the Sumitomo process mentioned above were independently investigated extensively by Sumitomo laboratories (Yamamoto *et al.*, 1969a, b; Komatsu *et al.*, 1973).

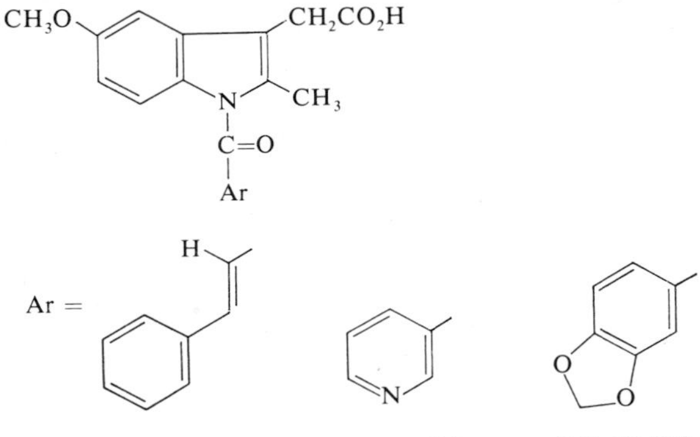

(**37**) Cinmetacin   (**38**) ID-133   (**39**) ID-955

The antiinflammatory and analgesic activities of these analogs range from $\frac{1}{10}$ to $\frac{1}{3}$ of those of indomethacin. Some changes of their overall pharmacological profiles were also observed.

Similarly, ureido (**40**) and urethane (**41**) analogs were obtained from reaction of the indole anion (**29**) with phenyl isocyanate or phenyl chloroformate respectively.

The free acid of (**42**) was independently investigated by us and by others as a weak prostaglandin synthetase inhibitor ($\frac{1}{150}$ × indomethacin) (Gryglewski, 1974).

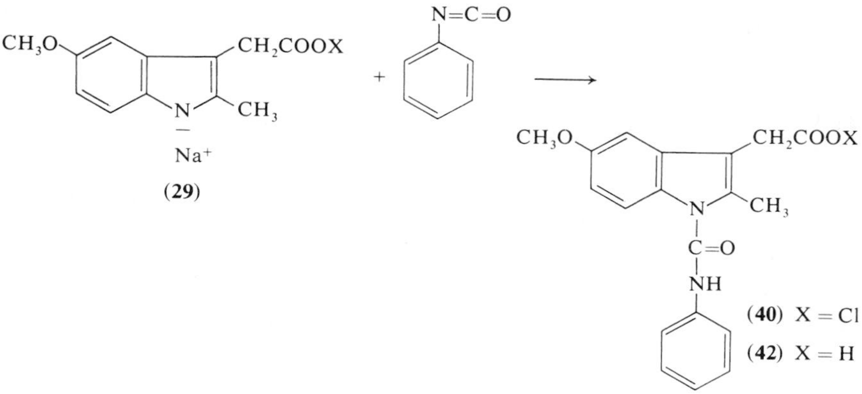

(29)

(40) X = Cl
(42) X = H

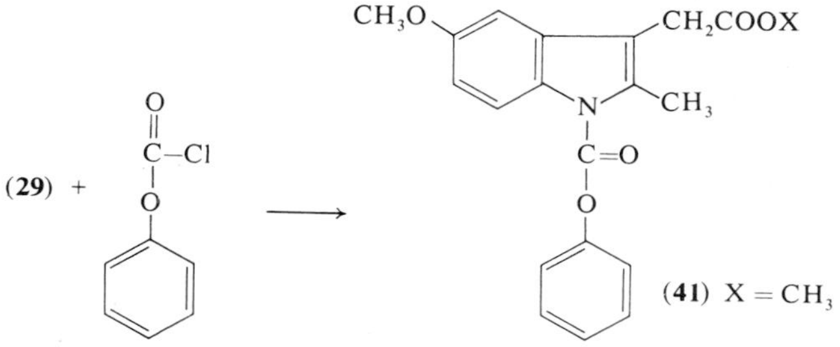

(29) +

(41) X = CH$_3$

4.1.4 Modification of indole ring substituents

To vary the ring substituents R' and R$_n$ as depicted in formula **44**, the usefulness of the Fischer reaction was again demonstrated:

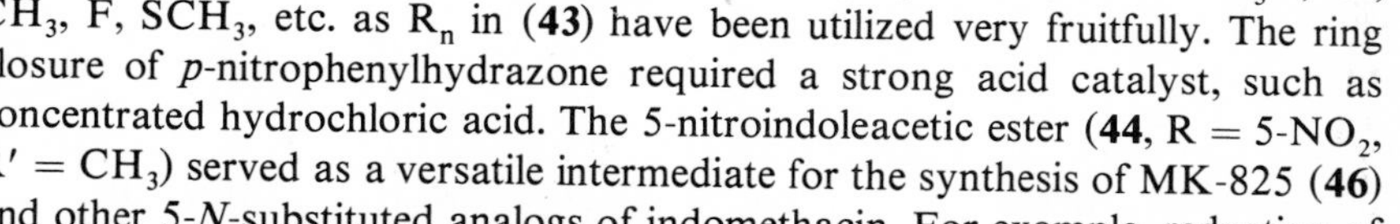

(43)   (44)

Various *para* and/or *meta* substituted phenylhydrazines with CH$_3$O, Cl, CH$_3$, F, SCH$_3$, etc. as R$_n$ in (**43**) have been utilized very fruitfully. The ring closure of *p*-nitrophenylhydrazone required a strong acid catalyst, such as concentrated hydrochloric acid. The 5-nitroindoleacetic ester (**44**, R = 5-NO$_2$, R' = CH$_3$) served as a versatile intermediate for the synthesis of MK-825 (**46**) and other 5-*N*-substituted analogs of indomethacin. For example, reduction of the 5-nitro group in **45** gave the 5-NH$_2$ analog, which was in turn converted to

the 5-CH$_3$CONH, CH$_3$N◯N-, (HOCH$_2$CH$_2$)$_2$N- and (ClCHCH$_2$)$_2$N-

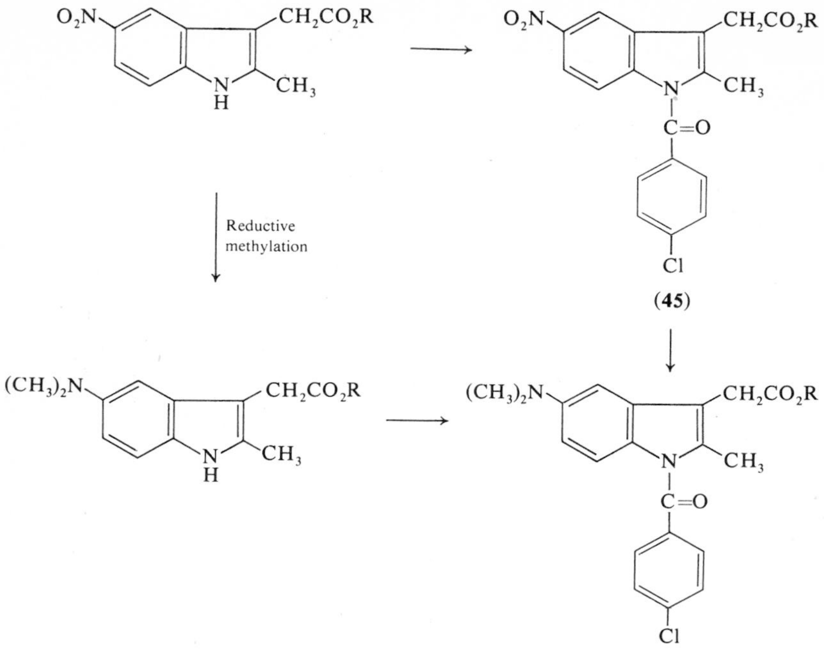

Reductive methylation

(45)

(46) MK-825   R = H

analogs. The last compound was synthesized as a potential alkylating agent with affinity for inflamed tissue. It might serve as an irreversible inhibitor of cyclooxygenase in the prostaglandin synthetase pathway.

The 5-cyano analog also showed good biological activity. Its reduction products, the 5-H_2NCH_2 and 5-$(CH_3)_2NCH_2$ derivatives were much less active.

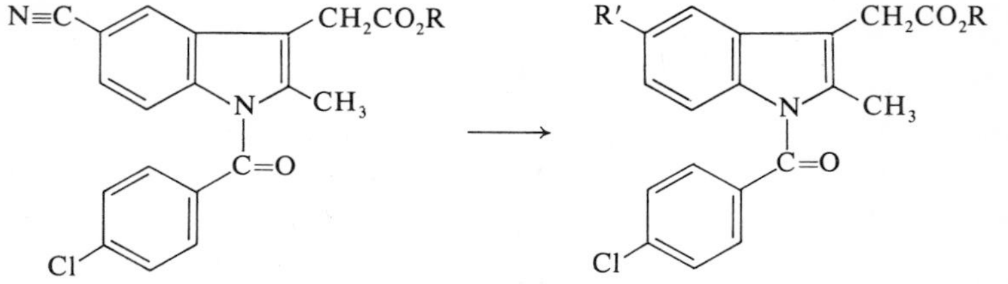

R = H; CH_3 R' = H_2NCH_2-; $(CH_3)_2NCH_2-$

The readily accessible α-ketoglutaric acid and substituted β-benzoyl-propionic acids also provided versatile indole intermediates when R' in **44** was CO_2H and substituted phenyl respectively. For instance, the 2-carboxylindoleacetic acid (47) was converted to the cyclic anhydride (48) and the ring was selectively opened to give a precursor (49) for 2-aminoindole (50) formation.

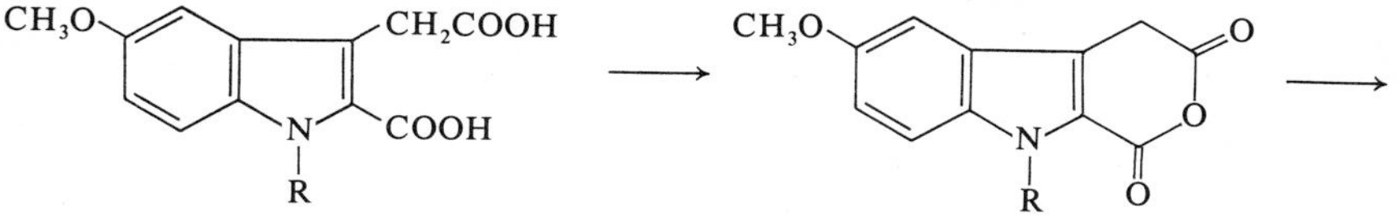

(47)   (48)

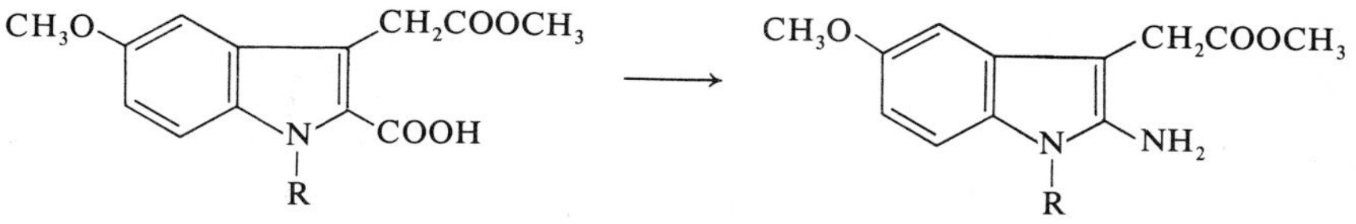

(49)   (50)

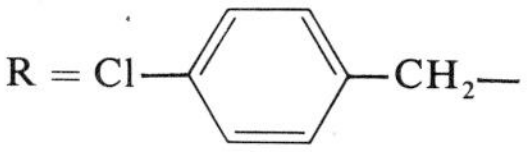

$$R = Cl-\!\!\!\left\langle\!\!\!\bigcirc\!\!\!\right\rangle\!\!\!-CH_2-$$

Another indole synthesis employed in this study was the Madelung reaction as illustrated by the preparation of 2-ethyl-5-methylindole (51). The side chain at C-3 was then added by the well-known gramine sequence via the 3-dimethyl-aminomethyl intermediate.

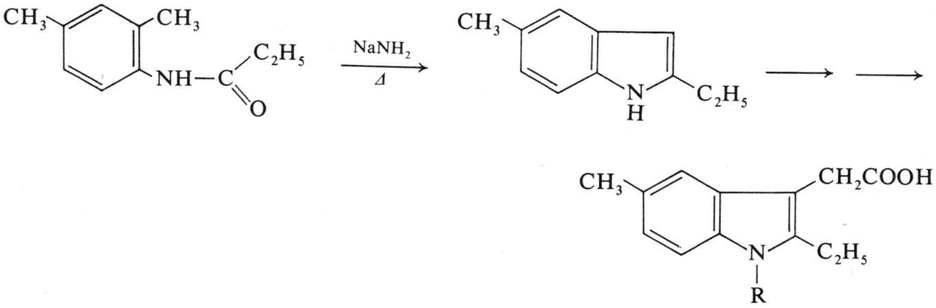

(51)

The synthesis of 51 and other 2-alkyl and 2-phenyl analogs has been described in considerable detail elsewhere (Walton et al., 1965). The 2-ethyl analog was nearly devoid of antiinflammatory activity but it was found to inhibit the growth of anaerobic bacteria and to have modest antitumor activity (Walton et al., 1965).

In the X-ray study of indomethacin, the phenyl ring in the N-p-chloro-benzoyl moiety is "cis" but not coplanar with the benzene ring in the indole nucleus (Kistenmacher and Marsh, 1972). Biphenyl analogs, such as the 7-phenylindoleacetic acids, were therefore investigated. The N-unsubstituted

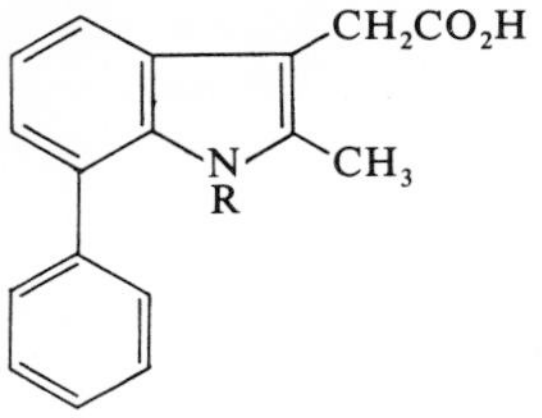

(52) R = H
(53) R = CH₃

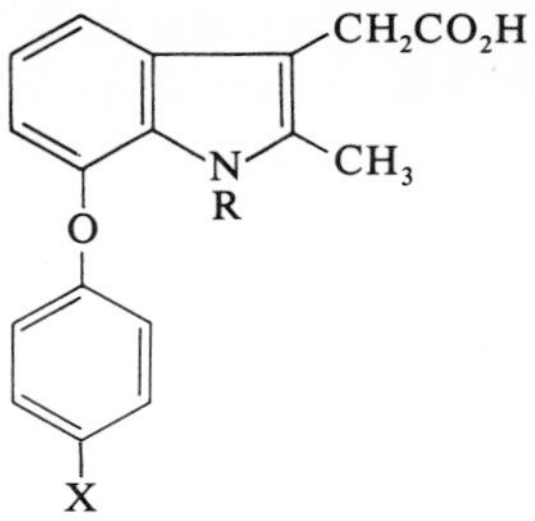

(54) X = H or Cl
      R = H or CH₃

analog (52) was comparable to phenylbutazone in the edema assay. The *N*-methyl homolog (53), having a greater degree of steric hindrance on the 7-phenyl substituent, was much less active. A small group of 7-phenoxy analogs (54) were also found to be weakly active only.

4.1.5 *Modification of the acetic acid side-chain*

In order to determine the optimal features of the acetic acid side chain, analogs with diverse stereochemistry and acidity were investigated.

Indoles bearing homologs of acetic acid, such as α-propionic, β-propionic and α-butyric at C-3 were readily obtained from the Fischer reaction using appropriate keto acid derivatives. With α,α-dimethyllevulinic acid the ring-closure was sterically hindered, giving only a small yield of the indole.

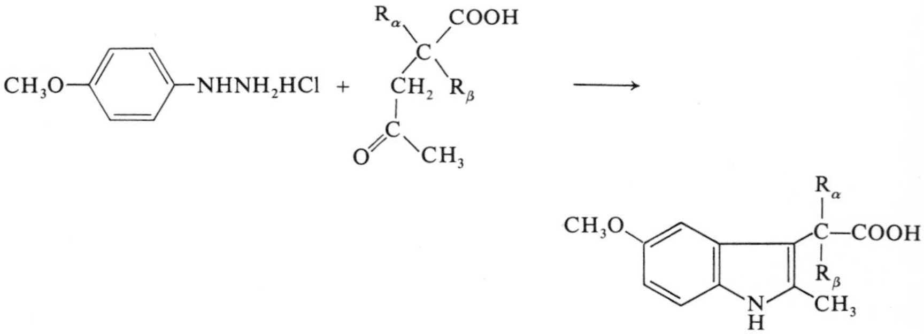

The Sumitomo process is also applicable to the synthesis of indomethacin analogs with a variety of alkanoic side-chains (H. Yamamoto and M. Nakao, U.S.P. 3 629 284) but no biological data on these homologs have been published.

Compared with phenylacetic acids, the α-methylene group in indole acetic acids is less reactive in base-catalyzed alkylation or acylation experiments.

Except in a few cases, direct alkylation or acylation at the α-position could be achieved only to a limited extent and under rather strenuous conditions. On the other hand, in the presence of sodium hydride or potassium t-butoxide, the enolate ion derived from a N-substituted 3-indolylacetic ester undergoes a condensation reaction with various active esters, such as formate, oxalate and trifluoroacetate, giving interesting and chelating intermediates bearing an α-carbonyl group (56).

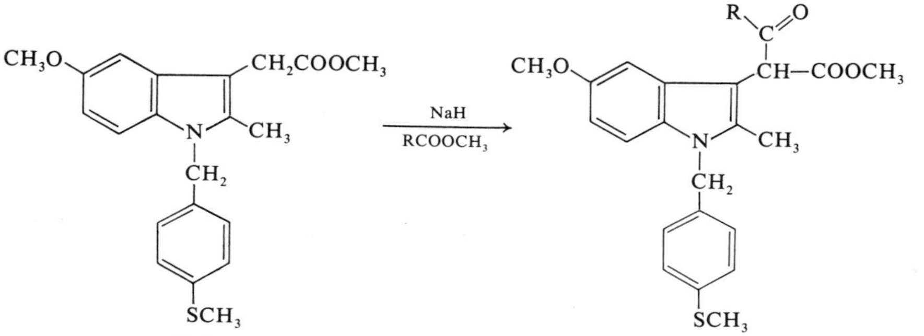

(55) $R = H; CF_3-; CH_3OOC-$ (56)

The 3-alkoxyoxalyl derivatives of indoles have been used extensively in the study of tryptamine derivatives (Heinzelman and Szmuszkovicz, 1963). In our studies, they also served as versatile intermediates for the synthesis of α-methylene (57), α-cyclopropylidene (58), α-amino (59) and α-acetoxy (61) analogs.

Due to the facile delocalization of electrons from the ring nitrogen at position-1 to C-3, an electronegative substituent at the α-position is a highly reactive as a leaving group. This is exemplified by the acid sensititivity of 3-indolylmethanol and by the facile polymerization of 3-indolylmethyl ethers (Henry and Leete, 1957) as well as by the nucleophilic substitution reactions of gramine. The delocalization of the electron pair on the indole nitrogen should be progressively minimized by N-alkylation and N-acylation, and this was demonstrated by derivative 61 with R = p-chlorobenzoyl. In contrast to analogs with a free NH group, the N-substituted 3-indolylmethanol (60) could be acetylated with acetic anhydride in pyridine to give the acetate as a stable derivative (61).

Among the α-substituents, an α-methyl group exhibited activity-enhancing properties for several active members of the series. The α-trifluoromethyl group was then given special attention because of its pronounced inductive effect resulting in an increased acidity of the weakly acidic side chain. In our first attempt to prepare this analog, a synthesis for α-trifluoromethyllevulinic acid was devised, but, unfortunately, repeated Fischer ring-closure experiments

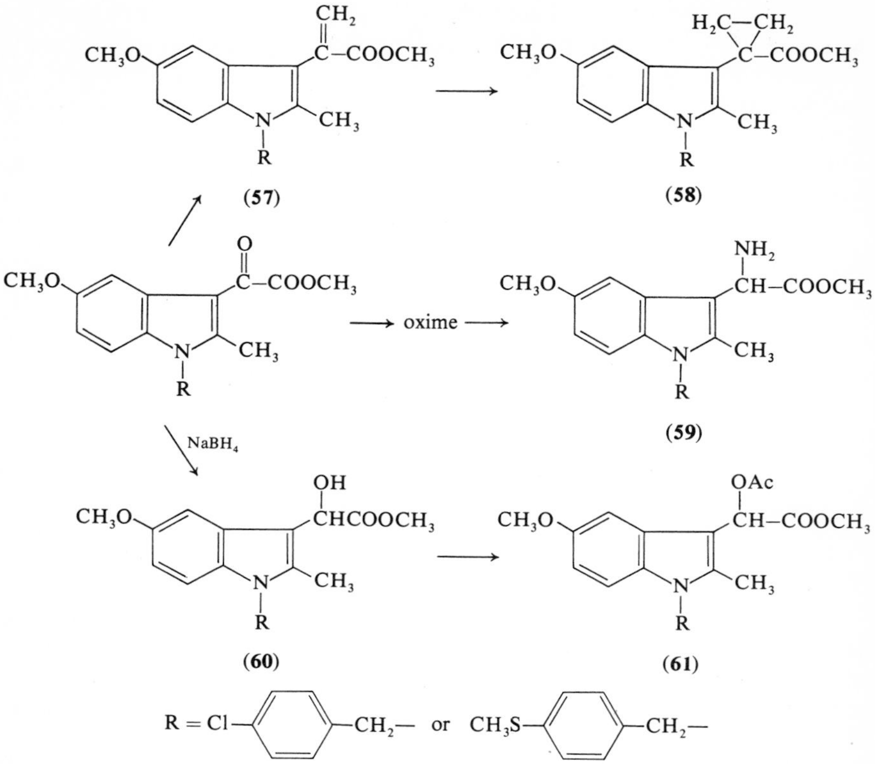

$$R = Cl-\!\!\left\langle\underset{}{\bigcirc}\right\rangle\!\!-CH_2-\quad \text{or}\quad CH_3S-\!\!\left\langle\underset{}{\bigcirc}\right\rangle\!\!-CH_2-$$

failed with this intermediate. Subsequently, taking advantage of the accessibility of 3-trifluoroacetylindoles, the desired compound (62) with an α-trifluoromethylacetic acid sidechain was constructed from the ketone via its glycidic ester. A multiple step sequence, carried out under mildly acidic or pyrolytic conditions, was necessitated by the tendency of the trifluoromethyl side chain to lose fluorine under hydrolytic conditions (Shen et al., 1962).

In the granuloma assay, the α-CF_3 derivative (62) was approximately $1\frac{1}{2}\times$ more active than the corresponding α-methyl analog.

To explore the effectiveness of various carboxyl equivalents, the gramine derivative was converted to the sulfonic (63) and phosphonic (64) analogs.

Other aliphatic side chains, known to be metabolizable to acetic acid in vivo, e.g. the aldehyde (65) (Glamkowski et al., 1973), alcohol (66) and amines (67) have also been synthesized for evaluation. Both the aldehyde (65) and its sodium bisulfite adduct (68) were almost half as active as indomethacin in the carrageenan edema assay.

The highly acidic tetrazole analogs were extensively studied by Bristol

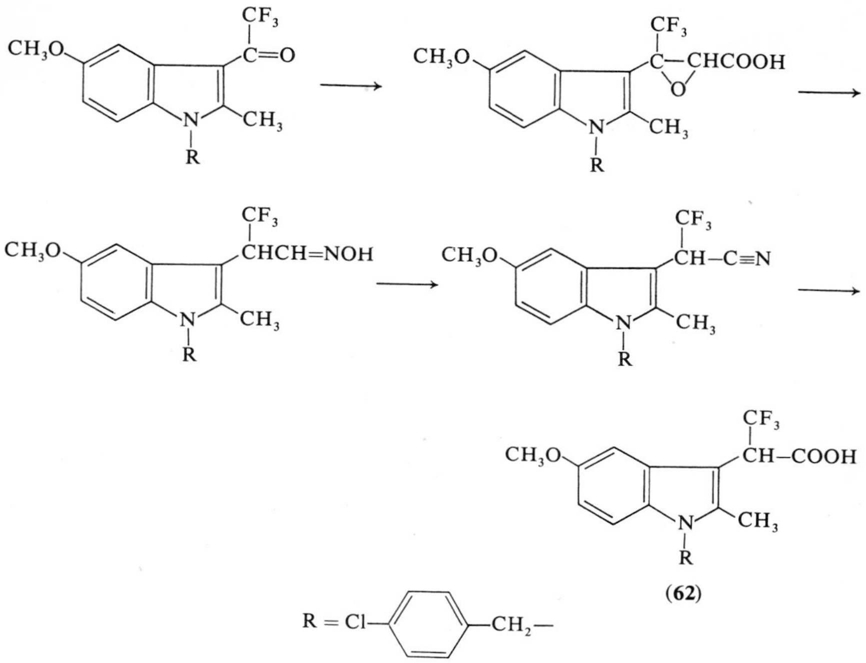

R = Cl—⟨benzene⟩—CH₂—

Laboratories (Juby and Hudyma, 1969). The structure–activity relationship in this series does not completely parallel with that of indole-3-acetic acids. The most active member, Intrazole (**69**, BL-R743), was one-sixteenth as potent as indomethacin in the carrageenan-induced rat paw edema test (Fleming *et al.*, 1969). It showed moderate clinical efficacy in rheumatoid arthritis and gouty patients (Roth and Englund, 1969; Steele and Phelps, 1971). Because of its longer serum half-life and platelet aggregation inhibitory activity it was also evaluated in man as a potential antithrombotic agent.

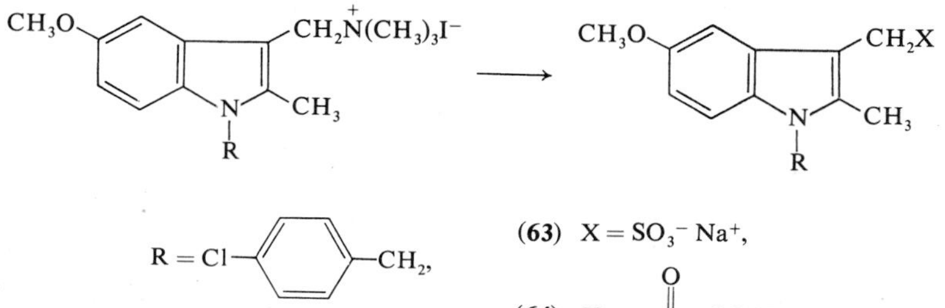

R = Cl—⟨benzene⟩—CH₂,

(**63**) X = SO_3^- Na^+,

(**64**) X = $-\overset{\overset{\displaystyle O}{\|}}{\underset{\underset{\displaystyle OH}{|}}{P}}-OC_2H_5$

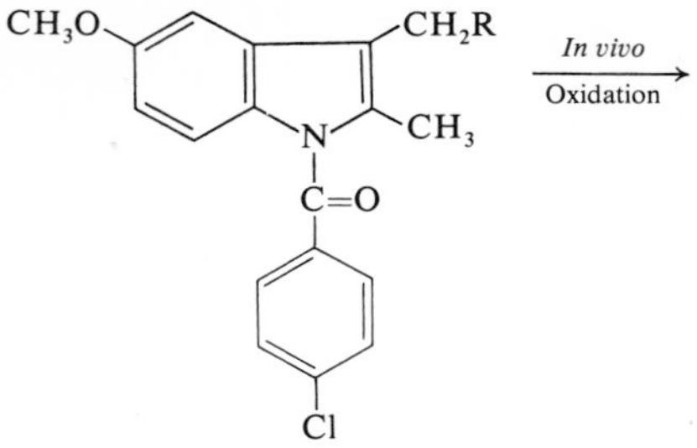

$$\xrightarrow[\text{Oxidation}]{\textit{In vivo}} \quad (1)$$

(65) R = CHO,

(66) R = CH$_2$OH,

(67) R = CH$_2$NH$_2$,

(68) R = CHSO$_3^-$ Na$^+$
        |
        OH

$$\xrightarrow[\text{NH}_4\text{Cl}]{\text{NaN}_3}$$

$$\xrightarrow[\text{ArCOCl}]{\text{2NaH}}$$

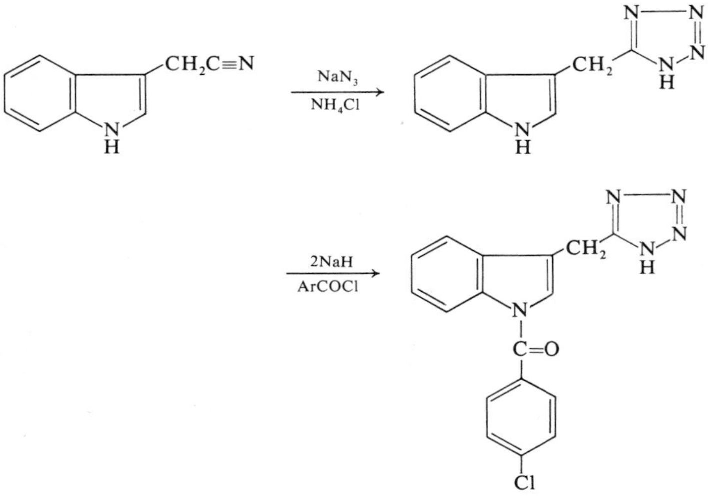

(69) Intrazole

The weakly acidic oximes (**70, 71**), enols (**72**) and sulfonamides (**73**) were also evaluated.

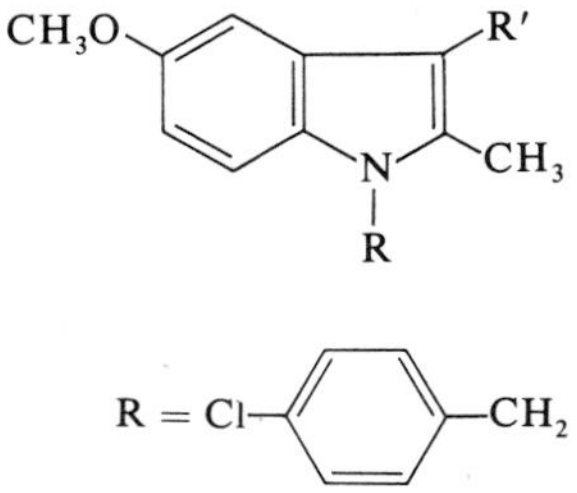

R = Cl—⟨ ⟩—CH$_2$

(70) R′ = —CH=NOH,

        CF$_3$
        |
(71) —C=NOH,

(72) —CH=C—CH$_3$,
        |
        OH

(73) —CH$_2$—CH$_2$NHSO$_2$CH$_3$

In general, these carboxyl equivalents, with varying degrees of acidity, were much less active in the antiinflammatory tests than were the corresponding acetic acids.

During these studies, 5-methoxy-2-methylindole (**74**) proved to be a versatile intermediate for structural modification at C-3. It could be readily prepared by the Nenitzescu reaction in fair yield (Nenitzescu, 1929).

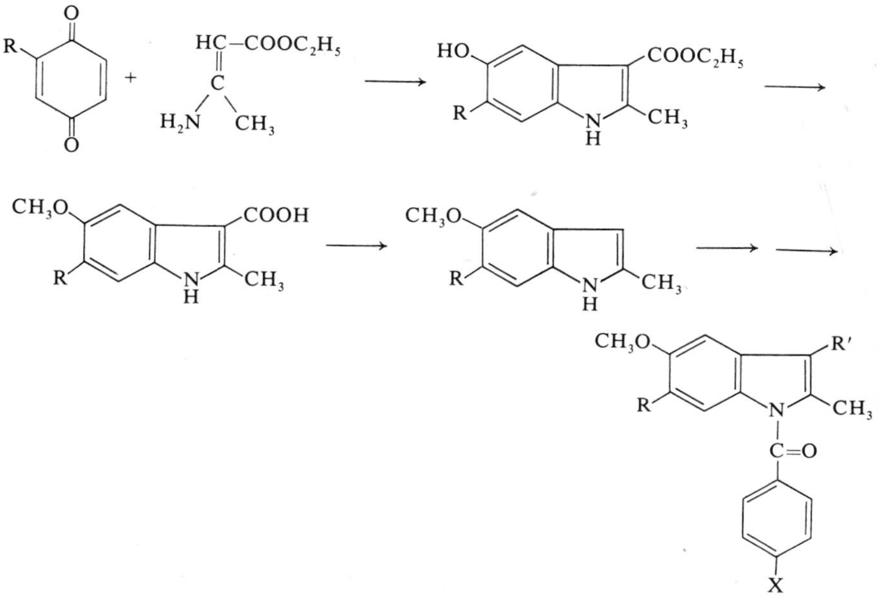

(**74**) R = H

The scope and the mechanism of this reaction have been studied very thoroughly in connection with the synthesis of mitomycin analogs. Starting with a 2-alkylated quinone, the corresponding 6-alkyl-5-methoxyindole was formed together with a minute amount of the 7-alkyl isomer (Allen *et al.*, 1966).

4.1.6   Position isomers

In our laboratory both the indolyl-1-acetic acid (**75**) and 2-acetic acid (**76**) analogs were found to be much less active than the corresponding indolyl-3-acetic acids.

The 3-benzoyl group was introduced by acylation of the Grignard derivative of 5-methoxy-2-methylindole (**74**). 3-Aroylindoles are fairly acidic and readily form sodio derivatives with sodium hydride. Alkylation with α-halo acetate followed by alkaline hydrolysis gave the position isomer of indomethacin (**75**). The 3-(*p*-CF$_3$ benzoyl) analog was prepared similarly.

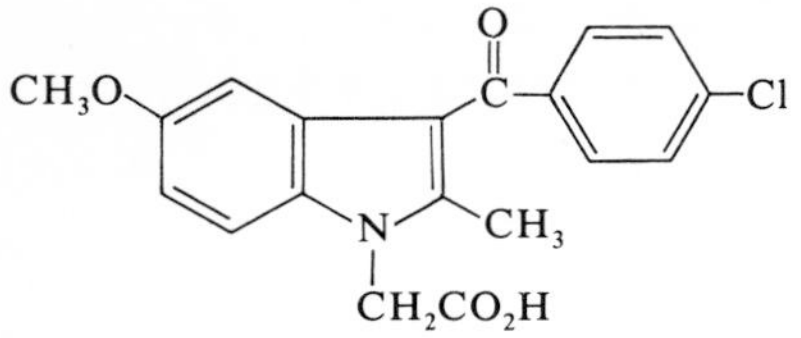

(75)

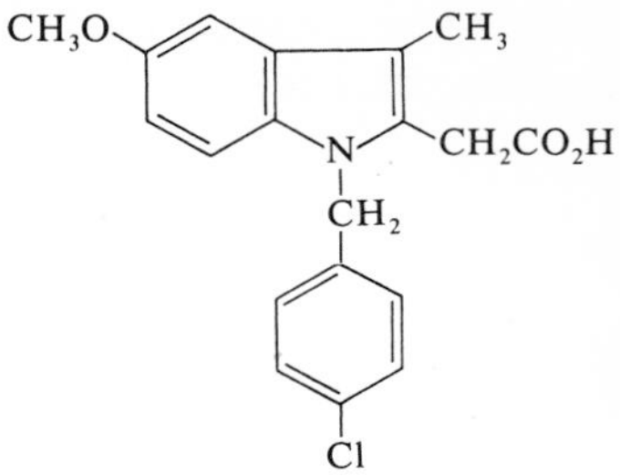

(76)

The 1-acetic acid series was also studied in the Geigy laboratory (Doebel, 1972). Both the 5-methoxy and the 6-methoxy (77) isomers were found to be inactive in the UV erythema and carrageenan edema assays. An homolog (78) was active at 100 mg kg^{-1}.

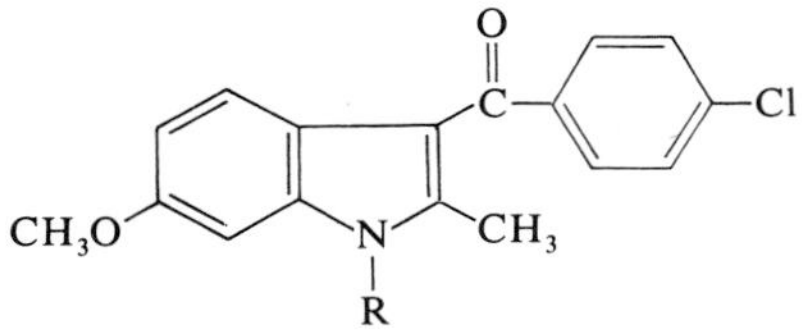

(77) R = CH$_2$CO$_2$H

(78) R = CH$_2$—CHCO$_2$H
             |
            CH$_3$

Very recently an extensive study of 3-aroyl indole-1-acetic acid analogs was reported by the Roussel-Uclaf laboratory (Allais *et al.*, 1975). The 6-methoxy analog (77, RU 3959) was found to have moderate antiinflammatory activity (1/20 × indomethacin) but with a moderately enhanced analgesia (1/10 × indomethacin) and less g.i. irritation. The clinical data on RU 3959 have not been published. The 6-Cl analog (RU 4452) is more potent (1/6 × indomethacin) in the antiinflammatory assay. In this study, 6-substituted-2-methylindoles were used as key intermediates.

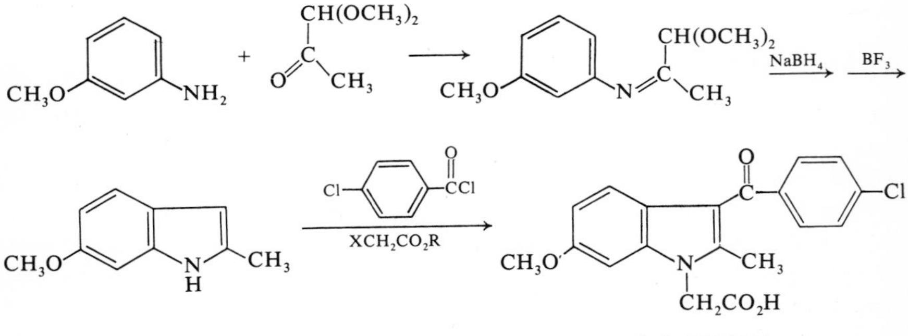

(77) RU 3959

4.1.7   Analogs with restricted configuration

It can be readily shown in a molecular model of indomethacin that both the flexible acetic acid side-chain and the N-p-chlorobenzoyl group retain some degree of freedom of rotation, even though a considerable amount of steric hindrance is imposed upon them by the 2-methyl group. An optimal conformation of this nonplanar molecule based on physical chemical studies will be discussed later. In addition to the flexible molecules, several analogs with specific configurations fixed by covalent bonds were synthesized and evaluated.

The p-chlorobenzoyl group in indomethacin is free to assume a conformation "cis" to either the benzenoid moiety of the indole nucleus of the 2-methyl group, but co-planarity with the indole ring is apparently inhibited. Nevertheless, a coplanar and highly conjugated isomer is easily obtained by the photochemical cyclization (79) of the o-iodo analog (78).

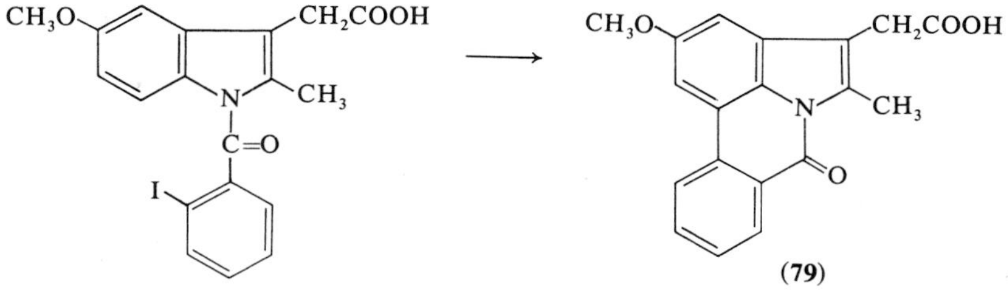

(78)   (79)

This class of compounds was independently studied later by Olson et al. (1974), but no significant antiinflammatory activity was found. The cyclized 2-keto analog (80) was also inactive. These results led to the conclusion that the coplanary and fully aromatic systems in 79 and 80 are considerably different, both sterically and electronically, from the optimal structural requirements for indomethacin analogs.

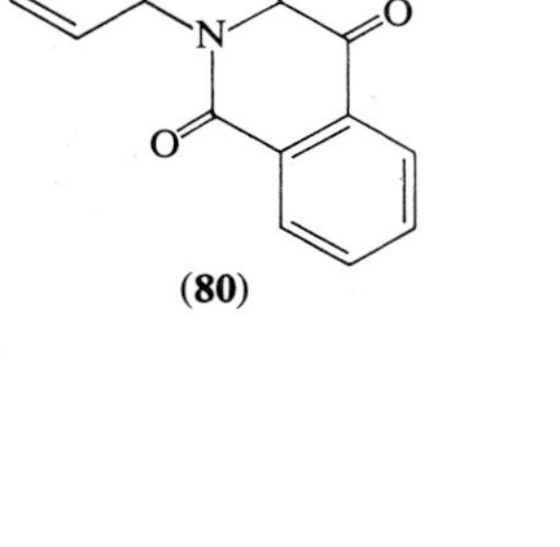

(80)

Attempts were also made to fix the spatial arrangement of the carboxyl group by cyclization of the side chains. The tetrahydrocarbazole analog (81) turned out to be essentially devoid of antiinflammatory activity.

(81) R = Cl—⟨ ⟩—CH$_2$

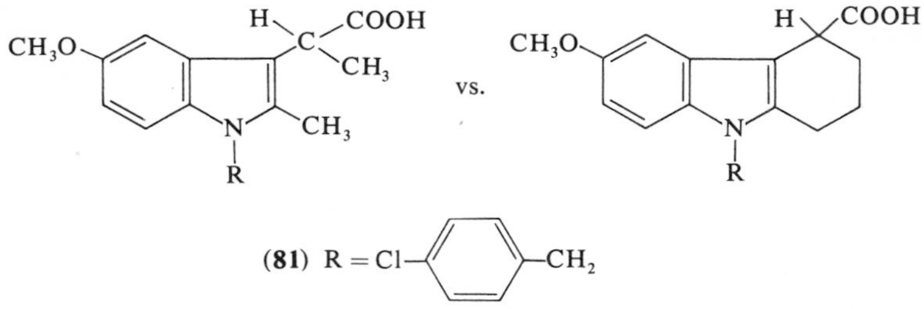

Another group of novel cyclic analogs was reported recently. Expansion of the 2,3-double bond in indomethacin to a cyclopropane ring markedly reduces antiinflammatory activity (Welstead *et al.*, 1974).

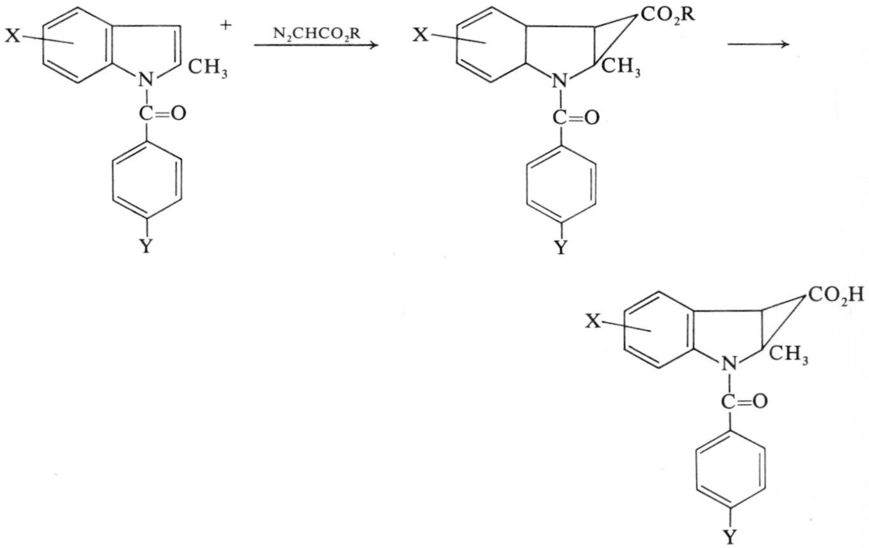

Interestingly, the exo 2-(*p*-chlorobenzoyl)-5-methoxy-1*a*-methyl-1,1*a*,2,6*b*-tetrahydrocycloprop[*b*]indole-1-carboxylic acid (82), upon melting, rearranges to indomethacin (1) in almost quantitative yield. As some C-2-modifications are not readily introduced by the conventional synthetic methods for indoleacetic acids, this indirect approach may provide a convenient alternative.

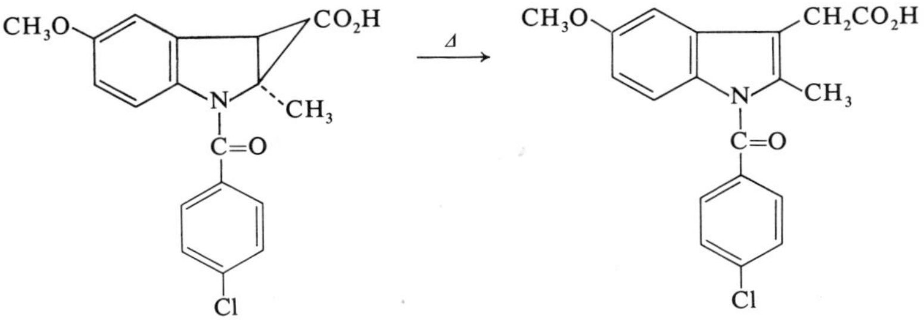

(82)   (1)

The lack of potency of these cyclopropyl analogs is consistent with our earlier observation that the 2,3-dihydro analog of indomethacin obtained from catalytic hydrogenation with platinum in acetic acid (B. E. Witzel, unpublished) and other analogs (e.g. **83** and **84**) are much less active. The structure–activity relationship in the dihydro series also appeared to be less well defined.

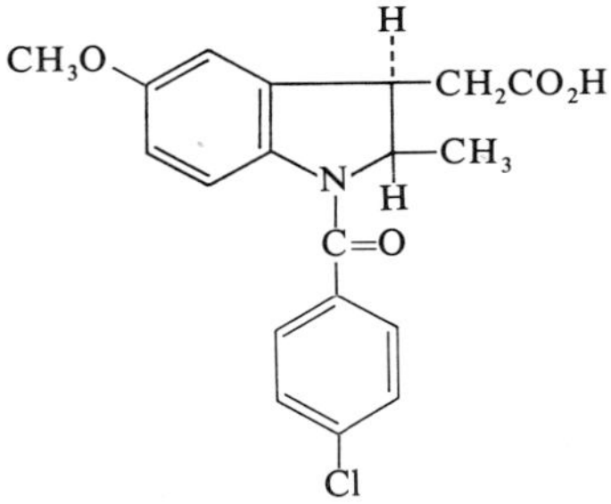

(83) 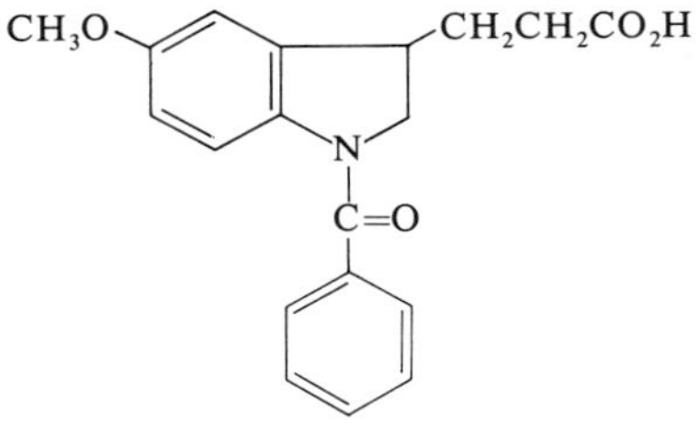   (84)

4.1.8 Synthesis of heteroaryl isosteres

As part of the comprehensive structure–activity relationship studies, a number of bicyclic ring-systems isosteric with indole were explored. Among these, the carbocyclic indene analogs with biological activity comparable to their indole isosteres were particularly noteworthy. The synthetic study leading to the discovery of sulindac (**2**) will be discussed in detail in the next section (4.2). Examples of heterocyclic isosteres studied include derivatives of benzimidazole (**85, 86, 87, 88**), benzimidazolone (**89**), phthalimidine (**90**), indazole (**91**), etc. Typical structural features are indicated by the following formulae:

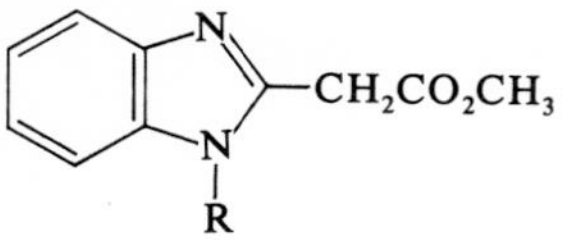

(86)

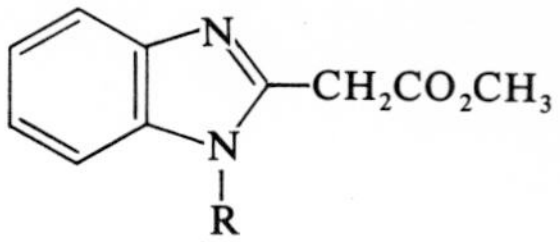

(85)

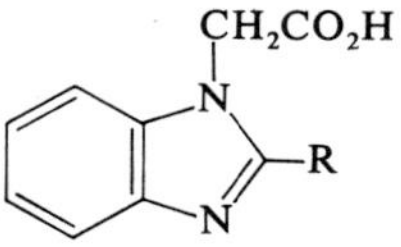

(87)

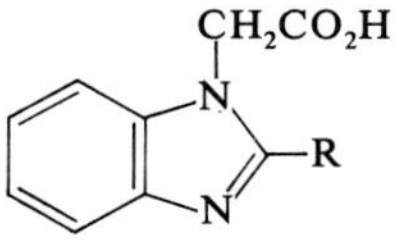

(88)

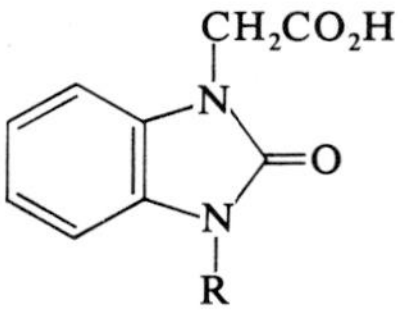

(89)

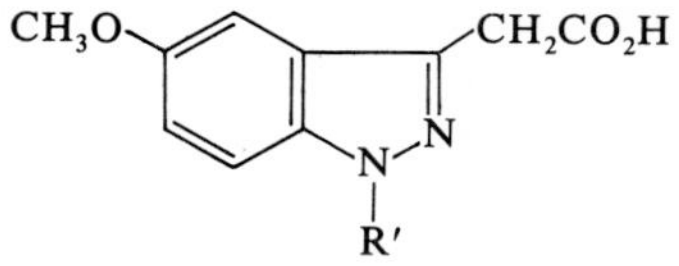

(91)

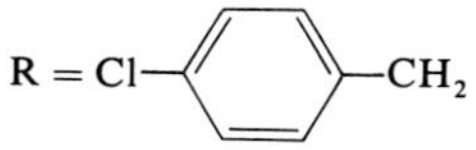

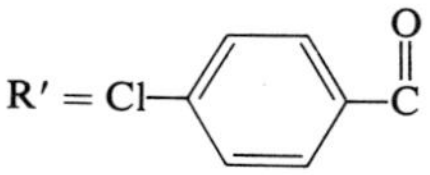

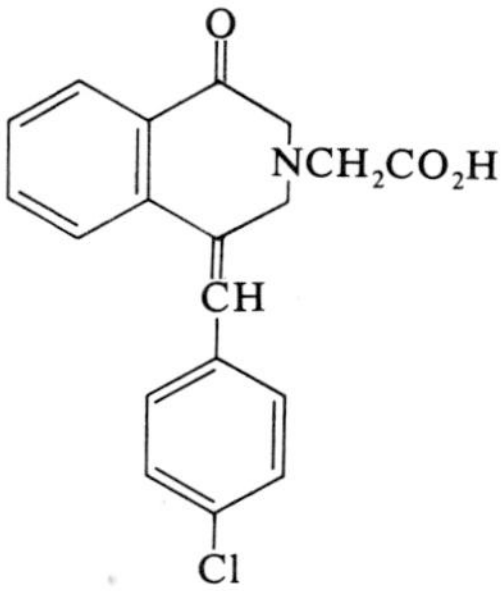

$R = Cl-\langle\rangle-CH_2$

$R' = Cl-\langle\rangle-\overset{O}{\underset{}{C}}$

(90)

The acetic acid analog (93) of the analgesic indazole, benzydamine (92), possesses a similar stereochemical arrangement as the 1-benzylindoleacetic acids, but it is only weakly active in antiinflammatory assays.

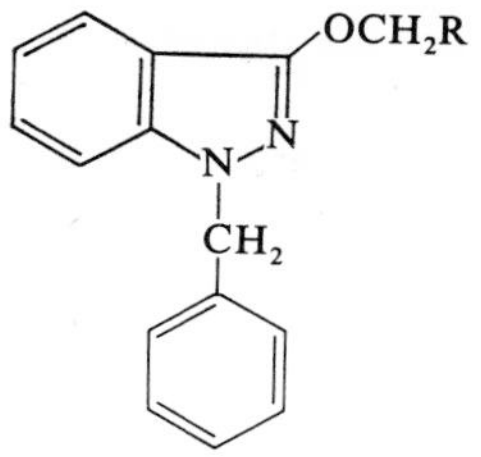

(92) R = CH_2CH_2N(CH_3)_2
(93) R = CO_2H, (benzydamine)

Both indolizine analogs (94, 95) were reported to be about 0·2 times the potency of indomethacin in the carrageenan edema assay (Casagrande *et al.*, 1971).

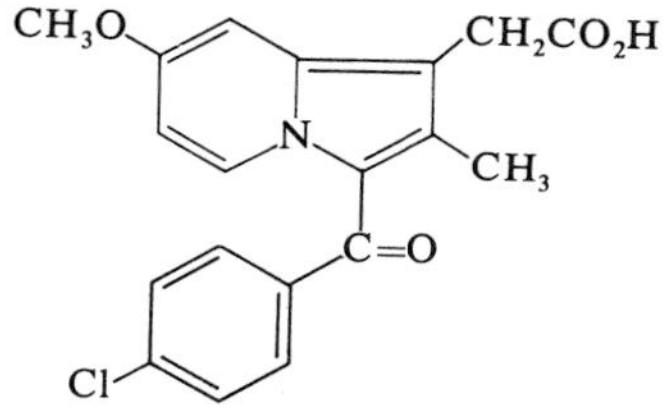

(94)

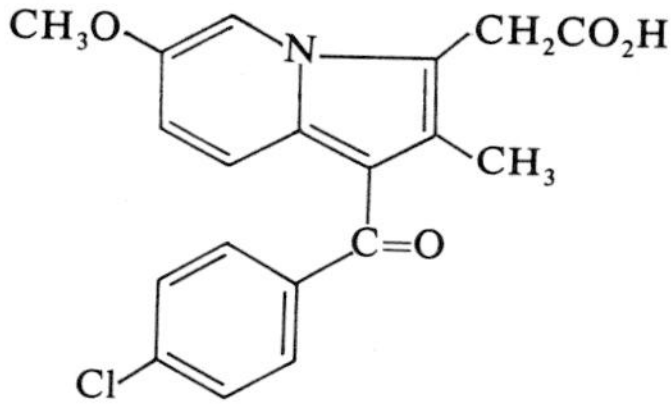

(95)

Most of the above heteroaryl isosteres were disappointing as candidates for extensive clinical developments. A group of pyrroleacetic acids, originally modeled after indomethacin but also bearing some structural features of potent phenylacetic acids, were investigated by Carson and Wong (1971). 5-Benzoyl-1-methyl-2-pyrroleacetic acid (96) (Tolmetin®) is about 0·4 times the potency of indomethacin in the carrageenan edema assay and about 0·14 times in the cotton pellet granuloma assay. It has been approved in the USA for the treatment of rheumatoid arthritis at 0·6–1·8 g d⁻¹.

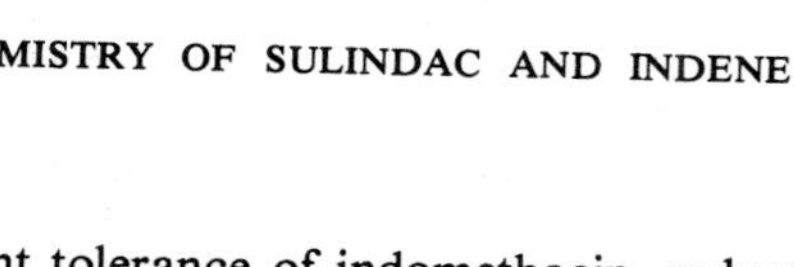

(Tolmetin®) (96)

4.2 SYNTHETIC CHEMISTRY OF SULINDAC AND INDENE DERIVATIVES

4.2.1 MK-715

To improve the patient tolerance of indomethacin, reduction of g.i. irritation and CNS effects are obvious goals. The g.i. side effect is readily measurable in acute or subacute animal models. However, the transient headache and some idiosyncratic reaction to indomethacin in certain patients are much more difficult to understand. In the absence of any biological rationale or laboratory models, it was hoped that a new analog without the indole nucleus might have less CNS effect in man.

In medicinal chemistry, a benzylidene indene molecule may be considered to be electronically isosteric with an *N*-acylindole. Molecular model studies also suggest much configurational similarity between the two molecules. After our initial study of the indene analogs was completed, this concept of isosterism was reaffirmed by the biological activity of the indene analogs of tryptamines (Winter and Gessner, 1968) by the X-ray studies of MK-715 (**97**) (Hoogsteen and Trenner, 1970) and indomethacin (Kistenmacher and Marsh, 1972), by the extrinsic Cotton effect in binding to serum albumin (Shen, 1972) and, most recently, by a CNDO/2 calculation (Gund and Shen, 1977). These will be discussed in greater detail later.

At the onset, the indene analog of indomethacin (**97**, MK-715) was synthesized by the following route (Shen *et al.*, 1967). Two geometrical isomers are formed with the *cis* isomer predominating.

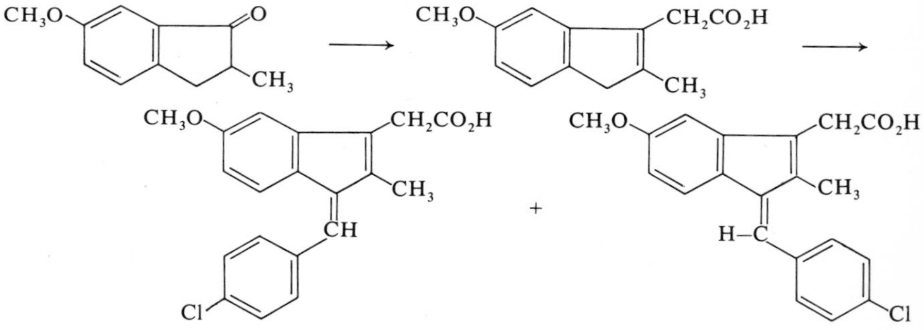

(**97**)	(**98**)
MK-715 (*cis*)	(*trans*)

The *cis* isomer (**97**) is five times more potent than the *trans* isomer (**98**) in the carrageenan-edema assay. Its overall efficacy was about $\frac{1}{4}$–$\frac{1}{2}$ as potent as indomethacin in several animal models as well as in a preliminary clinical study. At 200–400 mg d^{-1}, some antiarthritic activities were evident in a small group of patients. MK-715 appeared to be less irritating to the gastrointestinal tract and was free of any CNS symptoms. However, it was soon observed that crystalluria occurred at the higher dose levels (Sarett, 1971). The fine yellow crystalline precipitate in the urine was identified as MK-715 and its glucuronide (**99**) (Hucker, unpublished). Glucuronide metabolites are usually much more soluble in water than parent drugs. This is true for indomethacin (4·5 mg ml^{-1}) and its glucuronide (very soluble) but not for MK-715. Both MK-715 and its acylglucuronide are very poorly soluble (*c.* 0·04 mg ml^{-1}) in water.

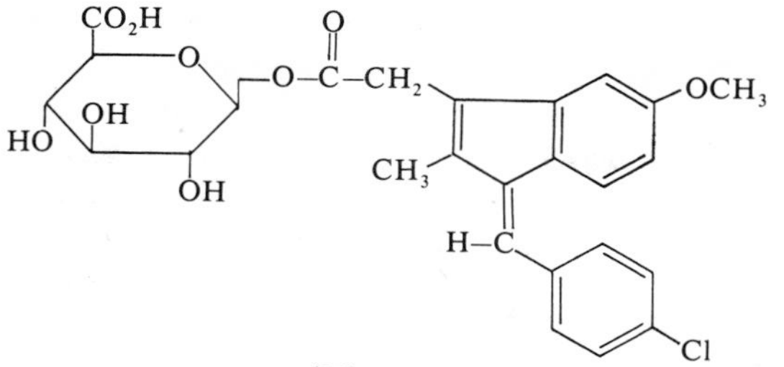

(99)

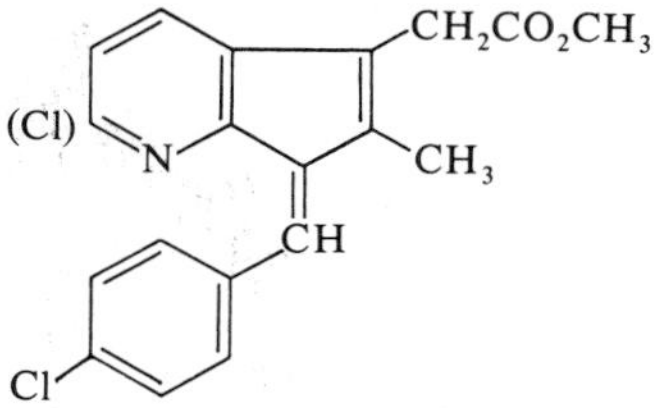

(100)

4.2.2 Sulindac and related compounds

In order to circumvent this problem, a synthetic effort was initiated to discover a more soluble and more potent congener. Several conventional approaches, e.g. introduction of hydrophilic substituents, and reduction of the rigidity of the molecule were examined. However, none of them met the required solubility enhancement. Some typical examples are shown below and most are much less potent than MK-715.

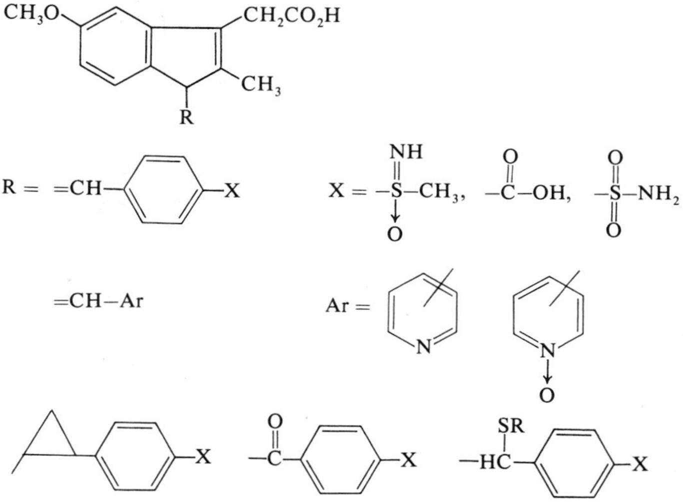

Several 7-aza analogs (**100**) were also synthesized for comparison. Being substituted 1,7-H-pyrinidine acetic esters, they were obtained only after the completion of a sequence of complex reactions (Greenwald and Shen, 1970). Some increase in aqueous solubility was realized but, as a group, they are much less active biologically than the corresponding indene congeners.

The most fruitful search was based on the characteristics of a p-methylsulfinyl substituent. Our study of indomethacin analogs has shown that a p-methylsulfinyl substituent is comparable to p-chloro in potency enhancement. In an earlier attempt to correlate physicochemical parameters with bio activities, it was noted that the *para*-methylsulfinyl group was capable of increasing the solubility of this class of compounds 10-fold and the water/lipid distribution coefficient almost 100-fold (Shen, 1967) (Table 19).

TABLE 19

Solubility-enhancing effect of a sulfinyl group

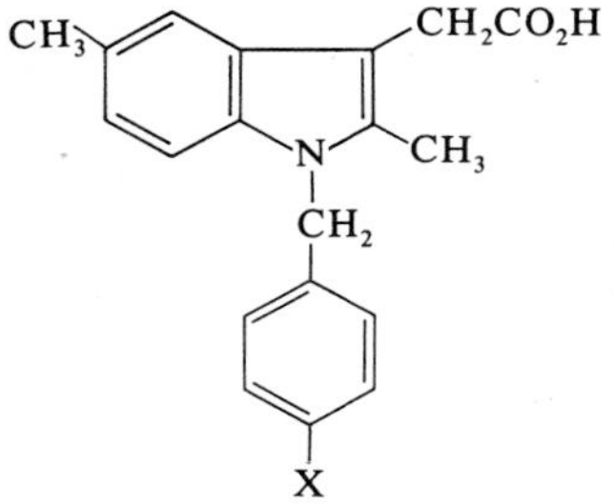

X	Solubility	$P_{(H_2O/Octanol)}$
Cl	0·4 mg ml^{-1}	0·010
SCH$_3$	0·3	0·016
SCH$_3$ ↓ O	4·1	0·94

Finally, it is well known that a p-methylsulfinyl group is readily oxidized *in vivo* by monooxygenases such as the liver microsomal cytochrome P450 to the sulfone and, to a lesser extent, the sulfonic acid. It is reversibly convertible to the sulfide, which in turn can be demethylated to the sulfhydryl derivative. The estimated solubility and antiinflammatory activity of these potential metabolites of an analog of MK-715 are indicated above. The formation of multiple metabolites not only minimizes the accumulation of any single metabolite beyond its solubility in the body, but, in this case, also results in an interesting pharmacokinetic pattern as discussed below. The p-methylsulfinyl analog of

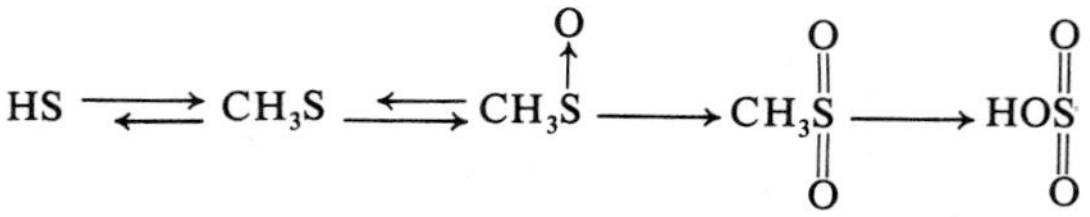

Activity	++	++	++	+	−
Solubility	+	−	++	+	+++

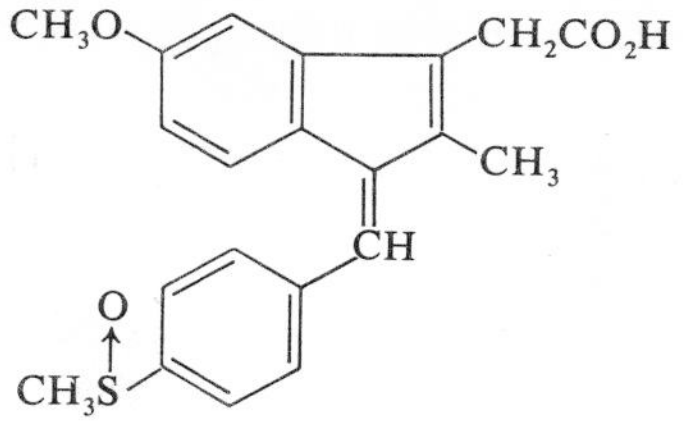

(101)

MK-715 (101) was first synthesized to verify these considerations. Indeed, the solubility was much improved from 0·04 mg ml^{-1} to 0·7 mg ml^{-1}, an almost 20-fold increase. However, the potency is slightly lower, c. 0·7×, than MK-715. Taking advantage of our previous structure–activity relationship concept of this type of compounds, a group of ring-fluorinated analogs was investigated next. The procedure used is exemplified by the preparation of sulindac (2) and its sulfide metabolite (102). The structure assignment of geometrical isomers relied primarily on NMR anisotropy. A consistent shift of the 2-methyl peak from 7·8τ (cis) to 8·1τ (trans) was observed in all cases (Table 20). Since the configuration of MK-715 was unequivocally established by its X-ray

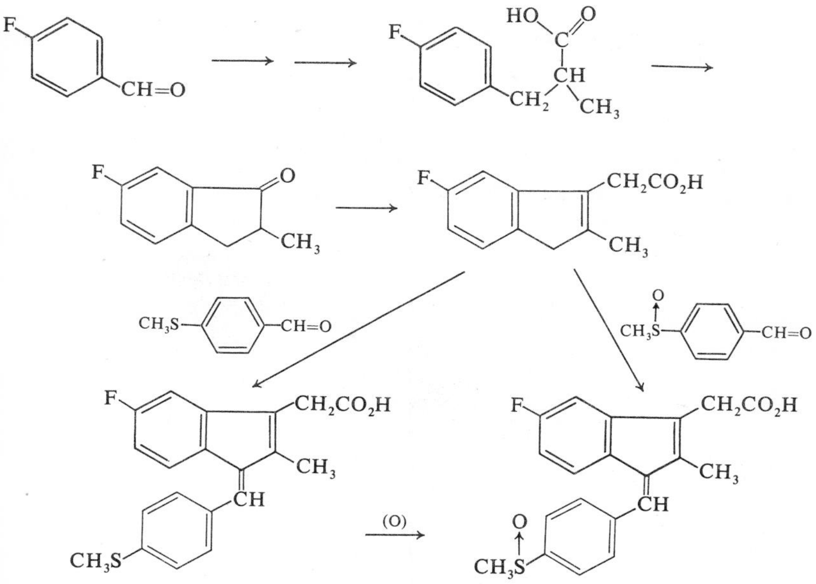

(102)   (2)

crystallography, the configuration of other geometrical isomers were assigned by correlation with MK-715 isomers. With 5-F, 5,6-diF and 6-F-5-CH$_3$O analogs, the *cis* isomers are formed predominantly in the aldehyde condensation step. However, in the presence of a 7-substituent, e.g. in the case of the 5,7-diF analog, the *trans* isomer is formed as the major product. The steric hindrance introduced by a 7-F group reversed the ratio of *trans/cis* isomers to 3.

TABLE 20

Structural assignment of geometric isomers by nmr anisotropy—Chemical shift of 2-CH$_3$

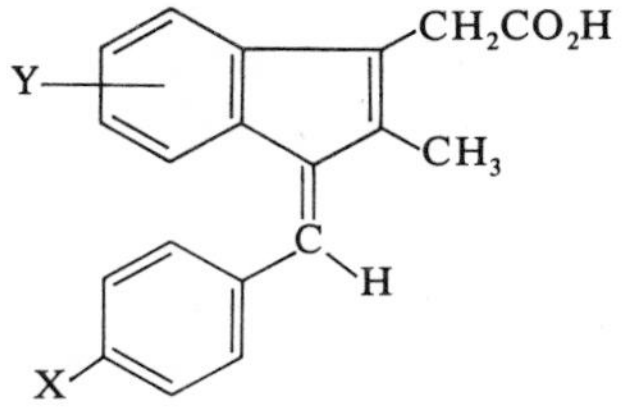

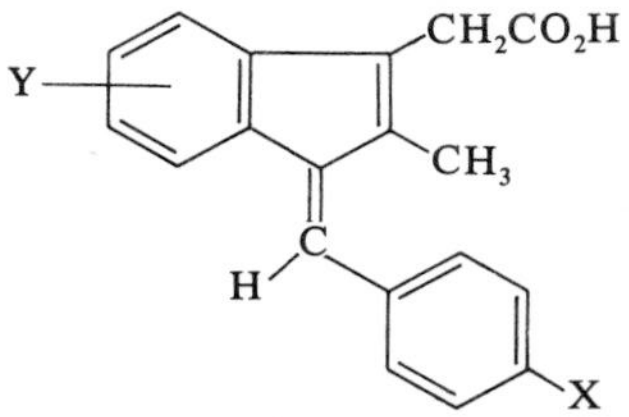

Y	X	*cis*	*trans*
5-CH$_3$O	Cl	7·8τ^a	8·1τ
5,7-diF	CH$_3$S, CH$_3$S → O	7·8	8·1
5-F	CH$_3$S → O	7·8	

^{a} Configuration established by X-ray crystallography.

The α-methyl homologs (**103**) of **2** and its sulfide metabolite were also synthesized in a similar manner. The *exo*-double bond isomers **104** (Y = F, X = CH$_3$S→O or CH$_3$S) were not detected in the above reaction sequence for **2**, but they have been synthesized by a different route (Shuman *et al.*, 1977) and found to be much less active in antiinflammatory assays. They rearrange readily to **2** and its sulfide metabolites, respectively, under mildly acidic conditions.

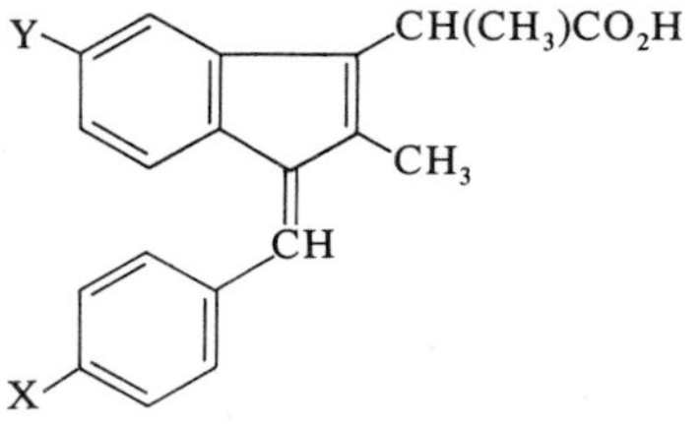

(103) 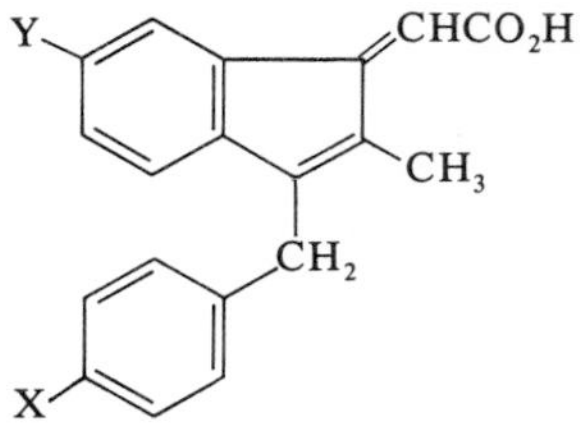   (104)

Among the more potent indene acetic acid analogs synthesized are 5-Cl, 5-F, 6-F, 5,6-diF and 6-F-5MeO. Their antiinflammatory-analgesic activities are either comparable to or better than indomethacin. On the whole, they are less irritating to the g.i. tract in acute assays. After substantial subacute safety evaluations, the 5-F analog appeared to have the optimal combination of efficacy and safety.

The methylsulfinyl group is tetrahedral in configuration and therefore asymmetric. The racemic mixture of the 5-F analog was resolved with (+)- and (−)-2-phenethylamine into two stable optical enantiomers with rotation of $[\alpha]_D^{27}$ (methanol) $+22\cdot6°$ and $-21\cdot2°$, respectively. Within the experimental error of animal assays, both isomers are comparable in biological activities. Presumably, both isomers are in equilibrium with the active sulfide metabolite *in vivo*. Consequently, the racemic mixture, analogous to sulfinpyrazone, is used as sulindac for clinical evaluation. Its pharmacological characteristics are described in detail in section 3 above. Sulindac is a yellow crystalline compound, m.p. 184–186°, with a pK_a of $5\cdot8 \pm 0\cdot5$. Its solubility in water at pH 6 is $0\cdot45$ mg ml^{-1}. It has a distribution coefficient $K_{(Octanol/H_2O)}$, $1\cdot52$ at pH $7\cdot2$. It absorbs uv strongly at λ_{max} 3270, 2850, 2580 (shoulder) and 2270 nm with A per cent 367, 417, 405 and 538 respectively.

To make certain that we had resolved the crystalluria problem in the laboratory, the potential metabolites of sulindac were synthesized for solubility determination in human urine. These studies are described in section 6.

5   Structure–activity relationship

In the course of our study of indomethacin, sulindac and related compounds, a total of 500 indole and indene derivatives and related structures were evaluated. In retrospect, the synthetic study followed many general principles often practiced in medicinal chemistry. Some of these were applied with success but many others were inexplicably disappointing.

In analyzing the structure–activity relationship, attempts were made at different times to correlate the physicochemical properties, e.g. pK, π, σ, etc. with inhibitory data in the cotton-pellet granuloma or carrageenan foot-edema assays. But no simple or significant correlations were obtained so far. Variation of the *in vivo* data was one major complicating factor. On the other hand, the *in vivo* data were consistent enough to establish certain prominent features in the structure–activity relationships, which appeared to be generally valid for all three major groups we studied, the *N*-benzyl- and *N*-benzoylindoles and the indene isosteres. The more potent compounds usually gave good dose–response curves in comparative studies. Thus, the identification of six clinical candidates in this series was able to follow a logical and progressive pattern.

The structures of six clinical candidates are shown below.

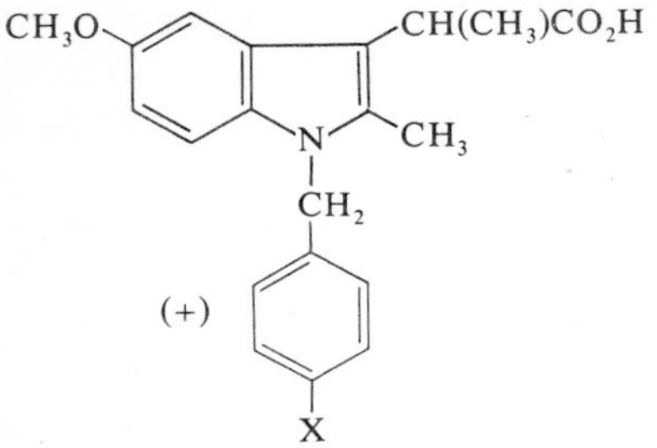

(1) MK-555 X = Cl

(2) MK-410 X = SCH$_3$

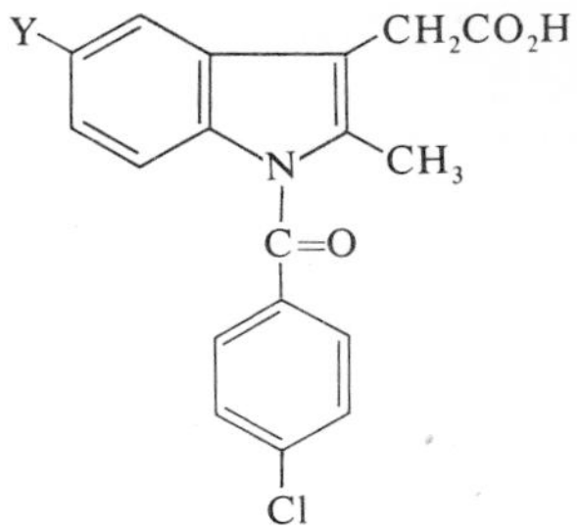

(3) MK-615 Y = (CH$_3$O)
　　　(Indomethacin)
(4) MK-825 Y = (CH$_3$)$_2$N

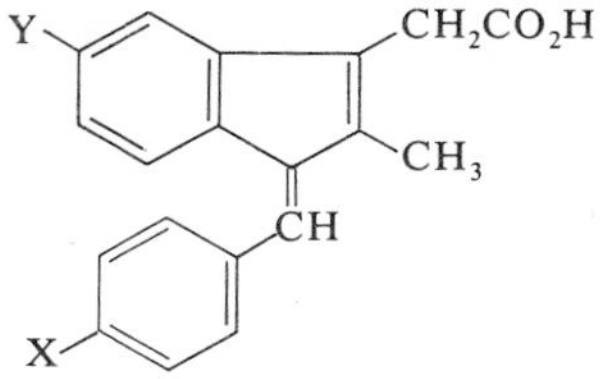

(5) MK-715 Y = CH$_3$O, X = Cl
(6) MK-231 Y = F, X = CH$_3$S→O
　　　(Sulindac)

Some medicinal chemical considerations involved in our comprehensive synthetic studies are outlined below.

i *Lead definition.* The process of selecting substituted indole acetic acid among a group of indole amides and amines as our lead is described in section 2. Suffice it to mention that the evaluation of various related indoles was much facilitated by the availability of indoles prepared previously in our laboratories for the serotonin antagonist program and the structure–activity relationship obtained therefrom.

The substituents which converted tryptamine to serotonin antagonists like bas (**105**), e.g. N-PhCH$_2$ > N-alkyl > NH; 2-CH$_3$ > 2H; 5-CH$_3$O, Me$_2$N, CH$_3$ > 5-H, also increased antiinflammatory activity almost in a parallel fashion when they were introduced to indole-3-acetic acid.

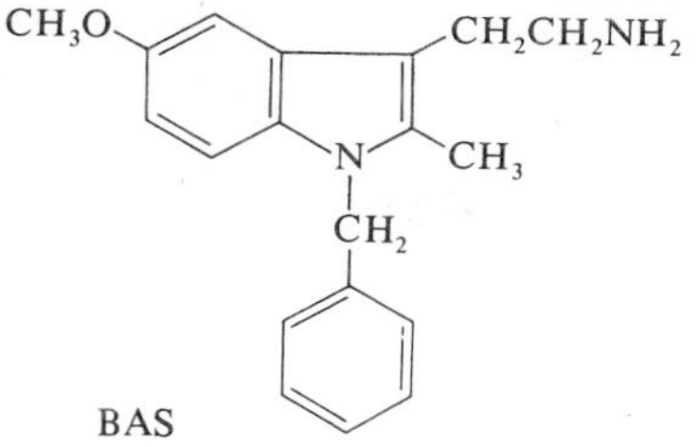

BAS (105)

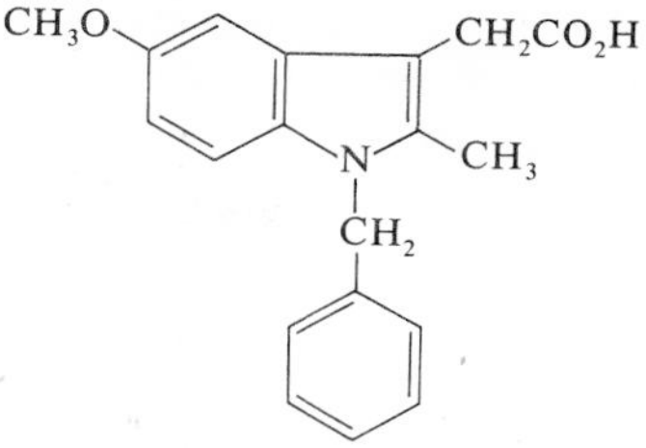

(8)

ii   *Model compounds.* As described earlier, *N*-alkylation and *N*-acylation of substituted indole-3-acetic acids often require protection of the carboxyl group first. Fortunately a consistent correlation of the potency of methyl esters with their corresponding free acids was observed early. The methyl esters are generally half as active as the free acid. The ethyl esters, for reasons unknown, gave irregular responses in rat assays. Using methyl esters as prototypes in our structure–activity relationship studies greatly simplified the task of chemical synthesis.

iii   *Minimum systematic structure modifications.* The lead has two aromatic moieties, an indole ring and a phenyl ring. In the late 1950s an attempt was made in our laboratories (Sarett, 1957, unpublished) to use three substituents, such as Cl, CH_3O and CH_3, to delineate the steric and electronic requirements at each position of the aromatic moiety in any lead. Fluorine was later added to this list. As a whole, this "minimal systematic variation" approach was highly effective in our study. The properties of Cl, F, CH_3O and CH_3 were later better defined in terms of their π, σ, dipole, etc. in the development of regressional analysis. It is of interest to see that these substituents were also favored as first-round structure modification in the Topliss tree approach (Topliss, 1975). At C-5 of the indole moiety, the initial finding of $CH_3O > CH_3 > H > Cl$ was later expanded to include other substituents to give a general order of

5-CH_3O
5-CH_3O–6–F > 5-CH_2=$CHCH_2O$– > 5-CH_3
5-F   5-$(CH_3)_2N$ 5-NH_2; NHAc; O〈   〉N–

                      > 5-H > 5-OH ≫ 5-EtO; $PhCH_2O$
                                        5-CH_3S; HS

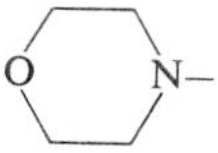

Representatives of these substituents gave similar activity-enhancing effects in the indene series.

iv   *Additivity of activity-enhancing effects.* The effects of activity-enhancing substituents are generally additive in antiinflammatory steroids (e.g. Δ' + (9α-F) + (16α-CH_3) + hydrocortisone = dexamethasone). Such additivity is not commonly encountered in other medicinal chemical studies, especially those dealing with smaller molecules (e.g. substituted salicylates, Shen, 1972). The molecular weight of indomethacin analogs are in the range of 350 and, fortunately, the activity-enhancing effects of such substituents as 5-methoxy, 2-methyl and *p*-chloro are compatible with each other and nearly additive. This additivity enabled us to evaluate the activity-enhancing effect of substituents individually or in model compounds before combining them into a more complex and often more active structure. For example, compound **29** was used extensively as a standard intermediate for the investigation of various *N*-alkyl and *N*-aroyl derivatives.

v *Parallelism of structure–activity relationships.* As the synthetic study progressed from *N*-benzylindoleacetic acids through *N*-benzoylindole acetic acids to benzylidenylindeneacetic acids, a selected group of substituents with widely different activity-enhancing effect was used in each series to check the parallelism of their structure–activity relationships. Within limits, this was true for all three series and greatly simplifies the need to reexamine many modifications found to be unattractive in one series or the other. In addition to their similarity in stereochemistry, the critical dependence of their substituents seemed to suggest that the active analogs in all three series may indeed share a common site of action with well-defined structure requirements for optimal interaction.

vi *Halogen-equivalents.* The activity-enhancing effect of a chloro substituent is probably most commonly encountered in any lead development. The exploration of various pseudo-halogens and chlorine-equivalent in the study of phenothiazine derivatives as CNS agents was noted with success in the 1950s. Application of this approach in our study was partially fruitful, especially at the *p*-position of the *N*-aralkyl or *N*-aroyl moiety. The p-MeS, MeSO, F, CF_3 analogs are also active compounds. Other chlorine equivalents in the phenothiazine series, e.g. $C\equiv N$, CH_3CO, $CONH_2$, OCF_3, $SO_2N(CH_3)_2$, etc. were not beneficial to indomethacin analogs. At the 4'-position of the *N*-benzyl, *N*-benzoyl or benzylidenyl group Cl or equivalents are clearly preferred in animal models.

$$Cl, F, CH_3S \gtrsim CH_3SO, SH > CF_3$$

Multiple substitutions in the phenyl moiety are less effective.

vii *Dihydro derivatives and vinylogs.* In medicinal chemistry the addition (dihydro) or subtraction (dehydro) of two hydrogen atoms and the insertion of a vinyl linkage (vinylog) occasionally yield an active compound with somewhat unexpected properties. Prednisolone (Δ'-hydrocortisone) and (di)hydro-chlorothiazide are notable examples. N-substituted, 2,3-dihydroindole acetic acids (**81**) are only moderately active as antiinflammatory compounds, which also displayed a different structure–activity relationship. A prototype in the vinylog series, N-cinnamylindole acetic acids was first checked by us and was found to be much less active than the corresponding N-benzyl analog. Later, the N-cinnamoyl analogs were studied by the Sumitomo laboratory independently. Their best compound, cinnametacin (**37**), was approximately $\frac{1}{3}-\frac{1}{10} \times$ indomethacin. In this case, the corresponding p-chlorocinnamoyl derivative was only poorly active. Obviously, the structure–activity relationships of these analogous series are divergent enough for the discovery of new active structures.

viii   *Carboxylic acid function.* Having concluded that the free carboxylic acid of the lead is likely the active moiety, we attempted to enhance the acidity of the weakly acidic ($pK_a \sim 6$–$6\cdot5$) indole acetic acid group by F, CF_3 and other electronegative substituents. Chemically, the preparation of indomethacin analogs with F or CF_3 at C_2 or the α-methylene position required much synthetic investigation. Other acid-equivalents, ranging from feebly acidic oximes to the highly acidic tetrazole ($pK_a \sim 4$) were also investigated by us and by others. In difference with the phenylbutazone and sulfinpyrazone series, no apparent correlation of pK_a with antiinflammatory activities was observed. Only the tetrazole analog intrazole (**69**) was found by the Bristol group to have moderate antiinflammatory activities (Juby and Hudyma, 1969). Unlike the carboxylic acids, the tetrazole is not readily conjugated *in vivo* and gives a prolonged serum half-life.

ix   *Attempted analgesic enhancement.* The analgesic effect of non-steroid anti-inflammatory agents has been characterized as mainly peripheral and likely mediated through the inhibition of prostaglandin synthesis. As prosta-glandins are considered to be modulators of the tissue sensitivity to pain stimuli, any blockade at this site would not significantly affect the CNS response. In an attempt to elevate the ceiling of the analgesic action of indo-methacin analogs, several amino-alkyl side chains, such as $R_2N(CH_2)_{2-3}$, were used to replace the substituents at N, C-2, C-3, C-5 and the *para* position of the N-benzoyl group in indomethacin or MK-715. Unfortunately, none of these hybrid molecules gave the desired combination of antiinflammatory and more potent analgesic activities.

x   *Acetic acid precursors.* Certain aliphatic substituents at C-3, e.g. $CH_2CH{=}O$, CH_2CH_2OH, $CH_2CH_2NH_2$, CH_2CO_2R, CH_2CONH_2, etc. are oxidized or hydrolyzed *in vivo* to the acetic acid side chain. These metabolic precursors might have different pharmacodynamic characteristics and possibly altered activity and toxicity profiles. In this case only the aldehyde precursor and several ester derivatives of indomethacin, e.g. $-CO_2CH_2CH_2NHAc$ and $-CO_2CH_2Ch_2CH_2OH$, were fully active in animal models. No really significant improvement on the gastrointestinal effects was observed with these derivatives.

xi *Stereochemical considerations*. The progression of *N*-benzyl to *N*-benzoyl for indoleacetic acids and then to benzylidenylindene acetic acids was accompanied by an increase of conformational rigidity towards a hypothetical

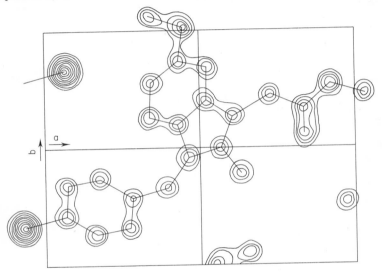

FIG. 2. X-ray structure of MK-715.

optimal configuration. The *N*-benzyl group is relatively free rotating, subject to slight steric interference by the C-2-methyl and C-7-hydrogen. This steric effect is more pronounced in the *N*-benzoyl series. X-ray crystallographic study, NMR and CNDO/2 calculations showed that the N-benzoyl group is slanted away from the C-2-methyl group and out of the plane of the indole ring. Similar configuration was found with the rigid benzylidene indene system as in sulindac (Fig. 2). The preference for this non-planar configuration was again indicated by a marked reduction in potency of fused-ring analogs (**79, 80**) which have a planar configuration. Position isomers such as **75, 76** and **77** were also much less active.

The most critical stereochemical requirement resides with the absolute configuration of the α-methyl acetic acid side chain. Although neither indomethacin nor sulindac possesses an α-methyl substituent, the α-propionic acids in this series are generally comparable to the corresponding acetic acids in potency within a factor of 2 or 3. From the *in vivo* data it was recognized early that only the (+) *S*-isomers are active. This general rule was verified in the *in vitro* prostaglandin synthetase assay (Shen *et al.*, 1974). Recent CNDO/2 calculations showed that the carboxyl group assumes a "down" configuration (Gund and Shen, 1977). The correlation of bioactivity with the absolute configuration (+) *S* is particularly good if the energy barrier for free rotation of the carboxyl group is more than 0·8 kg mol^{-1} as in indomethacin. It was noted that the active *S* configuration is identical with the configuration of the active enantiomer of plant growth regulators, the auxins (Shen, 1972).

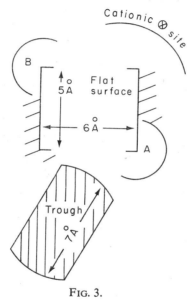

FIG. 3.

xii *Hypothetical receptor site.* Although the sites and mechanisms of action of nonsteroid antiinflammatory agents of the indomethacin type are still far from understood, the well-defined substituents and stereochemical requirements of indomethacin analogs prompted one of us to consider a hypothetical receptor contour (Fig. 3) in 1964 as a working model for the synthesis of other active structures *in this series* (Shen, 1964). The discovery of several active substituted phenylacetic acids, with potency comparable to or greater than indomethacin in animals, clearly indicated that this hypothetical receptor contour is by no means exclusive or limiting. Nevertheless, it inspired the development of some newer agents (e.g. Carson *et al.*, 1971; Kramiya *et al.*,

1975). It remains a useful working model for specific site of action of indomethacin, such as the prostaglandin cyclooxygenase, which exhibited a parallel structure–activity relationship with that summarized above. Several attempts have been made to estimate the conformation of the substrate (arachidonic acid) or product (prostaglandin G_2) of this enzyme for possible structure correlation with its potent inhibitors. A recent calculation (Gund and Shen,

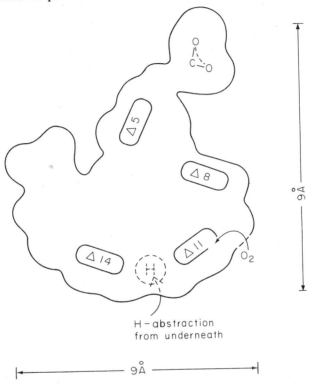

FIG. 4. The binding site of fatty acid substrate and inhibitors of prostaglandin synthetase.

1977) has refined the hypothetical binding site for arachidonic acid and indomethacin to that shown in Fig. 4.

The purification of cyclooxygenase has only recently been described (Hayashi *et al.*, 1976). In the absence of any receptor preparations, the interaction of indomethacin analogs with a biopolymer, human serum albumin, was explored by us several years ago (Shen, 1972). The binding of drug molecules by serum albumin is a familiar problem in many pharmacokinetic studies. The ability of serum albumin to stabilize and transport biological mediators, such as the labile tromboxane A₂ (Svensson *et al.*, 1976), may be of some significance in inflammation also. Considering albumin as a model of bio-polymers or drug receptors, we have examined the binding of indomethacin congeners to albumin by their extrinsic Cotton Effect. As shown in Fig. 5, the similarity of the CD spectra of indomethacin and MK-715 is contrasted with that of flufenamic acid. Most interestingly, albumin binding was specific enough to

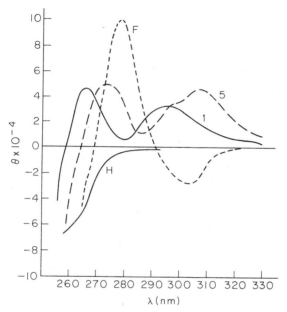

FIG. 5. Binding to human serum albumin (extrinsic Cotton Effect). H, human serum albumin alone; F, flufenamic acid; 1, indomethacin; 5, indene isostere.

distinguish the absolute configuration of the α-methylacetic acid side chain of a part of *S* and *R* enantiomers of MK-410 and their *p*-methoxy analogs.

These studies provided spectroscopic data to confirm the stereo and electronic similarity between these isosteres and analogs. On the other hand, because of the theoretical complexity involved in interpreting the change of Cotton Effect following the binding of a chiral molecular with albumin, only a qualitative or semiqualitative conclusion can be made. The p-MeO analog of MK-410 is much less active than MK-410, the similarity binding clearly showing that albumin binding was not a major factor influencing the anti-inflammatory activities of these compounds.

xiii *Evolution of clinical candidates.* In the process of improving the lead, the chemical study progressed from an *N*-benzylindole-3-acetic acid to the *N*-benzoyl series (indomethacin) and finally to the benzylidenylindene series (sulindac). Two clinical candidates were investigated in each series. Our major goals at different stages were, respectively, verification of the experimental models (MK-555, MK-410), potency enhancement (indomethacin), and reduction of side-effects (MK-825, MK-715 and sulindac). The progression of these compounds provided clinicians some perspective regarding both efficacy and tolerance of this class of antiarthritic agents. It also became apparent that laboratory animals were more responsive to these drugs, especially in acute assays, both in potency and in side-effects, when compared with man. On the other hand, the *relative* potency and safety of candidates within this series correlated well with their clinical performances. This correlation formed a rational basis for selecting the clinical dosage of some of the later clinical candidates.

The study of MK-825 was our first attempt to use possible differences in drug distribution and metabolism to alter the CNS side-effect of indomethacin in man. The development of sulindac started out with certain metabolic considerations to circumvent crystalluria. The fascinating pharmacodynamic pattern later evolved in animal and clinical studies further contributed to its successful b.i.d. dosing schedule. The lack of *in vitro* PG-synthetase inhibition and local antiinflammatory activity of sulindac established its prodrug status and provided some insight to its relatively low g.i. irritating property.

xiv *New drug as a research tool.* The introduction of a new drug like indomethacin signified the completion of one phase of medicinal chemical study but also made available a new research tool for biochemical pharmacological investigations. Numerous attempts were made to identify the mechanism of action of nonsteroidal antiinflammatory agents by studying the inhibitory actions of indomethacin, often at high levels of $0 \cdot 1-1$ mM. Attention was drawn to the pathological roles of proteases, lysosomes, leukocyte chemotaxis, cell membrane interactions, etc. The recent finding of prostaglandin synthetase inhibition by indomethacin at its therapeutic concentrations not only indicated a plausible mode of action but also suggested new biomedical applications which may respond to prostaglandin deprivation. Perhaps more importantly, the use of indomethacin has elucidated the physiological role of the transient and very low concentration of prostaglandins in many experimental systems. It is anticipated that these new understandings may yet bring forth new biological breakthroughs. Thus, the introduction of a new drug may also signify the beginning of a new phase of medicinal chemical research.

6 Metabolism and drug interactions

The study of drug metabolism has assumed increasing importance within the past few years. The distribution, excretion, pharmacodynamic activity and duration of action of a drug are affected by the chemical and physical transformations of the compound that occur in the body after its ingestion or injection. Determination of the fate of a new compound is preferrably undertaken early in the course of the study (Baer, 1972). It is an aid to the medicinal chemist in designing and developing leads (Clarke, 1972). It helps in understanding the pharmacological actions of a new compound and in anticipating interactions with other drugs (Stripp and Gillette, 1972). It provides indispensable information to the pharmaceutical chemist in devising proper dosage forms (Heimlich, 1972) and the clinician testing a new drug needs to know what to expect in the way of bioavailability, duration of action, route of excretion, variability of metabolism among species, and interactions with other drugs and with other substances naturally occurring in the body or in food (Lemberger, 1972). Variability of responsiveness among human subjects to drugs depends upon many factors, such as differences in drug metabolizing enzymes, exposure to environmental chemicals, and substances present in the digestive tract after ingestion of certain foods (Pantuck *et al.*, 1975).

6.1 METABOLISM OF INDOMETHACIN

The metabolic fate of indomethacin and several of its analogs has been studied in several laboratories. In preliminary studies of the urinary metabolites of ^{14}C-indomethacin in several species, Harman *et al.* (1964) described two metabolites: *N*-deschlorobenzoyl-indomethacin (**14**, metabolite II) and *O*-desmethyl-indomethacin (**106**, metabolite III). They were excreted both as the unconjugated form and as the glucuronide conjugate; indomethacin itself, either free or conjugated, was metabolite I. There was a remarkable diversity of metabolic fate in different species. Urinary elimination of II-glucuronide was especially important in the monkey and the guinea-pig, though III-glucuronide was also found in these species. In the rabbit, metabolite III was not found in the urine, and the most important excretory product was indomethacin glucuronide. No indomethacin, either free or conjugated, was found in rat urine, and only about half of metabolites II and III were excreted in conjugated form.

These workers reported a virtual absence of urinary excretion of indomethacin or any of its metabolites by the dog, and the absence of the drug in any form except indomethacin glucuronide in human urine. Their conclusions regarding excretion in man were based on rather limited data, and more recent investigations have revised the picture (Duggan *et al.*, 1972). Duggan's results demonstrated that the major pathway for catabolism of indomethacin in human subjects is demethylation followed by deacylation, though deacylation may occur without demethylation. Less than one third of an administered dose is excreted as indomethacin, and only about half that is in conjugated form. Total fecal excretion, ranging from 21 to 42 per cent of the dose, was almost entirely unconjugated desmethylindomethacin (**106**) or desmethyl-desbenzoyl-indomethacin (**107**).

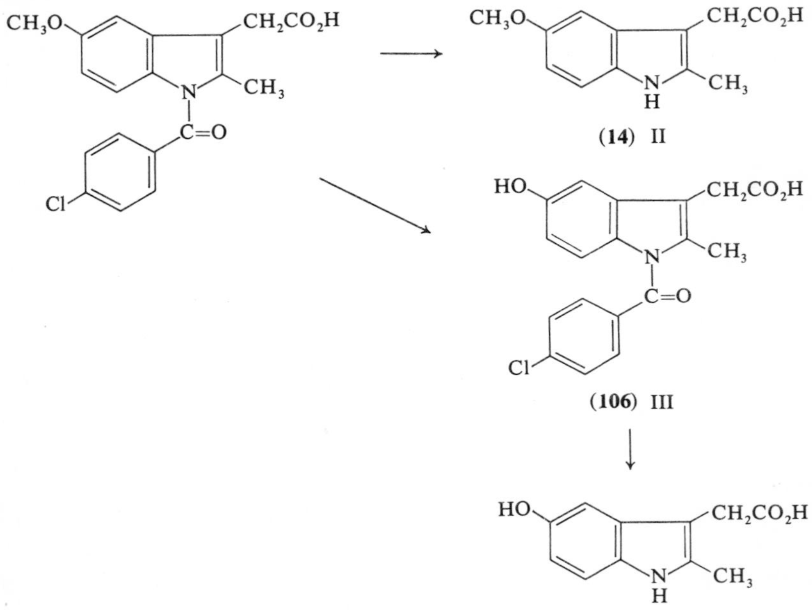

Data by Duggan and coworkers relating to absorption after oral ingestion agreed with previous conclusions of Hucker *et al.* (1966). Duggan found absorption to be rapid initially, then to continue at a lower rate for about 5 hours. Total urinary recovery in human subjects over a 48 h period was about 60 per cent and did not differ significantly whether the drug was ingested orally or injected intravenously. The data agree reasonably well with Hucker's finding of 54 per cent urinary recovery in 24 hours. It was concluded that indomethacin was nearly completely absorbed from the g.i. tract. After absorption, it is firmly bound to nondiffusible constituents (plasma protein). Hucker *et al.* (1966) found 90 per cent of the compound to be bound in human plasma and 94 to 98 per cent in dog plasma, depending on the procedure used.

Data by Hucker *et al.* (1966) and by Yesair *et al.* (1970) indicated a plasma half-life for indomethacin varying considerably according to the species and the route of administration. Plasma half-life after intravenous injection ranged from 20 minutes in dogs and guinea-pigs to 4 hours in rats. After oral ingestion, the range was from 90 minutes in dogs and monkeys to 4 hours in rats, with about 2 hours in man. Duggan *et al.* (1972) found the drug to disappear rather rapidly initially after intravenous injection in humans, with half life of 18 minutes, then more slowly after the first hour or so, with half life of 3·24 hours. They did not publish figures for oral administration, but the data shown in their Fig. 2 permits one to estimate a half life of slightly over 1 hour.

More recent investigations have revised these estimates. Work by Emori *et al.* (1973, 1974) indicates that the disappearance of indomethacin from plasma follows a biexponential pattern, with half-life of about 1 hour during the initial phase. After about 3 hours, a second phase exhibits a half life of about 9 hours. The second phase appears to be highly variable according to Alvan *et al.* (1975) and Kwan *et al.* (1976). Additional references are listed in Kwan's paper. Useful tissue levels of indomethacin can be maintained with three oral doses daily (Duggan *et al.*, 1972). Concentrations of indomethacin in all body compartments fall rapidly after withdrawing the compound. In this respect, indomethacin behaves differently from phenylbutazone, which has a biological half-life of about 3 days in man, and in some subjects rather high plasma levels may be found a week or more after the last dose (Burns *et al.*, 1953).

After absorption, indomethacin appears in the blood stream as unchanged compound firmly bound to plasma protein. It can be extracted by heptane after acidification of the plasma, then returned to an aqueous phase by shaking in alkali and determination can be made by spectrophotofluorometry (Hucker *et al.*, 1966). Increased sensitivity is reported for a specific mass fragmentographic method (Palmer *et al.*, 1974). Varying amounts of the compound, depending upon the species, are converted in the liver to the glucuronide, either before or after *O*-demethylation or *N*-deacylation or both. Unlike phenylbutazone, indomethacin appears not to induce enzymes which hasten its own metabolism (Alvan *et al.*, 1975).

Hucker and co-workers (1966) described an enterohepatic cycle for indomethacin in the dog. Nearly all the compound reaching the liver was converted to the glucuronide and excreted in the bile. Freed of its conjugation in the small intestine again, the compound could be absorbed to repeat the cycle. The cycle was not broken until the drug had been excreted in the feces. Subsequent investigators confirmed the existence of this cycle and noted considerable variation among species in its importance in the overall metabolic disposition (Yasair *et al.*, 1970; Duggan *et al.*, 1975). According to the latter, the extent of enterohepatic cycling is related to the sensitivity of each species to the production of intestinal lesions.

Duggan and co-workers (1972) thought that enterohepatic recycling of unchanged indomethacin seemed not to occur in man to any significant degree. They related this to the relatively low incidence of intestinal lesions in human patients. The side effect of dyspepsia frequently mentioned in clinical reports is probably usually unrelated to the severe lesions seen in those animals exhibiting the enterohepatic cycling to a marked degree, such as the dog and the rat. However, a severe g.i. reaction has been occasionally seen in human patients, and Alvan et al. (1975) thought that the second or *beta* phase of the plasma decay curve with its highly variable slope indicated that enterohepatic recycling does occur in man. Additional evidence for the recycling has been discussed by Kwan et al. (1976) and by Emori et al. (1974). Alvan and Kwan agreed on the complete bioavailability of indomethacin when taken orally in capsules, but they differed somewhat on bioavailability from rectal suppositories, obtaining estimates of 100 and 80 per cent, respectively.

The minimal plasma level of indomethacin needed for antiinflammatory action has not been determined. In the reports by Hucker and Duggan (see above), the highest plasma concentrations determined after various oral doses in human subjects were proportional to dose. The peak level after the usual therapeutic dose of 25 mg was $0 \cdot 8$ μg ml^{-1}. Steady state plasma concentration after multiple dosing was on the order of $0 \cdot 5$ μg ml^{-1} in Alvan's study (1975). Hence, it seems likely that plasma levels of less than 1 microgram per ml suffice to produce an antiinflammatory effect. Most of the antiinflammatory studies in animals have been performed in rats, but the only data on plasma concentration in that species were obtained after the high dose of 10 mg kg^{-1}, which yielded a peak plasma level of $45 \cdot 2$ μg ml^{-1} (Hucker et al., 1966). Since this dose is two orders of magnitude greater than that required to demonstrate antiinflammatory activity in the granuloma inhibition test (Winter and Risley, 1965), there is no adequate basis for estimating minimal plasma levels needed for such activity.

There is evidence that antiinflammatory compounds act at local sites, whether the drug is a steroid (Dougherty et al., 1958) or nonsteroid (Wilhelmi et al., 1959). Hence, plasma level is important only insofar as tissue level is dependent upon it. Duggan et al. (1972) in their analysis of the inter-relationships of indomethacin concentration among the various compartments of the body, concluded that although plasma concentrations rise and fall rather rapidly after each of three 25 mg doses commonly given daily, drug levels in a hypothetical organ build up more gradually, vary less during the day, and decay over a much longer time than concentrations in either the central (plasma) or peripheral compartment.

Indomethacin entered synovial fluid of arthritic patients, the peak concentration appearing about an hour after plasma peak (Caruso, 1971; Emori et *al.*, 1973, 1974). Equilibrium between plasma and synovial fluid was established about 3 hours after a single dose. The synovial concentration then fell less rapidly for the next hour than did the plasma level, so that from about the 5th to 9th hour, synovial fluid concentration was slightly higher than plasma level. Hucker and Hoffman (1971) presented evidence of concentration in inflamed tissue of rats of the indene analog of indomethacin (see section 6.3.1 below), and mentioned that they have unpublished data that indomethacin is similarly concentrated in an inflamed area.

6.2   METABOLISM OF AN ANALOG OF INDOMETHACIN

The 5-dimethylamino analog of indomethacin, MK-825 (**46**, Table 3) is a more polar compound that indomethacin, with different ionization characteristics and increased water solubility. The metabolic study (Hucker and Hoffman, 1971) established that the compound was handled in the body like indomethacin in several important respects, but there were several interesting differences. Both compounds were about equally well absorbed after oral administration, and equally bound to plasma proteins. The rate at which the compound was metabolized and disappeared from the plasma, however, was different. MK-825 was metabolized more rapidly than was indomethacin in man, with a plasma half life of only 1 hour, but the opposite was the case in dogs, where the new compound had a half life of about 4 hours, compared with 90 minutes for indomethacin.

In both dogs and humans, a major metabolite of MK-825 not described in the indomethacin studies was *p*-chlorohippuric acid. This metabolite was derived from hydrolysis of the *p*-chlorobenzoyl group and conjugation with glycine. It was excreted in the urine. The difference in metabolism was especially striking in dogs. Whereas urinary excretion of indomethacin or its metabolites was almost nil in dogs, and recovery was practically entirely from the feces, about one-third of an administered dose of MK-825 was recovered from the urine of dogs within a 3-day period, and about half the dose from the feces. Apparently, enterohepatic recycling in the dog is as important for MK-825 as for indomethacin, since about 95 per cent of an administered dose appeared in the bile either as either free drug or glucuronide conjugate within a 6-hour period. The compound must have been removed from the enterohepatic cycle thereafter, since about one-fourth of the administered dose appeared in the urine the first day. This probably accounted for the lessened toxicity in dogs, compared with indomethacin; studies for assessment of safety indicated that daily administration to dogs for 26 weeks at a dose of 13·5 mg kg^{-1} d^{-1} produced less severe gastrointestinal lesions than 8 weeks of indomethacin at 2 to 5 mg kg^{-1} d^{-1}.

6.3   METABOLISM OF SULINDAC AND ITS ANALOGS

6.3.1   *Metabolism of MK-715*

The metabolic fate of the indene isostere of indomethacin, MK-715 (**97**), as described by Hucker and Hoffman (1971), resembled rather closely that of indomethacin. Some differences observed may be attributed to the chemical stability of the *p*-chlorobenzylidene bond and the poor aqueous solubility of the indene analog. Both were well absorbed from the intestinal tract, readily conjugated with glucuronic acid, metabolized at about the same rate in rats, were widely distributed in the tissues with no marked tendency to be concentrated in any one tissue, and the proportion excreted in the bile of rats was about the same for both. *O*-demethylation occurred with both compounds, but no cleavage of the benzylidene group took place. Possibly influenced by its low solubility, final excretion of MK-715 in rats was predominantly in the feces, with only about 10 per cent of a dose appearing in the urine; in contrast, radioactivity of a labelled dose of indomethacin appeared amost equally in urine and feces. A significant degree of concentration of the drug appeared in inflamed tissue, as measured by radioactivity in the feet of rats injected with brewers yeast in the subplantar tissues. In dogs, excretion patterns of MK-715 and of indomethacin were similar.

The similarity in the metabolism of indomethacin and of MK-715, especially the excretion patterns in dogs, was reflected in the fact that in long-term toxicity tests, gastrointestinal lesions were the principal findings with both compounds. However, the doses needed to produce g.i. lesions were so much higher for the indene compound that it appeared to have about a ten-fold greater safety margin than did indomethacin. In human trials the glucuronide conjugate of MK-715 proved to be relatively insoluble in human urine, and crystalluria appeared in some subjects. This finding prompted a discontinuance of the trials, and a search for a compound with improved solubility but otherwise similar properties.

6.3.2   *Metabolism of sulindac*

The search mentioned above led to the discovery and development of MK-231, sulindac. The metabolic rationale considered in the design of sulindac is described above in section 4.2. The methyl sulfinyl group was expected to be metabolized to its sulfide and sulfone derivatives. The verification of this supposition and other findings in laboratory and clinical studies may be summarized as follows:

After oral ingestion of sulindac, enormous differences were found among animal species in plasma concentration of sulindac and metabolites as judged by total radioactivity. For example, 1 hour after 10 mg kg^{-1} of labelled drug, plasma radioactivity in rats was about 44 μg ml^{-1}, compared with 0·8 μg ml^{-1} in dogs receiving the same dose—more than 50-fold difference. Although plasma levels of indomethacin, MK-825 and MK-715 were also higher in rats than in dogs, the differences were much smaller than for sulindac (Hucker *et al.*, 1966, 1971; Hucker and Hoffman, 1971). Dogs gave markedly different responses to the different compounds; 10 mg kg^{-1} of indomethacin yielded plasma levels nearly twice as high as did 20 mg kg^{-1} of MK-715, and about 20 times as high as did 10 mg kg^{-1} of sulindac. It is of interest to note that these differences in plasma levels are roughly parallel with the observed potency of these drugs in the dog synovitis assay.

Smaller differences were seen in human subjects, and both indomethacin and sulindac seem to be well absorbed from the gastrointestinal tract. In fasting subjects, Duggan *et al.* (1972) found about 0·8 μg ml^{-1} 1 hour after 25 mg of indomethacin, while Hucker *et al.* (1973) reported 1·3 μg ml^{-1} 1 hour after 50 mg of sulindac. In five separate clinical studies, a minimum of approximately 88 per cent of oral dosage is absorbed. The major biotransformations involve irreversible oxidation of the sulfoxide group of sulindac to sulfone (**108**) and a reversible reduction to the sulfide (**102**). All three compounds are found in the plasma (Fig. 6). A minor urinary metabolite, the dihydroxylated derivative **109**, has also been identified. These relationships are as follows:

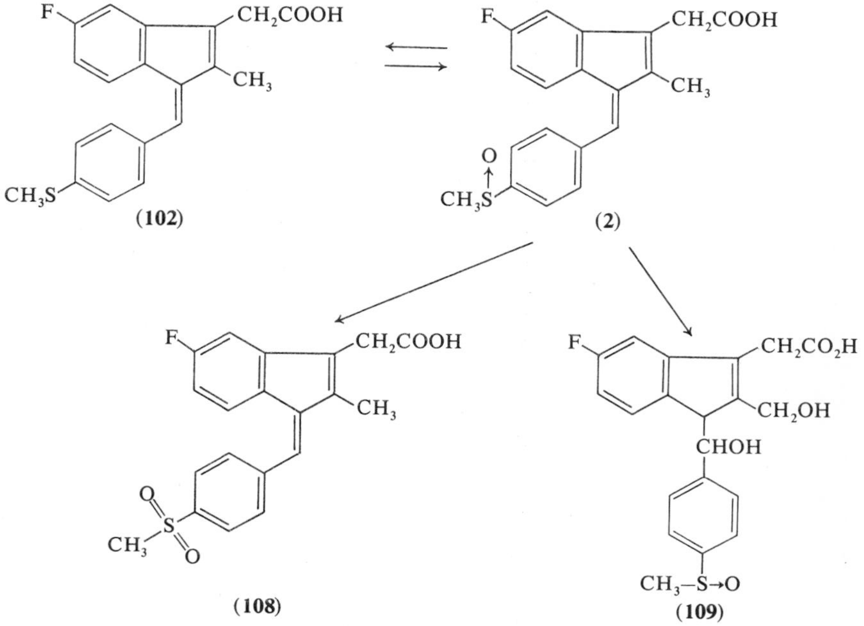

The major urinary metabolites are sulindac (**2**), the sulfone (**108**), and their glucuronides. In general, at 100, 200 and 400 mg d^{-1} dosage levels, the sulfone (**108**) and its glucuronide comprise the major constituents in urine, c. 28 per cent, while the sulindac and its glucuronide correspond to c. 20 per cent of the

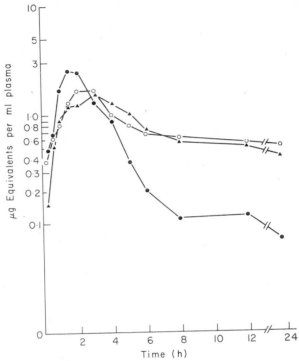

FIG. 6 Mean plasma levels of metabolites of sulindac: sulfoxide, ●; sulfide, ○; sulfone, ▲.

dose. No more than a trace amount of the insoluble sulfide metabolite (**102**) and its glucuronide has been detected in urine samples of man as well as five animal species: rat, dog, guinea-pig, rabbit and monkey.

In plasma, unlike urine, the concentration of sulfide, sulindac and sulfone are all comparable. It is a striking feature of the disposition of the compound that the substantial plasma level of the less soluble sulfide is not reflected in the urine. Interestingly, the sulfide and its glucuronide are excreted in the bile only to a minor extent also. A significant amount of sulfide in the fecal recovery is presumably formed by the reduction of sulindac by colon and fecal contents, and probably not by the ileal content (Duggan et al., 1977a). A summary of the urinary and fecal recoveries of these metabolites is shown in Table 21.

In the plasma, the bioactive sulfide metabolite (**102**) has an apparent half-life of 18 hours. Following twice daily dosage of sulindac for 5 days, at 400 mg day^{-1}, plasma levels of sulfide approach an apparent steady state. The level of sulindac increases 1·4-fold whereas the level of sulfide metabolite plateaus at 2·7-fold. Consequently, no steady accumulation of the sulfide metabolite after chronic administration is expected.

TABLE 21

Recoveries of sulindac and metabolites in man (average of six human subjects)

	Dosage (mg)		
	100	200	400
Urinary excretion (0–96 h) (mg equiv)			
Sulindac			
Free	6·7	14·4	25·6
Conj	13·4	24·9	55·2
Sulfone			
Free	4·7	8·8	15·2
Conj	25·6	46·7	84·1
Unknown	12·7	26·0	37·6
Total	51·7 (51·7%)	97·6 (48·8%)	176·9 (44·2%)
Fecal excretion (0–96 h) (mg equiv)			
Sulindac	0·94	2·2	3·2
Sulfone	11·7	19·4	35·3
Sulfide	11·1	20·4	37·3
Unknown	4·6	7·2	16·2
Total	28·3 (28·3%)	49·2 (24·6%)	92·0 (23·0%)

The metabolizing enzyme(s) responsible for the reoxidation of the sulfide metabolite to sulindac has not been identified, but cytochrome P-450 is probably not involved. A likely candidate is a monooxygenase in the microsomal fraction of liver which carries out the sulfoxidation of aromatic sulfides (Prema and Gopinathan, 1976). The enzyme is a flavoprotein, containing a non-heme iron, requiring NADPH for its activity and not inhibited by SKF 525A. The sulfoxidation is mediated through the formation of superoxide anions (O_2^-) (Prema and Gopinanthan, 1974). It is of interest to note the biochemical similarity of this monooxygenase and prostaglandin cyclooxygenase which is inhibited by the sulfide metabolite.

6.3.3 *Sulindac as a prodrug*

In a variety of assays for antiinflammatory, antipyretic and analgesic activities Van Arman *et al.* (1976) indicated that the sulfone metabolite is inactive. The sulfide metabolite is generally about twice as potent as sulindac itself following oral administration. However, when the two drugs are applied locally, e.g. in the topical mouse ear assay and the dog synovitis assay, sulindac is much less active than the sulfide (Duggan *et al.*, 1977c) (Table 22). Similar difference in potency was observed in the topical treatment of ocular inflammation in rabbits (LeDouarec, unpublished). In *in vitro* tests for effects on aggregation of human platelets, or the inhibition of prostaglandin synthetase, sulindac is

TABLE 22

Sulindac as prodrug

	Sulindac (prodrug)	Sulfide metabolite (active species)
In vitro assays		
PG synthetase inhibition ID_{50} (μM)	inactive	2·2
Platelet aggregation versus arachidonic acid ($\mu g\ ml^{-1}$)	inactive	32
Platelet aggregation versus ADP ($\mu g\ ml^{-1}$)	inactive	0·5
Topical administration		
Intrasynovial (canine synovitis) ED_{50} (mg kg^{-1})	6·4	0·1
Mouse ear inflammation	6·2	
Ocular inflammation (rabbits)	weakly active	active
Relative potency in *in vivo* models ED_{50} (mg kg^{-1} po)		
Platelet aggregation (guinea-pig), 1 h	0·8	0·2
Urate synovitis (canine), 2 h	45	5·3
Antipyresis (rat), 2 h	2·9	0·5
Carrageenan paw edema (rat), 3 h	5·5	2·3
Cotton pellet granuloma (rat), 7 days	5·4	>3·4
Adjuvant arthritis (rat), 14 days	0·55	0·36
Correlation of drug concentration versus response		
Synovial fluid concentration in urate synovitis	none	good
Plasma level in carrageenan edema	poor	good

inactive, while the sulfide metabolite is nearly as active as indomethacin. These results suggest that sulindac is active *in vivo* only because it is metabolized to the sulfide. In other words, sulindac could be characterized as a prodrug. Additional evidence for this view is seen in the relation between pharmacological activity and areas under the plasma curves of time–concentration. The correspondence is reasonably close for the plasma sulfide curve, no matter which form (sulfoxide of sulfide) is given, but drug activity is unrelated to the plasma sulfoxide curve.

These studies further showed that sulindac has a relatively long duration of action; this, too, may be related to conversion to the sulfide, for Hucker and co-workers (1973) reported the half life of the sulfide to be about twice that of the sulfoxide in the rat, and even longer in the monkey and man. According to Duggan (1976) the capacity for net conversion of sulindac to its active metabolite the sulfide is higher for man than for the other species examined, and hence the prodrug concept for sulindac is particularly applicable to the human. The long half life of the sulfide metabolite in man made it possible to maintain high plasma levels of drug with oral administration only twice daily. In subjects receiving twice daily doses of 200 mg, samples taken 12 hours after each dose exhibited evidence of accumulation during the first days, but a steady state had been reached by the sixth day. The accumulation was less marked for the sulfoxide, but for both forms the findings were in marked contrast with the metabolic behavior of indomethacin.

In view of these findings, the rationale for developing sulfoxide as the drug of choice instead of the sulfide may not be immediately apparent. However, it is common knowledge that gastrointestinal intolerance is a limiting factor in the use of antiinflammatory compounds (see sections 3.4.2 and 3.4.3). Sulindac has markedly less gastrointestinal toxicity than does indomethacin (see sections 3.4.5 and 3.5.4). Sulindac, then, provides a theoretical advantage in that the drug is absorbed through the gastrointestinal mucosa before it is in an active form. Antiinflammatory activity is so closely linked with g.i. intolerance that some have suggested that both effects may involve the same intrinsic mechanism, probably the inhibition of prostaglandin synthetase (Vane, 1974). The rationale for the selection of a prodrug is equally valid, however, whether that is so or not.

Most antiinflammatory aryl acids undergo enterohepatic recirculation either unchanged or in the form of glucuronide conjugates. The latter may be cleaved in the intestine to liberate the free drug again. The continuous exposure of intestinal wall to these agents probably contributes to the development of lesions. Hucker et al. (1973) estimated that about 17 per cent of an administered dose of sulindac was recovered from the feces in human subjects. Rats and dogs excreted nearly all the compound in the feces, and when sulindac was administered intravenously to rats, 86 per cent could be recovered from the bile within 24 hours. In spite of this enterohepatic recycling, however, sulindac has a low order of toxicity in both rats and dogs. Evidence by Duggan (1976) suggests that the major biliary metabolites are the inactive sulfoxide, sulfone and their conjugates, the active sulfide has a low biliary clearance. The reabsorption of the sulfoxide sustains the plasma level of the sulfide metabolite.

The pharmacodynamic pattern of sulindac is illustrated by the following diagram. It is of interest to note that the gastrointestinal tract is only exposed to the inactive sulindac and sulfone metabolite, thereby minimizing any local irritations.

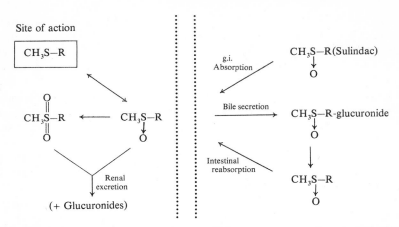

A summary of experimental data identifying the sulfide metabolite of sulindac as the active species *in vivo* (Duggan *et al.*, 1977) is tabulated in Table 22.

6.4 CHEMICAL PROPERTIES OF METABOLITES

6.4.1 *Indomethacin metabolites*

The facile oxidation demethylation of indomethacin *in vivo* to give the 5-OH analog (**106**) can readily be matched by a one-step acid-catalyzed cleavage *in vitro*. Treating indomethacin with boron tribromide in methylene chloride at room temperature for 3 hours gives **106** in 70 per cent yield (Witzel, unpublished). Under the conditions used, the hydrolysis of the *p*-chlorobenzoyl group is largely avoided. To obtain the deacylated metabolites simple hydrolysis under alkaline (e.g. 1 N NaOH, room temperature a few hours) or acidic conditions of indomethacin or **106** will suffice.

The acyl glucuronide of indomethacin (110) is highly water soluble and chemically labile. The ester glycosidic linkage, like the N-p-chlorobenzoyl group, is easily hydrolyzed in either acidic or alkaline medium.

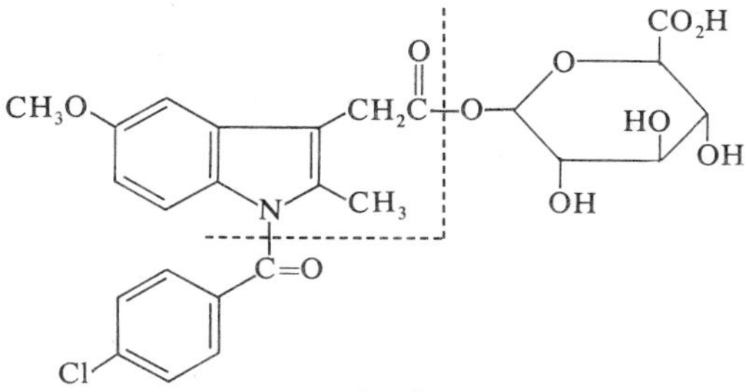

(110)

For this reason special synthetic procedures had to be developed for the preparation of acyl glucuronides. Indomethacin glucuronide was initially isolated and identified as its fully acetylated methyl ester (111) (Harman et al., 1964). An authentic sample was prepared by coupling indomethacin with the methyl ester of tri-O-acetyl-D-glucuronyl bromide (Strachen et al., 1964).

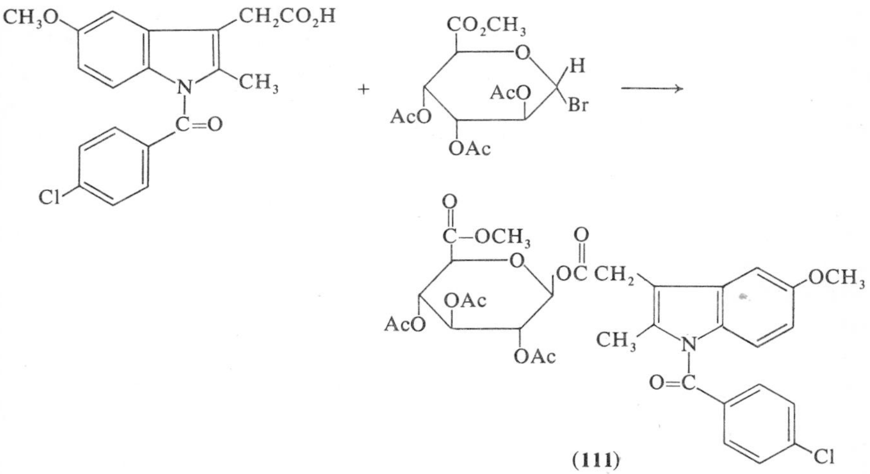

(111)

Later, a new synthetic procedure for the synthesis of acyl glucuronides in general was developed in our laboratory (Bugianesi and Shen, 1971). Using a new intermediate of D-glucuronic acid (112) with β,β,β-trichloroethyl as protecting groups, the unsubstituted indomethacin glucuronide is obtained by deblocking under nonhydrolytic conditions.

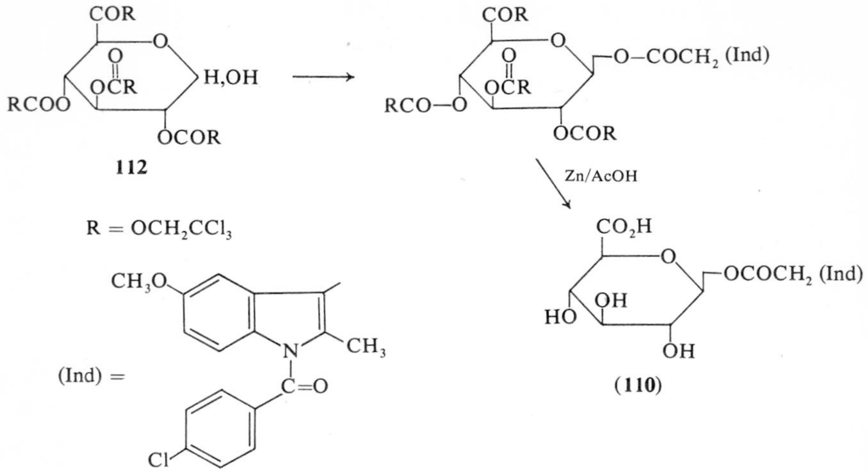

112

R = OCH$_2$CCl$_3$

(Ind) =

Zn/AcOH

(110)

6.4.2 Sulindac metabolites

The sulfide and sulfone metabolites of sulindac were synthesized in the original structure activity relationship study by the general method described in section 4.2.2. The glucuronide of these metabolites were prepared for solubility determinations. As the benzylidenyl linkage in sulindac and other indene analogs is nonhydrolyzable, it was possible to carry out a preferential hydrolysis of a fully protected glucuronide intermediate to give a small, though adequate, yield of glucuronide metabolites (**113**) in our study (Jones *et al.*, 1977).

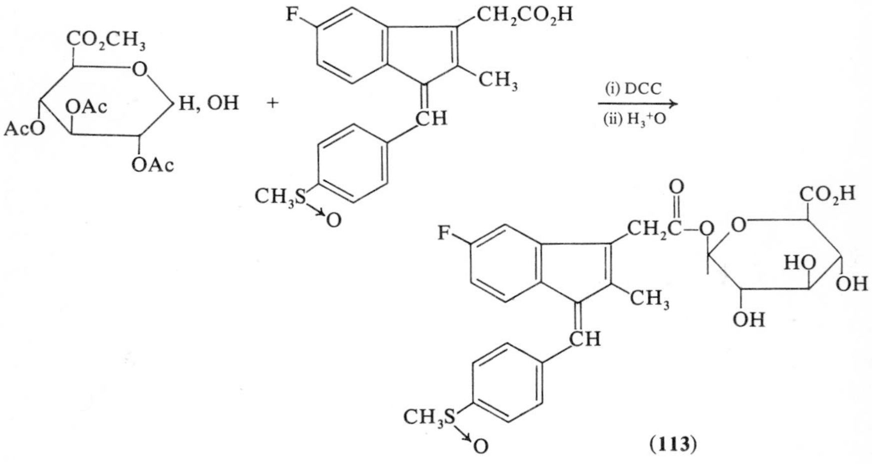

(i) DCC

(ii) H$_3$$^+$O

(**113**)

6.5 DRUG INTERACTIONS INVOLVING INDOMETHACIN AND ITS ANALOGS

Modification of the effects of a drug by prior or concurrent administration of another is all too frequently overlooked as a possibility when medications are prescribed. An understanding of possible drug interactions is important in view of multiple therapies often employed and the increasing potencies of new drugs. Drugs may interact in many ways, and the net result of the interaction may be described by such terms as summation, addition, synergism, potentiation and antagonism. Such effects may be brought about by modification of absorption, alteration of transport systems, displacement from binding sites, effects on drug metabolizing enzymes, changes in excretion patterns or rate of excretion, etc. Not all of these factors have been thoroughly explored with regard to indomethacin and its analogs, but several drug interactions involving indomethacin have been described, and some controversial findings have been reported.

6.5.1 Indomethacin–steroid interactions

Interactions between indomethacin and corticoadrenal steroids have received considerable attention. When the compound was first subjected to large-scale clinical trial, many of the patients receiving indomethacin were already using steroids and several of the reports of the trials mentioned a reduction of steroid dosage after introducing the new drug into the therapeutic regimen. This effect was referred to as "steroid sparing" (Smyth, 1968). It has been postulated that indomethacin might displace steroids from tissue and plasma binding sites, thus freeing the steroids for exhibiting their antiinflammatory action. Such an effect was proposed by Brodie (1965) as the mode of action of nonsteroid antiinflammatory compounds, including indomethacin.

Brodie's hypothesis had the merit of stimulating research on the question, though the bulk of the evidence soon rendered it untenable. The hypothesis seems to be based on reports by Maickel et al. (1965, 1966, 1969) that nonsteroid antiinflammatory compounds displace corticosterone from plasma binding sites. The observations of these workers, however, were made in animals receiving doses of drugs sufficiently high to produce nonspecific toxic effects which might stimulate the production of steroids by the adrenal cortex.

Domenjoz (1966) concluded that phenylbutazone action does not depend upon activation of the pituitary-adrenal mechanism, and Smith (1966) after an exhaustive survey of the literature emphatically rejected the view that adrenal hormones have anything to do with therapeutic actions of salicylates. Indomethacin exhibits antiinflammatory activity when it is added directly to the site of inflammation, and is also active in adrenalectomized animals (Winter et al., 1963). Several other investigators have demonstrated local or topical activity of indomethacin (see section 3.1.2). If steroids were released by the presence of indomethacin, one would expect thymus involution and body weight gain retardation in young rats (very sensitive indicators of corticoadrenal function), but these effects do not occur (Winter et al., 1963; Winter, 1965). Other experiments performed in our laboratory (Winter et al., 1968) showed that indomethacin is active in adrenalectomized rats in the virtual absence of circulating corticosterone, and that indomethacin in concentrations exceeding therapeutic levels does not affect in vitro binding of corticosterone in rat plasma or of cortisol in human plasma.

Other publications relevant to this question include the following: Riesterer and Jaques (1967) and Shanahan (1968) confirmed the local antiinflammatory action of indomethacin. In the latter study, the ED_{50} of indomethacin (defined as the dose producing at least 25 per cent inhibition of carrageenan induced edema in 50 per cent of the animals) was 7 μg per paw when injected directly into the inflamed tissue of the rat's paw. Not only was the action of the nonsteroid compound accomplished without intervention of the adrenals or the transport of steroid by the plasma, but in its local effect indomethacin proved to be several times as potent as cortisol or even dexamethasone similarly administered.

Gupta et al. (1969) demonstrated that indomethacin 6 mg kg^{-1} intraperitoneally did not affect the concentration of corticosterone in rat plasma. Even more significant was the report by Jansen et al. (1970) that therapeutic doses of indomethacin yielding plasma levels of drug of 0·8 μg ml^{-1} on the average in human subjects not only did not decrease plasma binding of cortisol but for a short time after administration of indomethacin there was sometimes actually an increase in bound cortisol. In vitro binding of cortisol in human plasma was not altered by concentrations as high as 20 μg ml^{-1}. Experiments in guinea-pigs by Jansen and Schou (1971, 1972) demonstrated that indomethacin in doses as high as 100 mg kg^{-1} for 3 days or 20 mg kg^{-1} day^{-1} for 3 weeks did not affect cortisol levels in plasma, plasma ultrafiltrate or skin, nor did it affect the plasma half life or apparent volume of distribution of 4-^{14}C-labelled cortisol. The authors concluded that their results did not support the concept of a displacement of cortisol from binding sites as a possible mechanism for activity of nonsteroid antiinflammatory drugs.

The results of Stenlake et al. (1971) showed that a variety of nonsteroid antiinflammatory drugs, including indomethacin, had no effect upon protein binding of cortisol in the plasma of either normal subjects or patients with rheumatoid arthritis. In some subjects, plasma cortisol was allowed to remain at endogenous levels, and in others, it was raised by the administration of labelled cortisol. In some of the in vitro tests, the nonsteroid compounds were added to bring plasma level up to four times usual therapeutic concentrations.

Lowry et al. (1973) measured corticosteroid production by isolated cells from the adrenal cortex of rats. Indomethacin in a concentration of 10 μg ml^{-1} did not affect steroid output by the cells, nor did it interfere with responses to adrenocortical stimulating hormone (ACTH) from human pituitary glands.

As discussed in section 7.9.3, from the mechanism of action point of view, the blockade of arachidonic acid supply by corticosteroids and the inhibition of cyclooxygenase by indomethacin and aspirin may produce a sequential inhibitory effect in theory at least.

6.5.2 Indomethacin: anticoagulant interactions

Another drug interaction which has led to some confusion in the literature relates to the displacement from plasma binding sites of anticoagulants by nonsteroid antiinflammatory compounds. Such displacement, when it occurs, increases the amount of free anticoagulant compound and may lead to hemorrhagic complications. It has long been known that this is one of the occasional hazards of phenylbutazone therapy. Hoffbrand and Kininmonth (1967) noted such complications in a patient while on phenylbutazone. The same patient had previously had indomethacin. The authors, though carefully pointing out that the complications had not occurred while the patient was on indomethacin, speculated that indomethacin *might* produce a similar effect by analogy with phenylbutazone.

Hoffbrand and Kininmonth's paper has been widely cited by subsequent authors, frequently misquoted, the statements enlarged upon, and gradually what started out as a speculation became stated as a "fact". Among the papers listing indomethacin as increasing the anticoagulant response due to displacement from binding sites are those by Hussar (1967, 1969), Morelli and Melmon (1968), and Formiller and Cohon (1969), using the Hoffbrand–Kininmonth paper as "authority". The supposed effect has also been incorporated in reference books, such as "Remington's Pharmaceutical Sciences", and the "Handbook of Drug Interactions" edited by E. A. Hartshorn (Hamilton Press, Hamilton, Illinois). Papers by Vessell et al. (1975) and by Winter (1969) list additional references.

On the other hand, several clinical studies pointed out that indomethacin had no effect upon the action of anticoagulants when given to patients during anticoagulant therapy. Such studies include those of Müller and Zollinger (1966), Frost and Hess (1966), Müller and Herrmann (1966) and Gáspárdy et al. (1967). The subject was critically studied by Vesell et al. (1975) in controlled double blind tests in human subjects receiving indomethacin and warfarin concurrently. Their results clearly showed that indomethacin did not alter hypoprothrombinemia induced by warfarin, nor was there any effect upon plasma warfarin concentrations or upon prothrombin times. Their conclusions were the same as those of the other clinical investigators mentioned above;

namely, that indomethacin does not interact in a clinically significant fashion with warfarin, and that it may be safely administered to patients on warfarin therapy. Odegaard (1974) did, however, report a small group of patients which apparently exhibited a small but statistically significant change in "Thrombotest" values.

The apparent lack of clinically significant effect of indomethacin on warfarin pharmacodynamics may be regarded as surprising in view of the protein binding properties of the compound. Hucker *et al.* (1966) showed that indomethacin binds to plasma protein over a wide range of concentrations. Mason and McQueen (1974) determined that the binding is to albumin and that at physiological concentrations the affinity is firmer than previously thought. Solomon *et al.* (1968) claimed that warfarin can be displaced by indomethacin in *in vitro* studies, but Vesell *et al.* (1975) pointed out that Solomon's results were obtained under highly unphysiological conditions. Solomon dissolved the indomethacin in 0·1 N NaOH, so the observations were made on indomethacin derivatives of unspecified chemical structure, rather than on indomethacin itself.

Vesell speculated that the indomethacin–warfarin interaction might be complex, consisting of two actions having opposite effects, since the net effect was a lack of change in prothrombin time or plasma warfarin concentration. There seemed to be no experimental proof or disproof of this speculation. It has also been stated that the binding of warfarin at its primary site may cause significant changes in protein structure so that additional (secondary) binding sites are formed. Mason and McQueen (1974) suggest that indomethacin may have the same action and that both drugs are bound at the same sites.

None of these authors seem to have considered the possibility that under the usual clinical circumstances plasma levels of indomethacin do not become high enough to displace a clinically significant amount of anticoagulant compound even though such a possibility might theoretically exist. Plasma levels of phenylbutazone (Burns *et al.*, 1953) after administration of therapeutic doses to human subjects are higher than those of indomethacin by several orders of magnitude. Such high levels of indomethacin cannot be safely achieved, and one can only speculate whether changes in warfarin pharmacodynamics would be seen under such circumstances.

An analogous situation is that of displacement of thiopental. Aspirin and phenylbutazone administered to rats which had just regained the righting reflex after an anesthetic dose of thiopental returned the rats to a sleeping condition (Chaplin *et al.*, 1973) by displacing thiopental from plasma binding sites so that the level of free thiopental was increased. Indomethacin showed the same ability as aspirin and phenylbutazone to displace thiopental at the same *in vitro* concentrations, but it could not be shown to reinduce thiopental sleep in mice. Phenylbutazone at 50 mg kg^{-1} intravenously reinduced sleep in 40 per cent of the animals, but 50 mg kg^{-1} of indomethacin under the same conditions was lethal. Such a dose is well within the range often used to demonstrate anti-inflammatory activity of phenylbutazone, but far above the doses of indo-methacin.

The quantitative and molecular aspects of drug protein binding were discussed in detail at a recent symposium (Anton and Solomon, 1973). These physical and biochemical studies should provide a rationale basis in further consideration of any clinical effects.

6.5.3   Indomethacin–probenecid interactions

Skeith *et al.* (1968) observed that administration of probenecid doubled the blood levels of radioactivity in patients receiving labelled indomethacin. The effect was attributed to a reduction in renal tubular secretion. However, the rate of plasma level increase and the concentrations achieved suggest that this might not be the sole mechanism involved. Yesair *et al.* (1970b) obtained comparable results in rats. According to their data, when a large dose of probenecid was given intravenously 3 hours after indomethacin—while the indomethacin plasma level was falling—there was a significant rise in indo-methacin concentration. This result, if confirmed, suggests a continuing (perhaps even increased) absorption of indomethacin accompanied by a fall in renal excretion. The net effect was the opposite of the action of salicylate on blood level of indomethacin; the authors suggested that salicylates might inhibit intestinal absorption while increasing biliary and fecal excretion.

Brooks *et al.* (1974) confirmed Skeith's findings in human patients, and further reported that the increased blood level of indomethacin produced by the indomethacin-probenecid interaction resulted in improved therapeutic activity in patients with rheumatoid arthritis without a corresponding increase in side effects. The significance of this seemingly paradoxical finding requires further elucidation. Duggan *et al.* (1977b) showed that probenecid depresses the biliary clearance of indomethacin in dogs and monkeys. The possible correlation of this depression with intestinal tolerance was considered.

6.5.4   Interactions between indomethacin and other nonsteroid anti-inflammatory agents

Interactions between indomethacin and other nonsteroid antiinflammatory compounds, especially aspirin, have received considerable attention and yielded some conflicting results. Optical studies of serum albumin binding sites by Chignell and Starkweather (1971) indicated that aspirin alters the molecular architecture of the binding sites for phenylbutazone and flufenamic acid. The effect was seen with acetylsalicylic acid, but not with salicylic acid. These authors did not include indomethacin in their study, but they found that the acetylation of the human serum albumin had opposite effects upon binding of phenylbutazone and of flufenamic acid, binding of the former being increased and the latter decreased.

According to Mason and McQueen (1974) indomethacin and phenylbutazone complete for the same binding site, and indomethacin not only displaces phenylbutazone because of its higher affinity, but in the presence of phenylbutazone, indomethacin binding is increased. Salicylate and ibuprofen, on the other hand, displace indomethacin even though they have lower affinity constants. This was interpreted by the authors on the assumption that salicylate and ibuprofen cannot attach to the primary binding site when it is occupied by indomethacin, so they attach to secondary sites, which in turn produces such structural alterations in the primary site that indomethacin is released.

Phenylbutazone at 50 mg kg^{-1} orally or intravenously in rats did not affect plasma levels of ^{14}C-indomethacin according to Yesair et al. (1970b) but salicylic acid significantly decreased ^{14}C concentration. This effect was accompanied by increased biliary and fecal excretion, so apparently bound indomethacin was released and then excreted in the bile. Although the results were obtained with high dose levels, the findings were consistent with those of Mason and McQueen mentioned above. The report by Hogans et al. (1971) is slightly at variance since, although aspirin reduced plasma radioactivity after ^{14}C-indomethacin, there was no increase in biliary secretion. In experiments by Jeremy and Towson (1970), when human subjects ingested 100 mg of labelled indomethacin, plasma levels of ^{14}C were lower if the subjects received large doses of aspirin for several days before the experiment. These results are not necessarily related to plasma binding, however, and can be interpreted as an effect upon intestinal absorption, as the authors pointed out. Another nonsteroid antiinflammatory compound, naproxen, is also displaced from binding sites by aspirin according to Segre et al. (1974), resulting in lower plasma levels and increased renal clearance, though the effect was said to be so small as to be of doubtful clinical significance.

Rubin et al. (1973) noted significant reductions in peak plasma concentration of either fenoprofen or indomethacin in the presence of aspirin in normal human volunteers. Total area under the time-concentration curve for indomethacin, however, was not uniformly reduced. A thorough study on the effect of aspirin on plasma concentration and physiological disposition of indomethacin has been conducted by Kwan and colleagues. Using the total area under the plasma concentration curve as the criterion of effect, Kwan found that a single 1·2 g dose of aspirin reduced the plasma level of indomethacin after a single 50 mg dose by 8 per cent, but daily treatment with aspirin for 1 week reduced plasma indomethacin by 20 per cent. Chronic aspirin also decreased renal clearance of indomethacin, as well as efficiency of gastrointestinal absorption; biliary clearance and enterohepatic circulation were increased.

Some investigators have obtained data inconsistent with the above reports. Champion *et al.* (1972) could not detect any difference in serum levels of indomethacin in either normal human volunteers or in arthritic patients in the absence of salicylate or after ingestion of 3·6 to 5 g of aspirin daily. Lindquist *et al.* (1974) gave 100 mg of indomethacin to human volunteers in the form of suppositories and followed blood levels for 8 hours. Serum concentration was unaffected by oral administration of 1 g of calcium aspirin whether given concurrently, before, or after indomethacin. The concentration curves of the two drugs were said to be independent of each other.

To complete the confusion, plasma levels of indomethacin in subjects receiving single doses of 100 mg were said to be significantly higher when buffered aspirin was given before and concurrently than when the indomethacin was given alone (Garnham *et al.*, 1974). The effect was seen 30 minutes and 1 hour after ingestion of indomethacin and seemed to be due to more rapid absorption in the presence of the buffered aspirin. The results seem to be the opposite of those reported by Jeremy and Towson (1970). An obvious difference in the two studies was in the use of buffered versus unbuffered aspirin, but the significance of this difference would become clear only after further exploration.

The subject of aspirin–indomethacin interaction in plasma binding sites is, of course, of clinical importance only if it is reflected in therapeutic actions. The report by Mainland and the Cooperating Committee of the American Rheumatism Association (1967) indicated that patients taking large doses of aspirin received little or no further benefit when indomethacin was added; the study did not include any patients on indomethacin alone. Brooks *et al.* (1975) also saw no clinical advantage of administering both indomethacin and aspirin, and indeed their patients preferred indomethacin alone to the combination.

Further clinical evidence along this line is scarce, but there have been a number of animal experiments in an attempt to find an experimental basis for the Mainland report. Mielens *et al.* (1968) reported that neither indomethacin nor phenylbutazone was additive to aspirin in the carrageenan edema assay. A similar result was obtained by Swingle and co-workers (1970) who found no combination of the three nonsteroid compounds gave an additive result with any of the others, though each of them was additive to steroids. Swingle *et al.* (1971b) also found diflumidone to be additive with steroids but not with indomethacin, aspirin, or phenylbutazone. Evidence of increased side effects of aspirin–indomethacin combination compared to indomethacin alone is scarce, but Shaw and Wischmeier (1973) found the combination to be more ulcerogenic in rats than either drug alone.

Van Arman *et al.* (1973) reported that aspirin antagonized indomethacin in adjuvant arthritis in rats. The antagonism was seen with remarkedly small doses of aspirin and was seen even if the aspirin was discontinued before instituting indomethacin treatment. In this study, a wide variety of drugs reduced the effect of indomethacin, small doses of aspirin prevented the effects of large doses of aspirin given later, and even small doses of indomethacin abolished the action of antiinflammatory doses of indomethacin given at appropriate times later. The results do not permit any simple explanation, nor is the application to the clinical situation apparent. Also, these authors found aspirin to antagonize cortisol, quite the opposite of findings which others had reported; however, experimental conditions were quite different. Previous reports of nonsteroid–steroid combinations had been concerned with acute tests (carrageenan edema inhibition) in contrast to Van Arman's arthritic rats.

According to Standish *et al.* (1972) even in acute tests one can observe either additive effects, antagonism, or no interaction between aspirin and indomethacin depending upon the dosage schedule, the model used, and the time of measurement of the effect.

About all that one can conclude about all these observations is that aspirin and indomethacin can interact, and that one must exercise caution in interpreting clinical results in cases where more than one nonsteroid antiinflammatory compounds are given at the same time. The circumstances under which antagonism, additive effects, or no interaction occur are far from having been elucidated.

Of the indomethacin analogs discussed in previous sections of this report, no data are available on their possible interaction with aspirin, except for one series of experiments with sulindac. In the paper by Van Arman and colleagues (1973) one way to demonstrate the inhibiting effect of a compound on adjuvant arthritis in the rat was to administer the drug on days—1, 0 and +1, with day 1 being the day of injection of adjuvant. If no further drug is administered, measurement of foot swelling on day 14 will show the inhibitory action of an active drug. Van Arman (in press, *Scand. J. Rheumat.*) has shown that sulindac exhibits the same interaction with aspirin in this test as seen with indomethacin and certain other antiinflammatory agents. For example, 0·5 mg kg^{-1} of sulindac on each of the 3 days mentioned, gave 57 per cent inhibition of foot swelling on day 14. When aspirin was administered together with the sulindac in doses ranging from 0·75 mg kg^{-1} to 6 mg kg^{-1}, inhibition ranged from 11 to 43 per cent, with no clear relationship between aspirin dose and degree of antagonism to sulindac. Strangely, perhaps, a higher dose of aspirin, 12 mg kg^{-1}, did not significantly alter the action of sulindac.

The finding with regard to sulindac–aspirin combination is in agreement with Van Arman's published data on various combinations of antiinflammatory compounds; namely, the antagonism shows considerable variability. In terms of biochemical mechanism of action of these drugs, the partial inhibition of the acetylation of cyclooxygenase by aspirin by indo-methacin (Stanford *et al.*, 1977) indicates that two drugs are competing for two related, or overlapping, but non-identical binding sites in cyclooxygenase. This kind of interaction may be only one of several involved in the overall biological efficacy of these drugs.

7   Mechanisms of action

7.1   INTRODUCTION

Investigations on the mechanism(s) of action of antiinflammatory drugs, both steroid and nonsteroid, have been stimulated at least in part by the hope that knowledge of the mode of action would help in the design of new and better drugs. Ideas in this active field of investigation have been subject to rapid change. The rapidly growing literature has stimulated several extensive reviews; recent volumes of the Annual Review of Pharmacology have included summaries by Paulus and Whitehouse (1973) and by Ferreira and Vane (1974), while Flower (1974) outlined certain aspects of the problem in Pharmacological Reviews. An excellent short summary is that by McQueen (1974). In the volume edited by Robinson and Vane (1974) on "Prostaglandin Synthetase Inhibitors", several papers are devoted to mechanisms, especially that by Vane (p. 155). Some follow-up investigations are described in the two volume "Advances in Prostaglandin and Thromboxane Research" edited by Samuelsson and Paoletti (1976). A comprehensive treatment is that by Hichens (1974).

Experimental activities aimed at producing a unifying biochemical concept to account for antiinflammatory activity have led to a variety of suggestions regarding possible modes of action. Under appropriate experimental con-ditions, active compounds have been found to stabilize plasma proteins, to possess important membrane stabilizing properties, and to inhibit the activities of various cellular or plasma enzyme systems. Among the latter effects, that on prostaglandin synthetase has received special attention in recent reports. Evidence in favor of such inhibition as an important mechanism of action has been presented in very persuasive terms, but in order to put it in perspective it should be considered against the background of other contenders for attention. There has been no lack of suggestions and hypotheses regarding mechanisms of antiinflammatory action. One of these, that of displacement of plasma corticosteroids, has been dealt with above (section 6.5.1) and will not be further discussed here.

7.2   UNCOUPLING OF OXIDATIVE PHOSPHORYLATION

The various antiinflammatory drugs, although they belong to different chemical classes, share certain biochemical properties. Among these is the

ability *in vitro* to inhibit the synthesis of compounds containing high energy
phosphate bonds without simultaneously depressing the oxygen consumption
of living cells. This dissociation of phosphorylation and oxidation is termed
"uncoupling". Pharmacologically active substances of many kinds are
uncoupling agents (Brody, 1955). Brody (1956) related uncoupling to toxicity
rather than to therapeutic activity, but Adams and Cobb (1958) suggested a
relationship between uncoupling ability and antiinflammatory activity. It may
be hypothesized that uncoupling could deprive inflamed areas of energy-
dependent processes needed to support the active metabolizing activities
sustaining the inflammation.

A correlation between antiinflammatory activity and uncoupling has been
claimed for such compounds as aspirin, phenylbutazone and indomethacin.
From such considerations, there arose the idea that antiinflammatory
compounds owe their therapeutic activity to their uncoupling ability, and
during the 1960s a considerable literature appeared on the subject. The concept
was especially developed by Whitehouse who has reviewed it in detail (1965).
There are, however, many instances in which the expected correlation is
absent, concentrations required to demonstrate the effect are high, and no new
therapeutic agents have been developed by following uncoupling as a lead.

More recently, attempts to explain antiinflammatory activity have taken
other directions, and interest in the uncoupling theory has diminished. Van den
Berg and Nauta (1975) examined a large series of 2-aryl-1,3-indandiones
which were more active uncoupling agents than indomethacin but which had
less antiinflammatory activity than phenylbutazone. Within the series, no
correlation between the two activities could be detected.

7.3 EFFECTS ON MEDIATORS OF INFLAMMATION

A traumatic disturbance producing inflammation activates a very complicated
process in which several stages may be distinguished. Ordinarily, the final stage
is repair of the injury and restoration of the injured tissue to a healthy state.
Antiinflammatory drugs are used to diminish the manifestations of the active
phases of inflammation, rather than specifically to promote the restorative
phase. Diverse traumatic stimuli produce inflammatory responses having much
in common, suggesting the release of common mediators. Much research has
sought to delineate these mediators, and the effects of drugs upon them.

The major attention of investigators has shifted from one mediator to
another as research has progressed. Vasoactive amines, especially histamine
and serotonin, were objects of special consideration in the early phases of work
on inflammation, followed by the kinins. Currently, the role of prostaglandins
and their reactive hydroperoxide intermediates is the focus of attention. This
historical succession coincides with the order in which mediators are released

during the development of inflammation produced by subcutaneous injection of carrageenan according to sequential analysis by Willis (1969) and by DiRosa et al. (1971). Several other mediators have been described but less well characterized chemically, such as "slow reacting substance in anaphylaxis" (SRS-A) and "lymph node permeability factor" (LNPF). For detailed discussion of mediators, the reader is referred to the volume edited by Spector (1964), and those by Spector and Willoughby and by Rocha e Silva and Garcia-Leme (references 64 and 65 in Ferreira and Vane, 1974).

Most investigators agree that vasoactive amines are involved in early stages of inflammation (carrageenan edema, for example) but antihistaminic drugs do not prevent the delayed phases of inflammation, nor are antiinflammatory drugs notable for antihistaminic activity. Cyproheptadine, a potent antihistaminic and antiserotonin agent, does not prevent carrageenan edema (Winter, 1965; Vinegar et al., 1969) nor does indomethacin inhibit serotonin edema (Winter, 1965). In high concentrations, indomethacin can inhibit in vitro release of histamine by histidine decarboxylase (Skidmore and Whitehouse, 1966a) but the hypothesis of Schayer (1963) that antiinflammatory action can be explained by inhibition of histidine decarboxylase has not met with widespread acceptance.

Bradykinin-induced bronchial spasms in the guinea-pig can be inhibited by nonsteroid antiinflammatory agents, but this action seems not to be correlated with antiinflammatory activity. Carrageenan edema, widely used for antiinflammatory screening, is suppressed by depletion of plasma kininogens (DiRosa and Sorrentino, 1970; Briseid et al., 1971), the amount of suppression being directly correlated with the degree of depletion. Edema induced by egg white or by dextran appears to be mediated by histamine and serotonin (DiRosa and Sorrentino, 1970). Indomethacin, highly active against carrageenan edema, is relatively ineffective against egg white or dextran edema (Winter, 1965).

In spite of an apparent correlation between the effectiveness of indomethacin and the importance of kinin mediators in diverse types of inflammation, antiinflammatory action cannot be fully explained on the basis of direct antagonism of kinins or by blocking their release. Indomethacin can inhibit some local effects of intradermal bradykinin, according to Pelczarska and Gieldowski (1970), but the action seems to be nonspecific, and the degree of activity of various compounds appears not to be correlated with antiinflammatory potency. Edema induced by injection of bradykinin in the rat's foot is not antagonized by indomethacin (Van Arman and Nuss, 1969), nor does indomethacin inhibit the permeability enhancing effect of bradykinin (Walters and Willoughby, 1965). It has been suggested that indomethacin may interfere with the activation of kallikrein (Miller and Melmon, 1972, quoted by McQueen, 1973), but Davies et al. (1966) found no effect upon the release of kinin as mediated by kallikrein. The latter is in accord with the findings of Van Arman and Nuss (1969). Rats with adjuvant arthritis exhibited high levels of plasma bradykininogen which was not affected by indomethacin in doses sufficient to control other manifestations of adjuvant disease. *In vitro*, neither bradykinin formation from plasma by trypsin nor kallidin formation by kallikrein were prevented by indomethacin (Van Arman *et al.*, 1968). It seems fair to conclude that an explanation of antiinflammatory activity was not found in these investigations.

Among the mediators of inflammation, prostaglandins have assumed such prominence in recent research that they will be discussed in a later section of this report (7.9).

7.4 STABILIZATION OF LYSOSOMES

The hypothesis that antiinflammatory activity should be related to lysosomal stabilization is based on the presumed capacity of lysosomal enzymes to produce tissue damage with resulting inflammation, release of chemical mediators, attraction of leucocytes and all the other sequelae relevant to inflammatory disease, acute or chronic. It follows that prevention of release of such destructive substances as lysosomal enzymes should lessen the manifestations of inflammation. Evidence that antiinflammatory compounds act in this way is, however, far from clear. Even the word "lysosome" seems to have different connotations for various investigators. Thus, McQueen (1973) defined lysosomes as "intracellular organelles taking the form of granules", while Paulus and Whitehouse (1973) regarded the lysosome as not really a body, but a part of a system; this system is a barrier—having some of the properties of a membrane—which limits accessibility of certain acid hydrolases to their substrates. Compounds or conditions which increase the activity of these enzymes in lysosomal preparations are said to labilize the membrane, while those which prevent the release of the active form of the enzyme are said to stabilize it.

It has been held that antiinflammatory steroids have the ability to stabilize lysosomal membranes while most nonsteroids do not. The literature has been reviewed in detail by Hichens (1974). Much of the renewed interest in nonsteroidal compounds as lysosomal stabilizers stems from the work of Ignarro (references in Hichens). More recent papers by Douwes (1974) and Nakanishi and Goto (1975) also claim lysosomal stabilization by indomethacin and other nonsteroidal compounds.

There are many inconsistencies in the data, however, and it is far from established that lysosomal stabilization offers a satisfactory explanation for the action of the drugs. Examples of contradictory findings are to be found in the *in vitro* studies by Ignarro (1971) and Ignarro and Colombo (1972). Lysosomes from guinea-pig polymorphonuclear leucocytes or from the livers of rats or rabbits were stabilized, while those from polymorphonuclear leucocytes of rabbits were labilized. Furthermore, the potency of various compounds in inhibiting enzyme release from guinea-pig PMNs was not parallel to their anti-inflammatory action. Such considerations led Ferreira and Vane (1974) to reject the lysosomal hypothesis.

Ignarro (1972) also described stabilization of rat liver lysosomes derived from animals which had received antiinflammatory compounds systemically. However, the *in vivo* activity was demonstrated only after doses known to be highly toxic to rats. Indomethacin was ineffective even when given as two oral doses of 5 mg kg^{-1} each daily. This is an amount many times higher than those needed to demonstrate antiinflammatory activity in rats. According to Pollock and Brown (1971) indomethacin and phenylbutazone are ineffective *in vivo* as lysosomal stabilizers at antiinflammatory doses. Ackerman and Beebe (1975) could demonstrate no effect of aspirin or indomethacin (even at the relatively high concentrations of 10^{-4} or 10^{-3} M) upon the release of beta-glucuronidase from guinea pig alveolar mononuclear cells in which lysosomal release was induced by phagocytosis of zymosan particles.

Paulus and Whitehouse (1973) have presented a thoughtful critique of reports on lysosomal stabilization, and the reader is referred there for discussion of many investigations not mentioned above. More recently, in their analysis of carrageenan induced inflammation, Vinegar and coworkers (1976) suggested that lysosomal enzymes are not the edema producing agents *per se*, but that they are responsible for activation of the prostaglandin biosynthetic pathway.

7.5 CELL MEMBRANE AND CELL MIGRATION EFFECTS

Lists of biochemical actions of antiinflammatory drugs have been presented in previous publications from our laboratories (Winter, 1971; Shen, 1972). Among these actions, cell membrane activity has received special attention from several investigators; indeed, it has been stated that ". . . when the final explanation for antiinflammatory drug action becomes available, it will resolve itself around the central theme of 'membrane stabilization'" (Glenn and Sekhar, 1971).

Actions on cell membranes may be related to the effects of the compounds upon protein stabilization, ligand interactions, cellular migration, and cell permeability. Reactions of antiinflammatory drugs with cellular membranes have been widely studied in the erythrocyte (Kahlben *et al.*, 1970; Görög and Kovacs, 1970; Glenn *et al.*, 1971; Brown *et al.*, 1971). Mizushima *et al.* (1970) sought to explain antiinflammatory activity on the basis of protein stabilization within the membrane. Indomethacin readily binds to plasma protein, and a small concentration of indomethacin added to a solution of plasma albumin confers such remarkable resistance to denaturation by heat that the reaction forms the basis of a proposed simple screening procedure for anti-inflammatory activity. Other serum proteins and other denaturing conditions yielded similar evidence of stabilizing activity of the compound (for reference, see Hichens, 1974).

Inflammation is generally accompanied by accumulation of leucocytes, both polymorphonuclear and mononuclear cells. A number of investigators have sought to demonstrate the ability of antiinflammatory compounds to decrease motility or prevent accumulation of such cells. Phelps and McCarty (1967) observed a decrease in motility of polymorphonuclear leucocytes (PMNs) in the Boyden chamber in the presence of urate crystals exposed to indomethacin, and suggested this effect as a mechanism of the action of the drug in gout. When DiRosa and Willoughby (1971) saw evidence of a parallelism between cell migration and swelling in carrageenan edema, they suggested that ability to provoke migration of leucocytes is a necessary attribute of a model of acute inflammation seeking to discover new antiinflammatory drugs.

On the other hand, the data of Van Arman et al. (1970a, 1971) and of Chang (1972) in dogs injected with urate crystals into the synovial space of the stifle joint, showed that indomethacin relieved the distress of the inflammation without affecting the number of leucocytes at the inflammatory site. Vinegar and co-workers (1976) also described reduction of carrageenan edema by indomethacin and aspirin without affecting neutrophil mobilization. In other experiments (Van Arman et al., 1970b) it was shown that indomethacin inhibits the Schwartzman reaction in rabbits without preventing the gathering of leucocytes at the reaction site. In all of these experiments, manifestations of inflammation were clearly not related to the accumulation of neutrophils. In human patients, Williamson and Holt (1968) found that treatment with anti-inflammatory drugs, steroid or nonsteroid, did not affect either total or differential cell count in synovial fluid.

The above evidence suggests that antiinflammatory action may not be primarily related to migration of PMNs. It has been suggested that active compounds may inhibit migration of monocytes. Accumulation of monocytes in certain types of inflammation has been linked with the release of prostaglandins (Willoughby and DiRosa, 1972; DiRosa et al., 1972). In the view of these investigators, monocytes are responsible for chronic inflammation, and in the models of inflammation used in their experiments the inhibition of prostaglandin release seemed to be secondary to inhibition of monocyte migration. Blackham and Owen (1975), however, regarded the action of anti-inflammatory drugs to be related to their ability to decrease the synthesis of chemotactic prostaglandins, leading secondarily to a decrease in numbers of migratory cells reaching an inflamed site. McCall and Youlton (1974) also suggested a PGE_1 mediated chemotactic mechanism as a point of attack by indomethacin, but later study (Ford-Hutchinson *et al.*, 1976) failed to confirm the chemotactic activity of freshly prepared PGE_1 solution at up to 100 mg ml^{-1}. The same group of investigators further showed that in an implanted sponge system the production of prostaglandins and the accumulation of leukocytes, including both PMN and monocytes, in the inflammatory exudates are separate events. The concentrations of indomethacin required to inhibit prostaglandin synthesis and leukocyte migration are 1 mg kg^{-1} and 3–6 mg kg^{-1} body weight, respectively (Walker *et al.*, 1976). When applied locally on the sponge before implantation, indomethacin is effective at 1 mg per sponge in inhibiting both processes.

Others have also seen evidence of cellular changes in inflammation which can be corrected by indomethacin. Hyaluronic acid is known to accumulate in inflamed joints, and indomethacin decreases the amount accumulated. The accumulation of hyaluronic acid is possibly stimulated by leucocytes, and Yaron *et al.* (1971) demonstrated such an effect of leucocytes on fibroblasts in tissue culture. This action of leucocytes could be abolished by indomethacin in a concentration well within the limits known to be present in body fluids after therapeutic doses. Williamson and Holt (1968) described alterations in staining reactions of leucocytes of patients responding favorably to indomethacin.

Other evidence of changes in surface properties of leucocytes under the influence of antiinflammatory drugs included the changes in the tendency of mononuclear cells to adhere to subcutaneously implanted glass or cellophane (DiRosa *et al.*, 1971b) and reduction by systemically administered indomethacin of the uptake of colloidal carbon by monocytes in animals deprived of PMNs (DiRosa *et al.*, 1971a). On the other hand, phagocytosis by PMNs is probably not affected by antiinflammatory drugs. Chang (1968) described suppression of phagocytosis of starch granules *in vitro*, but high concentrations of drug were required, and correlation between antiphagocytic activity and antiinflammatory potency was not impressive. According to Van Arman (personal communication) indomethacin does not suppress phagocytosis of crystalline sodium urate in the synovial fluid of the dog.

7.6 INHIBITION OF ENZYMES

Among the biochemical effects of antiinflammatory drugs, inhibition of various enzyme systems has long occupied a conspicuous place. In section 7.2, we discussed the uncoupling of oxidative phosphorylation. A corollary of the depression of the formation of high energy phosphate bonds is an inhibition of the biosynthesis of mucopolysaccharide. The enzymes involved in mucopolysaccharide biosynthesis are inhibited by antiinflammatory compounds, and those derived from connective tissue are more sensitive to such inhibition than are those from liver according to Bollet (1961).

The incorporation of ^{35}S, ^{32}P, ^{14}C-glucose or acetate into the polysaccharide of cartilage or other tissue has been used as a measure of metabolic activity susceptible to inhibition by drugs. Indomethacin in a concentration of 0·5 mM produced more than 50 per cent inhibition of ^{35}S incorporation into polysaccharide sulfate in cartilage slices *in vitro* (Whitehouse and Boström, 1965). Such a concentration is, however, several orders of magnitude higher than that encountered in body fluids after therapeutic doses.

Proteases from PMN and other inflammatory cells are involved in tissue destruction (Janoff, 1972), complement activation (Ward and Zwaifler, 1971) and stimulation of lymphocytes (Vischer *et al.*, 1976). Many polypeptides from a breakdown of tissue proteins, have a high degree of biological activity. Hence, inhibition of proteolytic enzymes might modify some of the manifestations of inflammation. Mörsdorf (1965) tested the ability of antiinflammatory drugs to inhibit the breakdown of rat paw homogenates by autogenous enzymes and found that the potency of several compounds in this assay paralleled their antiinflammatory activity. Indomethacin administered orally, however, did not inhibit edema induced in the rat's paw by trypsin (Domenjoz and Mörsdorf, 1965). Whitehouse and Skidmore (1965) proposed that certain enzymic reactions involved in inflammation depend upon the availability of epsilon-amino groups, and that antiinflammatory drugs inhibit these reactions by binding such groups. As an additional mechanism, they proposed (Skidmore and Whitehouse, 1966b) a competitive inhibition of certain enzymes such as dopa decarboxylase and chymotrypsin. Their data, however, indicated that the active compounds which they tested were effective only in unrealistically high concentrations, and there seemed to be no correlation between their *in vitro* activity and their known *in vivo* potencies. Indomethacin, in fact, failed to inhibit chymotrypsin, but was itself hydrolyzed by the enzyme.

Enzyme inhibition by antiinflammatory drugs at high levels and in a relatively nonspecific manner is probably related to the well-known binding of these compounds to proteins. As discussed by Hichens (1974) these studies have not yielded an explanation for the therapeutic value of antiinflammatory drugs. Recent studies of enzyme inhibition have centered upon enzymes involved in the synthesis of prostaglandins. The discovery that antiinflammatory compounds inhibit prostaglandin synthetase has given a whole new direction to the investigation of the mechanism of action of these drugs, and we shall devote a separate section of this review to this activity (section 7.9).

7.7 FIBRINOLYTIC ACTIVITY

Glynn (1963) produced a response resembling arthritis in rabbits by intra-articular injection of fibrin. The Glynn model is still sometimes used in research on synovial inflammation, but, owing to the amount of time and effort involved, has not been widely employed in assessing the activity of anti-inflammatory drugs. A reaction resembling rheumatoid nodules could also be produced by subcutaneous injection of fibrin. Glynn's work is one of a number of observations indicating a possible correlation between clotting mechanisms or fibrinolysis and joint disease. Glenn and Sekhar (1971) pointed out that all substances which promote clotting *in vitro* produce inflammation *in vivo*.

Some workers have suggested a possible correlation between anti-inflammatory and fibrinolytic activities of compounds. Roubal and Nemecek (1966) described fibrinolytic action of several compounds *in vitro*; indomethacin at concentrations on the order of 6×10^{-3} M produced complete lysis of a plasma clot. Similar activities were found for anthranilic acid derivatives (Gryglewski and Gryglewski, 1966). Von Kaulla (1967) suggested that indomethacin and similar drugs inhibit a plasma factor which prevents the activity of fibrinolytic plasma activator; thus freed, the activator induces fibrinolysis.

None of these studies has produced satisfactory evidence of a correlation between fibrinolytic activity and antiinflammatory potency. Indomethacin did not exhibit outstanding fibrinolytic activity compared to other compounds. A connection between this sort of activity and therapeutic effectiveness at useful concentrations has not been demonstrated.

7.8 SULFHYDRYL-DISULFIDE STABILIZATION

Gerber (1965) suggested that a metabolic defect might lead to an increased rate of disulfide-sulfhydryl (SS-SH) interchange in rheumatoid arthritis, with subsequent protein denaturation, inflammation, and antibody formation. Lorber (1966) reported a deficiency in SH groups in the sera of patients with connective tissue disease. Gerber *et al.* (1966, 1967) found that anti-inflammatory drugs accelerated the reaction between SH groups and 5,5'-dithiobis-(2-nitrobenzoic acid) (DTNB or Ellman's reagent), and suggested this as a possible basis of their therapeutic activity. Indomethacin (Gerber, 1966) was the most active of many compounds tested. The reaction of DTNB in plasma was presumably a measure of SH groups, and the increase in rate might be attributed to drug-induced changes in conformation of the plasma proteins. Suzuki (1966) suggested that enzymes which release bradykinin from its precursor bradykininogen attach the disulfide linkages within the precursor molecule, and antiinflammatory compounds might prevent release of bradykinin by preventing this reaction.

Oronsky *et al.* (1969) reported that the effectiveness of indomethacin or of aspirin could be diminished by adding a sulfhydryl donor (cysteine). Their criterion of inflammation was the increase in weight of cotton sponges during the first 24 hours after implantation. According to Swingle (1974), weighing the granuloma within 4 days of implantation measures mainly transudation and exudation, not the formation of new connective tissue.

Butler *et al.* (1969) reported a marked reduction in the rate of SS-SH interchange in rats with adjuvant arthritis as judged by changes in optical density between 1 and 2 minutes after adding DTNB. This abnormality was seen before signs of arthritis could be detected, and was corrected by steroid or nonsteroid antiinflammatory drugs.

The significance of these and other studies has been discussed by Hichens (1974). The rate of reaction of DTNB in plasma depends not only upon the concentration of SH groups, but also partly upon the concentration of free DTNB. DTNB, like antiinflammatory drugs, is extensively bound to plasma proteins, and when antiinflammatory drugs compete with DTNB for binding sites, the ratio of free to bound DTNB increases. The increase seen in the rate of reaction in the presence of antiinflammatory drugs, then, is not necessarily due to an increase in concentration of reactive SH groups, but to an increase in concentration of free DTNB. Indeed, Hichens found that the number of reactive SH groups as determined by the maximum extent of the reaction, was unchanged by the drugs.

In summary, it seems fair to conclude that stabilization of the SS-SH linkage has not been established as an explanation for the therapeutic effectiveness of antiinflammatory compounds.

7.9   PROSTAGLANDIN SYNTHESIS

Research reports, review articles, and symposium proceedings on prostaglandins are appearing at such a rate that entire books and even special journals are devoted exclusively to the activities of these pharmacologically potent lipids, and to the relationships between prostaglandins (PGs) and drugs, especially antiinflammatory compounds. Actions of indomethacin have figured prominently in these publications. In the review by Hinman (1972) he stated, "... it is no longer feasible to review the entire field in a single short paper". From the point of view of this present review, the value of these efforts has been in their contributions toward the understanding of how indomethacin and its congeners work, and conversely, the usefulness of these compounds in helping to elucidate the physiological importance of PGs.

Although PGs originally were named because they were assumed to be derived from the prostate gland, they have a wide distribution within the animal kingdom. PG synthetase activity has been found in all or nearly all mammalian tissues which have been investigated, as well as in certain other vertebrates and in several invertebrates (Christ and Van Dorp, 1973), but the highest enzymic activity is in the seminal vesicle (Sih and Takeguchi, 1973). New prostaglandins and related metabolites are continually being identified. In addition to the primary PGEs, PGF_as and PGAs, the reactive endoperoxides (PGG and PGH) and the newly discovered thromboxanes and prostacyclines (PGI_2) are of special interest to inflammation.

Summaries of the chemical syntheses and biosyntheses of the PGs include those by Weinshenker and Andersen (1973), Sih and Takegucki (1973) and by Samuelsson *et al.* (1975). Flower (1974) lists a number of reviews of the subject. The enzyme system acts with great rapidity, and PGs are formed from unsaturated fatty acids (arachidonic acid, for example) which in turn are formed from triglycerides by tissue lipases and from phospholipids by phospholipases (Bowery and Lewis, 1973). An outline of the synthetase pathway is shown below.

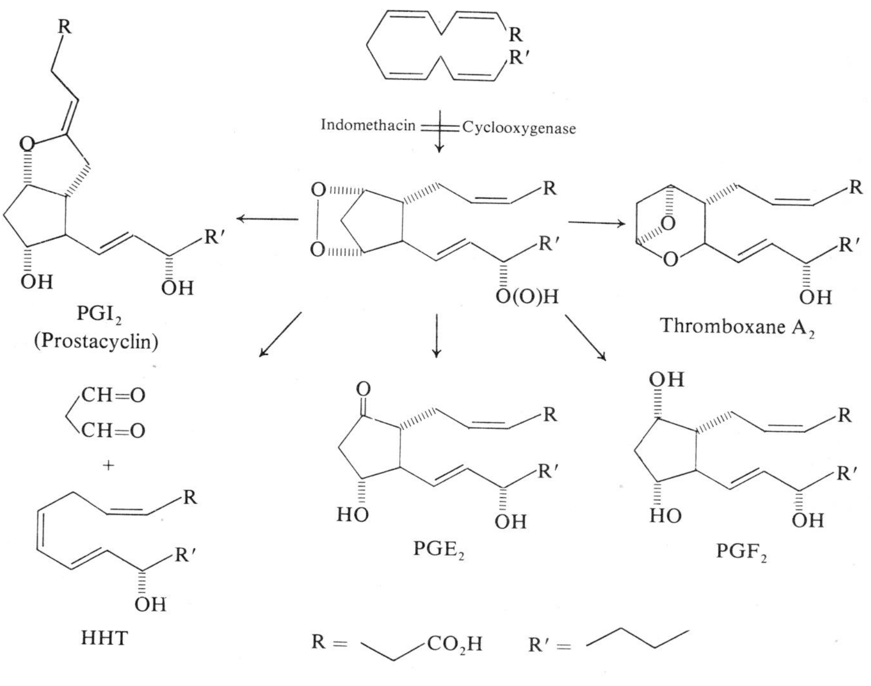

Stimuli which produce inflammation activate this system, and many studies have indicated that PGs and their biosynthetic intermediates can be inflammation mediators. Antiinflammatory compounds inhibit the conversion of unsaturated fatty acids to PG. It is on this basis that investigators working at the Royal College of Surgeons of England proposed the hypothesis which Ferreira and Vane (1974) summarized as follows: ". . . this enzyme effect is the mechanism of action of aspirin-like drugs." This thesis was developed in a long series of papers beginning with the publication by Vane (1971). Lists of these and other papers, as well as summaries of the hypothesis, have been presented in several reviews, such as that by Ferreira and Vane (1974) and Flower (1974), and in the volumes edited by Robinson and Vane (1974), and Samuelsson and Paoletti (1976).

Many of these papers refer to nonsteroid antiinflammatory compounds as "aspirin-like drugs" on the basis that they share the properties of analgesia, antipyresis, antiinflammation, and PG-synthetase inhibition. There is general agreement, however, that aspirin is not particularly potent in inhibiting the synthetase, and indomethacin is several orders of magnitude more active. Qualitative, as well as quantitative differences in their inhibitory actions on PG synthesis have also been noted (Stanford et al., 1977).

7.9.1   Prostaglandins as proinflammatory substances

Collier (1971) suggested that PGs may be considered as "local hormones"— humoral mediators which may serve some useful purpose when released in active form near their site of action, but producing undesirable effects if not promptly inactivated. Several lines of evidence indicate that PGs of either endogenous or exogenous origin induce inflammation. DiRosa et al. (1971a) presented data which strongly suggested that PGs are involved in carrageenan edema in rat's feet, though the release of PG did not occur in the absence of complement. According to Willis et al. (1972) PGE_2 has a role in carrageenan edema. Glenn et al. (1972) produced edema by injecting PGs into the tissue, the response varying both quantitatively and qualitatively depending upon the species of animal and the particular PG administered. PGE_1 was additive with several other inflammatory stimuli, though they did not rule out the possibility that the other substances might have induced release of endogenous PGs so that the combination was the equivalent of increasing the dose of PGE_1 injected. PGE_1 exhibited a bell-shaped dose response curve in the rat's paw, so that high doses failed to produce edema.

PGE_1 may also have been proinflammatory in the experiments of Thomas and West (1973) since it potentiated the vascular permeability effect of bradykinin in rat's skin, though it did not affect the actions of histamine, serotonin, or dextran. $PGF_{2\alpha}$ on the other hand, inhibited responses to all the non-PG mediators; it was not fully antiinflammatory, however, since it (like the other PGs examined) increased vascular permeability when used by itself.

Evidence is not lacking, however, that in some kinds of experiments, PGs may be antiinflammatory. Several investigators have noted suppression of adjuvant arthritis in rats by administering PGs, and according to Aspinall *et al.* (1973) the suppressant compounds include E_1, E_2, A_2 and $F_{2\alpha}$. Zurier and Ballas (1973) found histological evidence that injection of PGE_1 in adjuvant disease produced partial reversal of the inflammation. Both groups of workers suggested several possible explanations for the seemingly paradoxical effect of a proinflammatory substance ameliorating adjuvant disease, without expressing a preference for any particular explanation.

In human osteoarthritis, Robinson and McGuire (1974) reported evidence that PGE_2 is proinflammatory, promoting bone resorption. In addition, prostaglandins derived from rheumatoid synovia are capable of inducing bone destruction *in vitro* (Robinson *et al.*, 1975). Higgs *et al.* (1974) discussed the possible relationship of synovial PG release to the inflammation seen in rheumatoid arthritis. According to Hagenfeldt and Wennmalm (1975), rheumatoid arthritis is accompanied by accelerated biosynthesis of PGs, reflected by a significant reduction in free plasma arachidonic acid. Treatment with indomethacin led to a rise in arachidonic acid in arterial plasma. Moncada *et al.* (1974) argued in favor of the concept that synovial inflammation in animals induced by injection of carrageenan or urate is mediated by release of PGs into the synovial cavity. Direct injection of PGs into the knee joint of dogs produces inflammation (Rosenthale *et al.*, 1972). This effect has been related to the vasodilator activity of PGs (Grennan *et al.*, 1975), especially PGE_1.

Efforts have also been made to relate PGs to gouty arthritis. Denko (1974a) linked inflammation induced by monosodium urate crystals to PGE_1. In a subsequent paper (1974b) observations were extended to PGE_2, PGA_2, and $PGF_{2\alpha}$. Amounts as low as 1 ng enhanced the inflammatory action of urate, as determined by injection into the foot pad of rats deficient in fatty acids. The results can be interpreted as indicating that the inflammation induced by urate—and by inference, the arthritic symptoms of acute gout—may be related to the ability of the crystals to induce formation and release of PGs. Qualitatively similar effects were observed with all the PGs used.

It might be interesting to extend observations similar to those of Denko to crystal-induced synovitis in dogs as described by Phelps and McCarty (1966) or by Van Arman *et al.* (1970a). One observation by Denko showed that urate crystals which had been heated to 200°C did not stimulate release of PGs. Although the heat did not change the appearance of the crystals, Denko speculated that an electron shift might have occurred which changed the ability of the crystals to initiate action of PG-synthetase. Observations by Van Arman *et al.* (1974) may be pertinent; they related the ability of urate crystals to produce inflammation in dog's knee joints to the presence of adsorbed endotoxin. When extreme precautions were taken to assure that no endotoxin was adsorbed onto the crystals, injection did not produce the characteristic inflammatory reaction. Addition of *E. coli* endotoxin to such crystals, or even administration of the endotoxin by mouth, restored the proinflammatory effect of the urate.

Van Arman did not attempt to relate his observation to PGs, but all of these urate experiments taken together lead to the speculation that the combination of urate crystals and endotoxin may in some way activate PG-synthetase, and that application of heat, though producing no visible change in the crystals, may have inactivated the endotoxin so that PG synthetase was not activated. Even in the presence of crystals and endotoxin, inflammation might be prevented if the action of the synthetase were inhibited by antiinflammatory drugs. In addition to urate, deposits of pyrophosphate, calcium ortho-phosphate and hydroxyapatite have been identified in human cartilage. Hydroxyapatite, in particular, can cause an acute inflammatory reaction in animals and in man. Its potential importance to the etiology of osteoarthritis was discussed (Dieppe *et al.*, 1976).

Numerous other observations have sought to document the role of PGs in the signs and symptoms of inflammation. For a more complete survey of the literature, the reader is referred to other reviews, such as those by Ferreira *et al.* (1976), and a recent short review by Dunn *et al.* (1976).

7.9.2 *Platelets and prostaglandins*

Platelets adhere to the site of injury of blood vessel walls and form an aggregate (platelet thrombus) which is the initial physical barrier to blood flow out of the vessel. The aggregation is accompanied by a "release reaction"; platelet granule constituents, such as serotonin, are released which stimulate further aggregation so that the reaction is self-perpetuating. The second phase is inhibited by antiinflammatory drugs, with indomethacin being particularly potent. The mechanism by which this is brought about has received considerable attention (Kocsis *et al.*, 1973; Smith *et al.*, 1974.

The inhibition of the release reaction apparently has little clinically significant effect upon bleeding time or on the generation of thrombin (which comes at a later stage during hemostasis) in normal subjects, though large doses of aspirin may prolong bleeding time in hemophiliacs (Smith *et al.*, 1974).

Several suggestions have been made concerning clinical effects of the prevention of platelet aggregation by indomethacin, but relatively little that has met with widespread acceptance. Scheidt *et al.* (1974) suggested that this property of the drug might have a protective effect in cardiogenic shock, and Rubegini and co-workers (1975) suggested possible usefulness in prevention and treatment of thromboembolism. Such uses have not been established. On the other hand, inhibition of the adhesiveness and aggregation of platelets may lead to hemorrhagic complications in certain instances (Martyak, 1974). In this connection, it may be pertinent to recall that (contrary to what is often assumed) hemorrhagic complications due to displacement of anticoagulant drugs from binding sites is not a clinically significant effect of indomethacin (see section 6.4.2), although some antiinflammatory drugs have displacement effects at therapeutic doses.

Not all patients exhibit changes in platelet aggregation tests when they receive indomethacin (Ciavarelli et al., 1974). According to De Gaetano et al. (1974), those patients with chronic glomerular nephritis who did not respond by inhibition of platelet aggregation also did not respond by reduction in urinary excretion of an antigen related to fibrin. Formation of the antigen (presumably derived from fibrin) was inhibited only in those patients who were responders in the platelet aggregation tests. These workers did not establish a mechanism by which aggregated platelets might release an antigenic substance. According to Ellis et al. (1976) aggregated platelets produce substances which induce contraction of coronary arteries. The formation of these substances is blocked by indomethacin, and the effect seems to be related to the action of the drug upon PG-synthetase, since the spasmodic substance appears to be a PG cyclic endoperoxide.

The role of platelets in chronic inflammation is not clear (Paulus and White-house, 1973), and the results of Ubatuba et al. (1975) indicate that platelets do not contribute substantially to acute inflammation, at least insofar as the carrageenan edema model is concerned. They found in rats with platelets reduced to extremely low levels by injection of antiplatelet serum, carrageenan edema did not differ significantly from that elicited in normal animals, and indomethacin produced the same degree of inhibition in animals deprived of platelets as in normal rats.

7.9.3   Inhibition of prostaglandin synthesis

The brilliant investigations by Vane and his colleagues, beginning with the publication of a series of three papers in June, 1971, have led to a veritable explosion of reports from many laboratories, establishing beyond doubt that nonsteroid antiinflammatory compounds inhibit the synthesis of PGs, and supporting the hypothesis that this action is (at least in part) the basis for their activity. An especially concise and complete summary of the evidence for this theory has been presented by Vane (1974). According to this view, not only antiinflammatory activity, but also analgesia, antipyresis, and even many side effects are related to the inhibition of PG synthesis. Many excellent reviews have appeared; for example, Ferreira and Vane, 1974; Hichens, 1974; Flower,

1974; the latter also lists several reviews by Vane. A simplified diagram of the prostaglandin synthetase pathway is shown below:

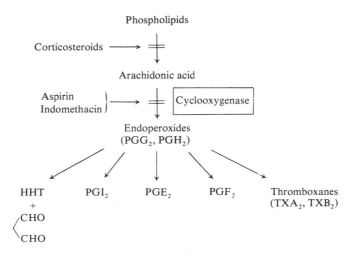

In addition to the inhibition of cyclooxygenase by aspirin, indomethacin and other nonsteroidal drugs, the antiinflammatory action of corticosteroids may be partly related to their blockade of the supply of the substrate, arachidonic acid, to cyclooxygenase. For example, hydrocortisone at a concentration of 5 $\times$ 10^{-6} M inhibited PG production by mouse fibrosarcoma cells (Tashjian *et al.*, 1975), and dexamethasone at 10^{-6} M blocked synthesis of PGE_2 and $PGF_{2\alpha}$ in human rheumatoid synovial tissue (Kantrowitz, *et al.*, 1975). Other independent studies related to these have also been reported (Gryglewski, 1976; Floman and Zor, 1976).

The blockade of the initial enzymatic reaction, either by steroids or by non-steroids, inhibits the production of the whole group of prostaglandins and their intermediates. Recent studies suggested that the chemically reactive and biologically potent thromboxane A_2 (Hamberg, *et al.*, 1975) and endoperoxide intermediates, PGG_2 and PGH_2 (Kuehl *et al.*, 1977) may play more important roles in the inflammatory process.

The irreversible inactivation of cyclooxygenase by aspirin is the result of a transacetylation reaction (Roth *et al.*, 1975). The chemically labile *O*-acetyl group in aspirin selectively acetylates a nucleophile at the active site of a functioning enzyme. The rate of acetylation is many times faster than the nonspecific acetylation of inactivated enzyme or other proteins by aspirin (Rome *et al.*, 1976). As mentioned above, the *N-p*-chlorobenzoyl group in indomethacin is also susceptible to nucleophilic attack. However, incubation of cyclooxygenase with indomethacin (**1**) and MK-825 (**46**), ^{14}C-labeled in the indole [^{14}C-2] and benzoyl [^{14}C-NCO] moieties respectively, does not yield any covalent bonded ^{14}C-label in the enzyme (Stanford *et al.*, 1977)

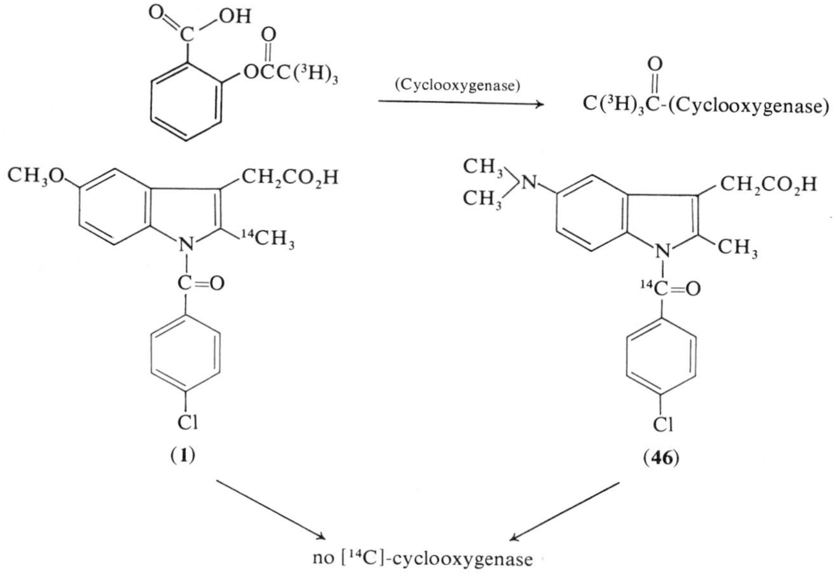

In other words, neither the indole moiety nor the *p*-chlorobenzoyl moiety is transferred through co-valent bonding to the enzyme. Under the conditions used, indomethacin behaves like a reversible inhibitor. Indomethacin, in spite of its low K_i, is only moderately effective in protecting cyclooxygenase from being acetylated by aspirin. Preincubation of cyclooxygenase with 1 μM of indomethacin, a concentration sufficient to inhibit the enzyme activity 90 per cent, only blocked acetylation by 200 μM of aspirin by 33 per cent. A second addition of aspirin completed the acetylation.

It would seem that the binding site of indomethacin and its close analogs is probably similar to, but is not identical with, that of aspirin.

Prior to the discovery of cyclooxygenase, a hypothetical "receptor contour" (Fig. 4) for indomethacin and close analogs was proposed on the basis of their structure-activity relationship (Shen, 1964). In the light of current understanding of cyclooxygenase action and additional X-ray data of newer prostaglandin synthetase inhibitors, the "receptor contour" has been redefined (Gund and Shen, 1977) (Figs 4 and 5). These contours seem to accommodate a large group of aryl acetic acids, reflecting the preferred stereospecificity of their α-methylacetic acid side chain, and are generally useful as working models for the synthesis of new cyclooxygenase inhibitors. Naturally, their true physical meaning, e.g. relationship to the active site of the enzyme, if any, remains to be shown. It may be mentioned that similar analysis of enzymatic mechanisms and computation of the stereochemistry of substrates, or their transition state, may facilitate the search for more selective inhibitors of thromboxane synthetase or other individual steps in the prostaglandin synthetase pathway. The *in vitro* synthetase inhibitory activity of indomethacin, sulindac and some related compounds is summarized in the following table:

TABLE 23

PG Synthetase inhibition and *in vivo* activities

	PG synthetase inhibition[a] ID_{50} μM	Carrageenan edema in rat ED_{50} mg kg^{-1}	Therapeutic dose in man mg day^{-1}
Indole series			
(1) Indomethacin	0·4	2·4	75–100
(46) MK-825	0·6	4	200
(32) MK-410	2·2	15	1000–1500
(32) MK-555	10	25	2000–3000
(106) Metabolite	1·5	*c.* 50	
(14) Metabolite	inactive	inactive	
Indene series			
(2) Sulindac	inactive	4	300–400
(102) Sulfide metabolite	2·2	2	
(108) Sulfone metabolite	inactive	inactive	
(109) Dihydroxy metabolite	inactive	—	
(97) MK-715	2	4	*c.* 400
Others			
(117)	0·6	*c.* 11	
(116)	3	9	
(114)	*c.* 3	—	
(115)	30	≥50	
(118)	13·5	>50	

[a] The PG synthetase inhibition assays of these compounds were carried out by Drs Ham, Humes and their associates in our laboratory using the sheep seminal vesicle system described in reference Ham *et al.* (1972).

As noted above, sulindac (2), as a prodrug, is not a synthetase inhibitor. Its sulfide metabolite (102), the active species *in vivo*, is nearly as potent as indomethacin *in vitro*. The preference for an α-propionic acid side chain with a sinister (S) absolute configuration, commonly true for many aryl α-propionic acids (Shen, 1972), is clearly shown by three pairs of S and R enantiomers in the indole series. The preference for a *cis* geometric isomer in the indene series in *in vivo* assays is confirmed *in vitro*. A general parallelism between *in vitro* and *in vivo* activities within the indole and indene series is also apparent. While the "receptor contour" above may indicate a broad tolerance for many aryl

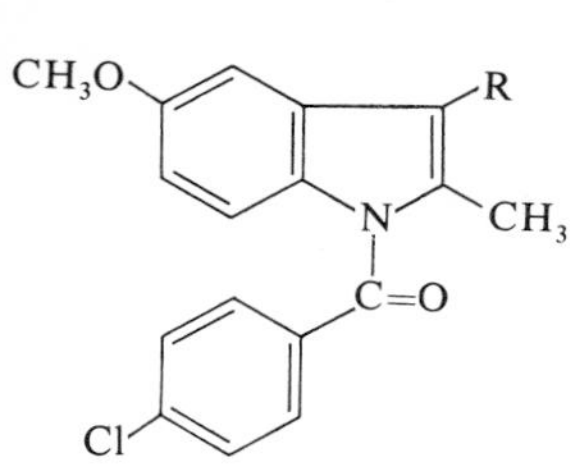

CH$_3$O— (ring) —R
—CH$_3$ (at 2-position), N
C=O
Cl— (benzene ring)

(114) R = CH$_2$CH$_2$OH

(115) CH$_2$CON(morpholine)O

NC— (ring) —CH(CH$_3$)CO$_2$H
—CH$_3$, N
C=O
Cl—

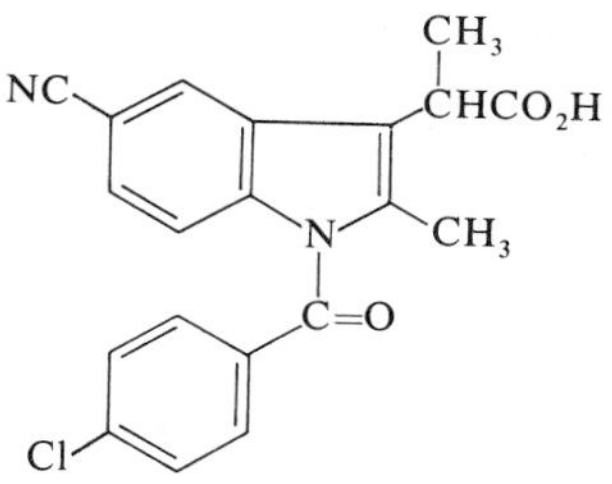

(116)

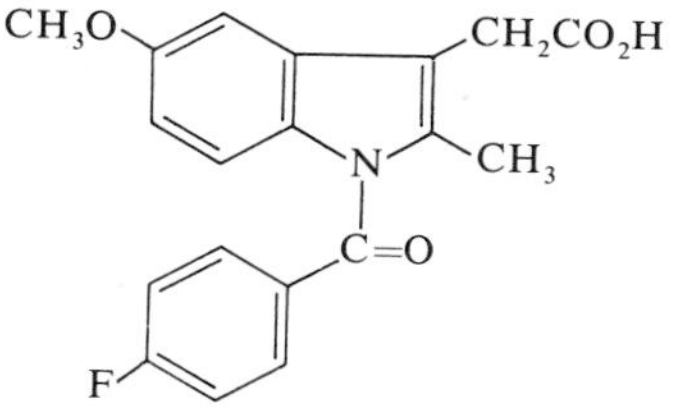

CH$_3$O— (ring) —CH$_2$CO$_2$H
—CH$_3$, N
C=O
F—

(117)

MeO— (ring) —CH(CH$_3$)CO$_2$H
—CH$_3$, N
CH$_2$
(−)
SCH$_3$

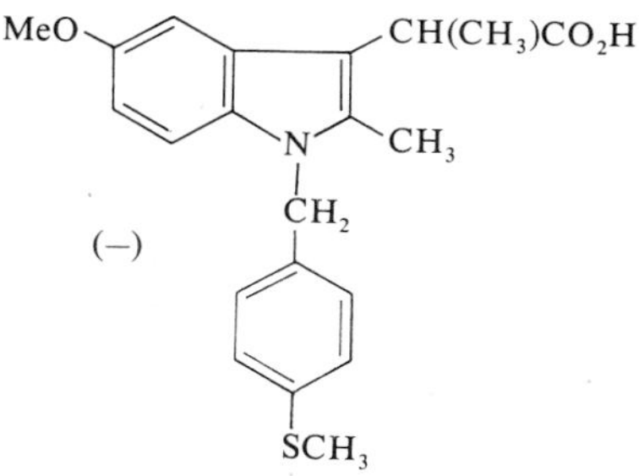

(118)

acidic compounds, the total lack of cyclooxygenase inhibitory activity of sulindac (2) and its sulfone metabolite (108), in contrast with the sulfide metabolite (102), demonstrates a very high degree of specificity at the *para* position indeed. Only CH$_3$S, but not CH$_3$S → O or CH$_3$SO$_2$, is tolerated at the binding site.

The inhibition of prostaglandin synthesis by indomethacin has been demonstrated in a variety of *in vitro* and *in vivo* systems. As shown in Table 24, the ID$_{50}$ value varies extensively in the literature. Factors such as tissue origin, enzyme preparation, concentration of substrate and cofactors, incubation time and other experimental conditions markedly influence the ID$_{50}$ value of cyclooxygenase inhibitors. Indomethacin is a substrate competitive reversible inhibitor, but it also causes a time-dependent, concentration-dependent, slow inactivation of the enzyme. Thus, in comparing the relative potency of different compounds, caution must be exercised if the ID$_{50}$ values are not obtained from the same assay.

In man, a 77–98 per cent reduction of the urinary metabolite, 15-keto-13,14-dihydroprostaglandin, was observed after treatment with 200 mg of indomethacin (Hamberg and Samuelsson, 1971). A comparative evaluation of aspirin and indomethacin on the production of prostaglandins by human platelets and synovial tissue (Patrono *et al.*, 1976) showed that both tissues are equally sensitive to inhibition by indomethacin. In contrast, human platelets are at least six times more sensitive to aspirin than synovial tissue. Similar conclusions were obtained by Majerus *et al.* (1977). Aspirin is 37-fold more potent in inhibiting the human platelet enzyme compared to that from sheep seminal vesicles. These data accord with the clinical observation that at their therapeutic dosage in arthritic patients aspirin has a longer-lasting and more profound inhibitory effect on platelet functions, e.g. aggregation, bleeding time, etc., than indomethacin.

An enzyme in the microsomal fraction of human and horse platelets which converts prostaglandin endoperoxides, PGG_2 and PGH_2, into the unstable thromboxane A_2 (TXA_2) was characterized recently (Needleman *et al.*, 1976). The endoperoxides and TXA_2 are many times more potent than PGE_2 in causing platelet aggregation. Indomethacin inhibits cyclooxygenase at <5 μg ml^{-1}, but >100 μg ml^{-1} is needed to inhibit the thromboxane synthetase (Moncada *et al.*, 1976).

Another novel enzymatic transformation of these endoperoxides to a new prostaglandin derivative, the bicyclic PGI_2 or prostacyclin (**119**), has generated a great deal of excitement in this field (Gryglewski *et al.*, 1976). PGI_2 is an unstable substance highly potent in preventing platelet aggregation and in relaxing some vascular smooth muscle. The conversion of endoperoxides to pro-aggregatory TXA_2 and the anti-aggregatory PGI_2 provides a homeostatic regulatory mechanism *in vivo*. The inhibition by aspirin, indomethacin and other antiinflammatory drugs of the formation of endoperoxides in effect blocks the formation of both pro- and anti-aggregatory mediators. Further clarification of these biological processes in inflammation and other circulatory diseases is obviously of interest.

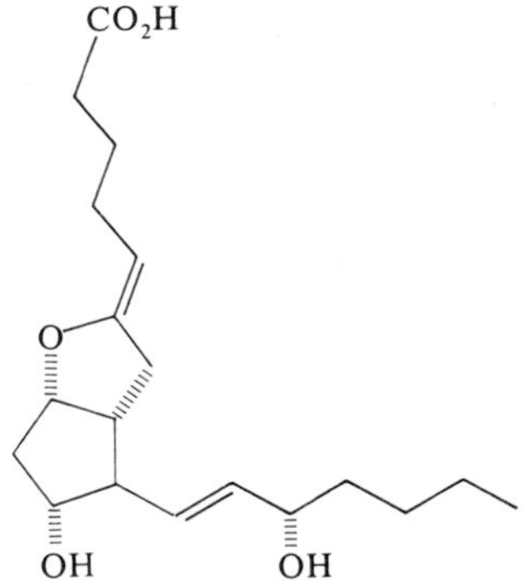

(**119**) (PGX, PGI_2, prostacylin)

Indomethacin has also been reported to be a moderate inhibitor of other enzymes involved in the metabolism of prostaglandins and cyclonucleotides. It inhibits 15-hydroxyprostaglandin dehydrogenase (PGDH), the catabolic enzyme of PGE and PGF, from several tissues and in a perfused rabbit lung system (Hansen, 1974, 1976). The *in vitro* inhibition of bovine lung PGDH by indomethacin is noncompetitive to PGE, with $K_i = 16$ μM. At higher concentrations, indomethacin has also been reported to inhibit the binding of PGE to high affinity binding sites of corpus luteum cell membranes (Rao, 1974) and thymocytes (Grunnet and Bojesen, 1976). It also inhibits cAMP phosphodiesterase at 10^{-4} M *in vitro* (Ciosek et al., 1974; Newcombe et al., 1974). These inhibitory concentrations are higher than that for cyclo-oxygenase. The physiological significance of these properties of indomethacin remains in question (Beatty et al., 1976).

7.9.4   *Prostaglandin regulation and inflammation*

Certain observations indicate that indomethacin and similar compounds do not directly antagonize the action of PGs. They include the following: PGE_1 or PGE_2 when injected into the knee joint of dogs produced incapacitation which was not prevented by indomethacin even in the high dose of 10 mg kg^{-1} (Rosenthale et al., 1972). Indomethacin 9 mg kg^{-1} did not prevent the action of PGE_1 in potentiating the vascular permeability effect of bradykinin or the inhibitory action of $PGF_{2\alpha}$ (Thomas and West, 1973). PGE_1 or PGE_2 or arachidonic acid produced fall in blood pressure and increase in heart rate in hypertensive rats; this action of arachidonic acid but not that of the PGs could be prevented by 2 mg kg^{-1} of indomethacin (Cohen et al., 1973). The contractile effect of arachidonic acid on smooth muscle from the rat's stomach was antagonized by indomethacin in a concentration of 10^{-6} M, but that of PGE_2 of $PGF_{2\alpha}$ was unaffected (Splawinski et al., 1973). Tolman and Partridge (1975), on the other hand, argued that nonsteroid antiinflammatory drugs have multiple interactions with PGs, and that not all the effects of these compounds are explicable on the basis of enzyme inhibition.

Efforts to demonstrate specificity of antiinflammatory drugs as PG synthetase inhibitors include experiments suggesting that almost all potent nonsteroid antiinflammatory compounds possess the property of synthetase inhibition, that a wide variety of compounds without antiinflammatory activity fail to inhibit PG synthesis, and that a correlation exists between inhibition of synthetase and of inflammation. These efforts have met with some success, considering the well-recognized difficulties in correlating *in vitro* and *in vivo* results, etc. These parameters were discussed in detail in the review by Flower (1974). The importance of pharmacokinetics was further analyzed by Brune *et al.* (1976). It seems that the accumulation of acidic drugs in inflamed tissue is a decisive factor favoring their *in vivo* antiinflammatory activities.

In general, correlation between inhibition of synthetase and of inflammation has been found to be good with potent acidic antiinflammatory agents, such as the analogs of indomethacin, but less good with moderately active nonacidic compounds. As indicated above, marked differences in sensitivity to inhibition by drugs have been recognized among enzymes from different tissues. For example, Tomlinson *et al.* (1972) found indomethacin to be 2140 times as potent as aspirin in inhibiting conversion of ^{3}H-arachidonate by enzyme from bull seminal vesicle, and Flower *et al.* (1972) reported indomethacin to be only about 100 times as potent as aspirin, using synthetase from dog spleen. These data were compared with the antiinflammatory activity of indomethacin in inhibiting carrageenan edema, about 23 times to 30 times aspirin in potency. Different sensitivities to indomethacin among PG synthetizing systems of diverse origins have also been noted by Bhattacherjee and Eakins (1974), Tolman and Partridge (1975) and Blackwell *et al.* (1975), cited in Table 24.

Compounds of fairly equal potency sometimes exhibit a different rank order in a test for edema inhibition than in synthetase inhibition; an example may be seen in data shown by Flower *et al.* (1972) in a table comparing meclofenamic acid, niflumic acid, and indomethacin. Within a series of indomethacin analogs, Ham *et al.* (1972) found rather good correlation between *in vitro* enzymic action and *in vivo* inhibition of carrageenan edema; correlation was also good when comparing groups of compounds, but within the fenemates correlation was not good. The latter may have been complicated by the fact that some fenemates inhibit other enzymes also (Shen, 1977).

Results reported by Lee (1974) indicate that PG-synthetase inhibition may not be the exclusive domain of antiinflammatory drugs. Psychotropic drugs, including both monoamine oxidase inhibitor antidepressants and tricyclic tranquilizers, compared favorably with the antiinflammatory compounds in enzymic activity. For example, phenelzine was an order of magnitude more potent than indomethacin while pargyline was about equal to aspirin against PG-synthetase derived from guinea-pig lung. Perhaps the psychotropic drugs examined by Lee also have antiinflammatory activity. Niemegeers *et al.*, (1964) examined a number of such compounds (and many others) in the carrageenan edema test; chlorpromazine was nearly twice as potent as phenylbutazone, while imipramine was equal to aspirin. Ordinarily, compounds classified as "antiinflammatory" are those which inhibit inflammation at doses not producing toxic, behavioral, or autonomic effects. It is possible that these are antiinflammatory agents possessing strong central nervous system properties which might or might not be related to their ability to inhibit PG synthetase.

It must be concluded that in the sum of these investigations, Vane's theory fares rather well. At least some PGs have inflammatory properties, indomethacin and other antiinflammatory compounds prevent PG biosynthesis at concentrations reasonably close to those which might be expected at active sites, and there is good correlation between anti-synthetase and anti-inflammatory activity among indomethacin analogs.

In addition to PG synthetase inhibition, it might still be possible to inhibit inflammation by blocking the events prior to or after the action of the enzyme.

TABLE 24

Inhibition of PG synthesis by indomethacin in various *in vitro* systems

Enzyme	ID_{50} (μM)	References
Bovine seminal vesicles	0·07	Dembinska-Kieć et al. (1976)
	0·6	Cushman and Cheung (1976)
	0·63	Vigdahl and Tukey (1975)
	1	Yanagi and Komatsu (1976)
	1·4	Horodniak et al. (1974)
	2·8	Horodniak et al. (1975)
	6	Ziel and Krupp (1975)
	6·5	Ku and Wasvary (1975)
	7	Tomlinson et al. (1972)
	7·5	Carminati and Lerner (1975)
	15	Adams et al. (1975)
	20	Deby et al. (1975)
Sheep seminal vesicles	0·45	Ham et al. (1972)
	0·5	Gaut et al. (1975)
Goat seminal vesicles	5·6	Wiseman et al. (1975)
Guinea-pig lung	0·6	Tolman et al. (1976)
Dog spleen	0·17	Flower et al. (1973)
Rabbit brain	0·6	Dembinska-Kieć et al. (1976)
	3·6	Flower et al. (1973)
Rabbit kidney	3·7	Blackwell et al., (1975)
	0·15	Dembinska-Kieć et al. (1976)
Rat platelets	2·2	Patrono et al. (1975)
Human platelets	1·3	Patrono et al. (1976)
Human synovium	0·003	Kantrowitz et al. (1975)
	0·5	Crook and Collins (1975)
	2·2	Patrono et al. (1976)
Human epidermal cells	3	Förström et al. (1974)

Silver and Smith (1975) outlined a possible sequence of events leading to PG release. It is presumed that some triggering event, acting as a stimulus for the inflammation, disturbs the cell membrane, resulting in activation of phospholipase so that membrane phospholipid is converted to the fatty acid which is the precursor of PG (arachidonic acid, for example). PG synthetase then converts the precursor acid to PG. The release mechanism of PGs after their formation is under investigation. Interference with any one of these steps might inhibit the release of PGs and hence inhibit inflammation before it got started. For example, stabilization of the membrane so that the initiating stimulus would fail to start the chain of reactions would stop the inflammation before it got well started. Such an action was proposed by Glenn *et al.* (1972).

The inhibition of PG production by corticosteroids mentioned above provides an example of similar nature. The steroids do not alter carrageenan-induced PG production in the rat according to Vane (1973). Nor do they inhibit PG synthetase in platelets (Smith and Willis, 1971), the perfused spleen (Ferreira *et al.*, 1971) or isolated microsomes (Flower *et al.*, 1972). Such results led Vane (1973) to state that antiinflammatory steroids do not act by direct synthetase inhibition. Corticosteroids are not phospholipase inhibitors either. Whether their blockade of the supply of arachidonic acid to cyclo-oxygenase is indeed related to some local change of membrane fluidity remains to be shown. The search for improved nonsteroid antiinflammatory drugs would probably not be well served by looking for more potent inhibitors of PG synthetase, since the compounds currently available are probably potent enough. Greater specificity of action directed at the metabolism of individual prostaglandins might improve safety and usefulness, but for better therapeutic control of the inflammatory response, the regulation of other mediators of inflammation and cellular processes should also be considered. New classes of antiinflammatory compounds must emerge from continued research on the mechanisms of inflammation, rather than from seeking compounds with the same actions as those already known.

7.9.5 *Other biological effects of prostaglandin synthetase inhibition*

Because of its extraordinary potency in inhibiting the biosynthesis of PGs, indomethacin has been widely used in investigations of the physiological functions of PGs. These biologically active lipids may act as local hormones or intracellular messengers in many tissues and organs (Kuehl *et al.*, 1973, 1974; Silver and Smith, 1975). Many detailed discussions on the importance of PGs in specific organs and systems are available. In a volume edited by Ramwell (1973) several investigators have discussed the functions of prostaglandins in autonomic neurotransmission, on homeostasis or renal function and blood pressure, in skin, lungs, in ocular pressure and eye inflammation, cardio-vascular activities, as well as various aspects of the endocrine system, especially those related to reproduction. A comparable series of reviews may be found in other volumes; for example, that edited by Bergström and Bernhard (1973). The series edited by Robinson and Vane (1974) includes discussion of effects of PGs on physiological function from the point of view of the contribution of PG synthetase inhibitors toward knowledge of PG function. The *Archives of Internal Medicine* devoted an entire issue (January, 1974, D. E. Wilson, ed.) to a similar series.

The role of PGs in reproduction has received special attention. This has been reviewed by Behrman and Anderson (1974) and by Behrman and Caldwell (1974) among others. PGs were originally discovered in the reproductive tract, and the earliest attempts at clinical use of PGs were as abortifacients. As summarized by Behrman and associates, PGs may act at several sites in the reproductive system, and their functions include stimulation of secretion of pituitary gonadotrophin, a probable role in ovulation, and in regulation of uterine motility. This field has attracted so much interest that one group was moved to comment that papers on PG function, many of them with a bearing on reproduction, appear on the average of more than one a day (Anderson and Speroff, 1973).

Since those reviews were written, the deluge of papers has continued. With the finding that PGs have so many important roles, it is not surprising that actions have been noted for indomethacin that were not apparent in the earlier work. On the basis of the importance of PGs for uterine contractions, several studies of the effects of indomethacin on labor have been undertaken. Among some of the recent ones at this writing: indomethacin was employed to stop uterine contractions in cases of premature labor (Zuckerman *et al.*, 1974). Normal parturition was blocked and gestation prolonged in rhesus monkeys by large doses of indomethacin (100 to 200 mg day^{-1} in animals 7·5 to 8 kg) (Novy *et al.*, 1974). Such studies may be taken to indicate that PGs are involved in the onset of labor, though there is no direct proof that this is so. Indomethacin has also been used to investigate the role of PGs in ovulation in the monkey (Wallach *et al.*, 1975).

Opposing results are sometimes obtained by investigators using different species or experimental conditions. Thus, using an estrogen to induce ovulation in sheep and indomethacin to block the estrogen-induced release of luteinizing hormone (LH), Carlson *et al.* (1974) concluded that PGs play an obligatory role in LH release, while Sundberg and co-workers (1975) found no evidence that PGs had any effect on LH-release from rat pituitaries *in vitro*, either under basal conditions or when stimulated by hypothalamic extract; curiously, indomethacin potentiated the effect of LH releasing factor. These results seem to be at variance with those obtained in intact rats, as discussed by Behrman and Caldwell (1974). According to the latter, indomethacin could inhibit ovulation in the rat if given at appropriate time prior to the expected release of LH. According to unpublished observations in Merck Institute (H. M. Peck, personal communication) a rather large scale study indicated that indomethacin, phenylbutazone, and aspirin administered twice daily to pregnant animals near term delayed the onset but not the duration of parturition in rats, but not in rabbits.

The potency of antiinflammatory compounds in inhibiting uterine motility *in vitro* follows to some degree their activity against PG-synthetase, which in turn bears a relationship to antiinflammatory potential. Accordingly, Lewis *et al.* (1975) proposed that inhibition of spontaneous contractions of the isolated rat uterus might be used to assess antiinflammatory activity of unknown compounds. The series of compounds upon which this proposal was based was too small to establish the validity of the proposal, and at least two of the compounds had a different rank order in the antiinflammatory test than in the uterine inhibitory assay.

Indomethacin has also been of value in the investigation of the role of PGs in cardiovascular and renal functions. Sympathetic nerve stimulation in the isolated perfused rabbit heart leads to release of norepinephrine; this release is apparently under control of PGs, at least to some extent. Adding indomethacin to the perfusate augmented the outflow of norepinephrine, even though the drug had no effect in the absence of nerve stimulation (Chanh *et al.*, 1972). This negative feedback of PGs as an important mechanism in control of sympathetic nerve activity was also discussed by Hedqvist (1973). The role of PGs in blood pressure regulation in renal hypertension was studied by Schölkens and Steinbach (1975) who found indomethacin to increase the development and course of the hypertension in rats.

These results are consistent with numerous reports of the importance of PGs in the regulation of renal blood flow. Indomethacin reduced the output of PGs into renal venous blood and prevented the increase in PG output generally seen when renal nerves were stimulated (Davis and Horton, 1972). The effect of indomethacin on renal PG and renal plasma flow is short lived (Solez *et al.*, 1974). The effects of furosemide and of ethacrynic acid on renal blood flow was considered to be mediated by PGs, on the basis of the inhibition by indomethacin of the increase in blood flow ordinarily produced by these agents (Williamson *et al.*, 1974, 1975). A recent study showed that pretreatment of rabbits with indomethacin 5 mg kg^{-1} reduced the elevation of urine flow, sodium excretion and plasma renin activity by furosemide 5 mg kg^{-1} (Oliw *et al.*, 1976). As the authors noted, the clinical significance of this drug interaction requires further studies in humans using the recommended dose of indomethacin (1–2 mg kg^{-1}).

Inhibition of prostaglandin synthesis produces constriction of the ductus arteriosus in normal fetal lambs *in utero*. In a recent clinical experiment, the closure of the ductus arteriosus in premature infants was completed by a single dose of 0·3 mg/kg or one or more doses of 0·1 mg kg^{-1} of indomethacin. At these levels, the renal function of infants was unaltered (Heymann *et al.*, 1976).

In spite of these effects upon renal blood flow and the increase in renal resistance after drug administration, indomethacin did not impair autoregulation of blood flow in the kidney as determined by changes in renal resistance after aortic constriction in intact anesthetized dogs (Venuto *et al.*, 1975). Also, indomethacin lacked the renal tubular effects of phenylbutazone upon water and electrolyte gradients and excretion (Bartelheimer and Senft, 1968; Heller and Tata, 1968).

7.9.6 Topical applications of indomethacin

Indomethacin has also been used to study PG synthesis in the skin. According to Greaves and McDonald-Gibson (1973) antiinflammatory drugs are less effective in inhibiting PG synthetase in skin than in other tissues. Even at the relatively high concentration of 0.28 mM, the compound produced only 34 per cent inhibition of the conversion of arachidonic acid to PGE_2 (but 64 per cent inhibition of $PGF_{2\alpha}$ formation) in a simple homogenate of human skin. Aspirin at double the concentration failed to inhibit formation of $PGF_{2\alpha}$ and was only slightly effective against synthesis of PGE_2. The results of Ziboh et al. (1973) were somewhat at variance with those of Greaves, since they found as high as 50 per cent inhibition of PGE_2 synthesis with indomethacin at a concentration of 6 μM. The studies were conducted with various centrifuged fractions of the homogenate.

The erythema seen after exposure to ultraviolet rays may also be related to PG synthesis. Inhibition of PG synthesis decreases and delays the erythema both in guinea-pigs and in humans (Snyder and Eaglstein, 1973); indomethacin is 45 times as effective as aspirin (Snyder and Eaglstein, 1974a). These findings are thought to support the idea of a role for PGs in mediation of sunburn, and lead to the possibility of the use of indomethacin in treatment of the effects of overexposure (Snyder and Eaglstein, 1974b).

Indomethacin is absorbed into the eye following topical application (Hanna and Sharp, 1972) and this fact has been used in the study of the relationship between PGs and ocular inflammation, as well as in observations on the antiinflammatory action of the drug in the eye. Although PG biosynthesis from arachidonic acid proceeds at a slower pace in ocular tissues than in some others, and the PG synthetase system is somewhat less responsive to indomethacin (Bhattacherjee and Eakins, 1974) there is substantial PG activity when uveitis is present, and the amount of PG correlates with the degree of inflammation (Eakins et al., 1972, 1973). The PGs released during ocular inflammation vary somewhat according to the species of animal used, but in general topical application of PGE_2 leads to miosis, vasodilatation in iris and conjunctiva, relaxation of the nictitating membrane, increased protein in the aqueous humor, and increased intraocular pressure (Neufeld and Sears, 1973). These effects are also produced by topical administration of arachidonic acid.

In tests by Podos et al. (1973) indomethacin was ineffective in antagonizing the actions of topically administered PGs, but pretreatment with the drug prevented the rise in intraocular pressure induced by arachidonic acid. In similar experiments, Conquet et al. (1975) determined indomethacin to be several times more effective when applied topically to the eye than when administered orally. Assay of drug concentration in the aqueous humor showed levels greater than 5 μg ml^{-1} after topical application of 0·5 mg of indomethacin, while plasma concentration was on the order of 0·2 μg ml^{-1}. After oral ingestion of the compound, on the other hand, concentration in the aqueous humor was only about 1/100th that in plasma. Such results imply that for some uses, topical application might produce antiinflammatory results at doses which could avoid systemic effects of the drug.

Experimental uveitis has responded favorably to indomethacin (Hanna and Keatts, 1967; Baldwin and Borgmann, 1970). Such findings have encouraged some clinical investigators to assess the value of indomethacin in the treatment of ocular inflammation. These studies will be discussed in a later section of this review (section 9).

7.9.7   Comment

The above is but a sampling of the vast and rapidly growing literature on the use of indomethacin in elucidating the physiological functions of PGs. The discovery of PGs and of their multitudinous activities is one of the most exciting developments in biomedical research within the past decade. Even at the present frantic pace of new developments, the full elucidation of the actions of these compounds and the realization of the therapeutic potential of the discoveries will undoubtedly require several years. In the furtherance of this quest, the inhibitors of PG synthetase, of which indomethacin is an outstanding example, will continue to play a fascinating and important role.

8   Pharmaceutical formulations

The effectiveness of a drug as a therapeutic agent depends not only upon the intrinsic pharmacological activity of the compound administered, but also on the bioavailability of the active substance. The variations in clinical results with different formulations is well illustrated by some of the early history of clinical trials of indomethacin.

In a previous section (see Tables 13 and 14) it was shown that the toxicity of indomethacin was approximately the same in rats by three routes of administration: oral, intraperitoneal and subcutaneous. In mice, intravenous, oral and intraperitoneal acute toxicity tests yielded data not differing significantly. In addition, in subacute tests in dogs (Table 17) intravenous or rectal administration produced about the same degree of toxicity as did similar doses administered by mouth. These studies indicated that the drug was about equally available to the organism regardless of the mode of administration. Caution must be exercised before transferring such data to man; this is emphasized by the finding in guinea-pigs in the same study (Table 14) showing that the drug was rather poorly available when administered orally in this species. The compound was given in an aqueous suspension in methylcellulose, a formulation which had proved adequate in the rats. It was not determined whether or not a different formulation would have given a different result in the guinea-pig.

In the early clinical trials of indomethacin, it soon became apparent that pharmaceutical formulation played an important role in consistency of therapeutic results as well as in incidence of side effects. Favorable results in the first informal trials were not always matched by reports received a bit later. It was soon concluded that a difference in formulation might account for the discrepancy. The very earliest trials were made with the powdered compound in gelatin capsules. These were soon replaced by compressed tablets, but subsequently it was found that tablets containing indomethacin harden on storage and have a variable dissolution rate; hence, drug absorption from the gastrointestinal tract was better and less variable from capsules than from tablets. This was confirmed in plasma level studies in several different clinical experiments (Paul et al., 1964; Ballabio and Caruso, 1964; Caruso et al., 1964).

The plasma level studies were confirmed by several clinical reports. Katz et al. (1965) observed a high incidence of gastrointestinal side effects with tablets containing indomethacin, but a subsequent publication from the same clinic (Pearson, 1966) noted that since switching to capsules their therapeutic results had been better and there was a notable reduction in side effects. Lövgren and Allander (1965), who had encountered a high incidence of peptic ulcers with indomethacin tablets, reported that a change to capsules permitted a lower dosage with a reduction of side effects. Other reports of reduction in incidence of severity of side effects with the use of capsules compared with the tablets include Paul et al. (1964), Michotte and Wanters (1964), Boardman and Hart (1964, 1967), Ballabio and Caruso (1964), Thompson (1964), Smyth (1965), and Wanka and Dixon (1964). Variations of effectiveness of antiinflammatory drugs correlated with physical form and with the vehicle have also been described in animal experiments (Glenn et al., 1967; Kaiser et al., 1967).

Since the above observations were made, orally administered drug is always given as a fine powder in gelatin capsules. Such capsules, stored in light-resistant containers, carry an expiration date of 5 years at room temperature (see NF XIII, p. 367ff). Suppositories are also commercially prepared. Kwan et al., (1976) have shown that indomethacin administered orally to human subjects in commercially available capsules has bioavailability equal to intravenously injected drug. When the commercially available rectal suppositories were used, absorption was more prompt but less complete than after oral ingestion, with about 80 per cent bioavailability.

8.1   INDOMETHACIN PREPARATIONS FOR LABORATORY USE

Indomethacin is a crystalline powder, odorless or nearly so, usually pale yellow, sometimes tan-yellow. Solvated crystals are white to lemon yellow, depending on the solvent used, but solutions are always yellow. The compound may exist in amorphous form, or in either of two crystalline forms. One crystalline form, designated as Form I, has a melting point of 160°C, while Form II melts at 153°C. Form I is the more stable, and on storage the other form gradually converts to it. Crystals may be obtained from methanol, tertiary butanol, methylene chloride, ether, acetone, dimethyl sulfoxide, or dioxane. Such crystals are solvated; that is, the compound is in combination with the solvent. Nonsolvated crystals may be obtained from ethylacetate or from 95 per cent ethanol.

Indomethacin is sparingly soluble in water, but solutions can be prepared with mild alkali, such as sodium carbonate or bicarbonate. Care must be taken in adding alkali; for example, the compound decomposes in a matter of seconds in $0 \cdot 1$ N NaOH. The decomposition products are p-chlorobenzoic acid and 2-methyl-5-methoxyindole-3-acetic acid (**14**). Neither of these products absorb light of the wave length of 318 nanometers (millimicra), as does indomethacin. Hence, the chemical integrity of the compound may be tested by testing for absorption at that wave length. For this purpose, a suitable solvent is phosphate buffer at pH 7. The absorptivity A (1 per cent, 1 cm) is approximately 175.

Table 25 shows the solubility of indomethacin at room temperature for several solvents, while Table 26 lists the solubilities of the compound in water at various pH values. The pK_a of indomethacin is $4 \cdot 5$. Some data on stability of indomethacin as related to pH and temperature are given in Table 27.

The authors have frequently been asked for instructions for the preparation of solutions or suspensions for use in animal experiments, so the following brief discussion may be helpful. The procedure depends upon the type of experiment. When we tested the antiinflammatory effects of indomethacin by applying the compound directly to cotton pellets to be inserted subcutaneously, a simple solution of the compound in alcohol or ether was added to a previously sterilized cotton sponge, then the solvent was permitted to evaporate before inserting the pellet (Winter *et al.*, 1963). Preparations for oral administration were sometimes prepared as follows: to a weighed sample of drug, we added $0 \cdot 5$ ml of dimethylacetamide (Eastman) and $1 \cdot 5$ ml of Emulphor 620 (Antara Chemicals Division of General Aniline & Film Corporation), then sufficient distilled water was added to bring the volume to 1 ml for each mg of indomethacin. This was a stock solution, and aliquots were used for making up the doses for each group of animals. The volume of solution prepared was sufficient for the day's experiments; fresh solutions were prepared daily, and unused solutions discarded.

TABLE 25

Solubility of indomethacin in various solvents at room temperature[a]

Solvent	Solubility (mg ml^{-1})
Methanol	18·5
Methanol 50%	0·4
Methanol 66%	2·1
Ethanol	35·0
Isopropanol	14·7
t-Butanol	3·77
Water	0·02
Dichloromethane	74·8
Trichloromethane	41·8
Tetrachloromethane	0·27
Ethyl ether	10·2
Acetone	131
Ethyl acetate	44·6
Tributyl phosphate	248
Benzene	5·0
Isooctane	5·0

[a] For the data in this and the other Tables in section 8, we are indebted to the laboratory of Pharmaceutical Chemistry, Merck Sharp & Dohme Research Laboratories, West Point, Pennsylvania.

TABLE 26

Solubility of indomethacin in water at various values of pH

pH	Solubility, mg per 100 ml
2·0	0·27
5·7	1·8
6·45	33·3
7·15	430

For subcutaneous injection, a solution can be made with the aid of sodium carbonate which will be stable for 24 hours if kept refrigerated. If freeze dried it can be kept for long periods. Examples of injectable solutions suitable for animal experiments are shown in Table 28. The exact procedure to be followed may be varied depending upon the final concentration of drug desired, but an example is as follows: for each 100 ml of final solution desired, prepare a solution of sodium carbonate monohydrate 300 mg in 80 ml of water for injection. Add and dissolve in the Na_2CO_3 solution, 800 mg of indomethacin, with agitation. Then add 100 mg of Emulphor EL 620. Add sufficient water for

TABLE 27

Stability of indomethacin in aqueous solution at
various pH values and temperatures

pH	Indomethacin half-life
12·0	About 1 minute at room temperature
10·0	1 to 1·5 hours at room temperature
9·4	0·38 hours at 50°C
8·14	3·13 hours at 50°C
8·0	195 hours at room temperature
7·57	6·83 hours at 50°C
6·61	47 hours at 50°C

injection to bring the final product up to 100 ml. The pH should be between 8·4 and 9·1. If sterilization is desired, the solution can be sterilized by filtration, but cannot be autoclaved. A millipore 0·22 micron pad with pre-clarification back-up filter will serve. If the solution is to be freeze dried, 2·5 g of mannitol may be added before bringing the mixture up to final volume. If it is desired to determine the chemical integrity of the preparation, absorptivity can be tested as mentioned above. Solutions can be diluted to desired strength by the addition of sterile water.

On an even more informal basis, solutions can be prepared by adding a suspension of indomethacin to a solution of sodium carbonate. There may be

TABLE 28

Examples of procedures that have been employed in preparing extemporaneous injectable solutions of indomethacin for administration to laboratory animals

Procedure A. 0·1 ml of this solution per 100 g body weight administers a dose of 8 mg kg^{-1} of indomethacin

Indomethacin	0·8 g
Sodium carbonate monohydrate	0·3 g
Mannitol^a	2·5 g
Emulphor EL 620	0·1 g
Water for injection q.s.	100　ml

Procedure B. 0·1 ml of this solution per 100 g body weight administers a dose of 3·58 mg kg^{-1}; for in vitro work, this stock solution diluted 100-fold yields concentration M^{-4}.

Indomethacin (M.W. 357·8)	358 mg
Sodium carbonate monohydrate	133 mg (or anhydrous 114 mg)
Water q.s.	100 ml

^{a} Mannitol may be added as bulking agent for cryodesiccation; may be omitted if solution is to be used same day.

For procedural details, see text.

some foaming, due to the reaction between the acidic moiety of the indomethacin and the carbonate, with the formation of sodium salt of indomethacin. If the solution is used promptly, pharmacological activity should not be affected, but solutions not used during the day's work should be discarded. Simple aqueous suspensions in methyl cellulose (sometimes used for intragastric administration to animals) should also be prepared fresh daily.

8.2 SULINDAC PREPARATIONS FOR LABORATORY USE

As sulindac is a stable organic acid, an aqueous solution can readily be prepared by dissolving the free acid, or preformed sodium salt, in dilute alkaline or butter solution at pH >7. The solubility of sulindac at 37° over pH range 5–6 is as follows:

pH 6	0.45 mg ml^{-1}
5.3 (human urine)	0.12
5	0.07

9 Clinical activities

9.1 SELECTION OF COMPOUNDS FOR CLINICAL TRIAL

As mentioned above (section 3.1, Table 3), no less than six compounds were selected for trials in human subjects during the course of these investigations. Some of the properties of these compounds have been discussed in previous sections; for their chemical formulae and biological properties see sections 3, 4, 5 and 6, and Table 3. The present discussion is concerned with the sequence of events leading to the selection of the particular compounds chosen.

The first compound submitted to clinical trial was the racemic form of compound **32**, which received the designation MK-555. It was selected because tests for antiinflammatory, analgesic, and antipyretic activities indicated that it was more potent than either phenylbutazone or aspirin. Preliminary clinical trials (unpublished) confirmed that MK-555 possessed activity, but it soon became apparent that greater potency would be desirable.

This finding was the first indication, amply confirmed by subsequent experience, that the inflammatory models in rats are particularly responsive to aryl acetic acids, and that experimental findings in rats exaggerate both their potency and their toxicity, when compared to their effects in human subjects. The rank order of activity of antiinflammatory compounds in man is in general reflected in the results of animal tests, but it is difficult to predict the human dose requirement on the basis of minimal effective doses in the rodent model. For example, in the subacute test for antiinflammatory activity—the granuloma inhibition test in rats—action of indomethacin could be detected at a dose as slow as 0.015 mg kg^{-1} d^{-1} (Winter and Risley, 1965), while a 70 kg human patient taking four 25 mg capsules daily is receiving 1.4 mg kg^{-1} d^{-1}.

When the dextrorotatory compound **33** became available, it proved to be several times more potent than MK-555 in animal tests. Under the designation of MK-410, it proved to be clinically active, but during the course of the trials, a still more effective compound came to light, MK-615, which received the generic name *indomethacin*. Initial clinical trials of indomethacin were performed with great caution because of the toxicity of the new compound in rats (section 3.5). Even in this species, however, the margin of safety (ratio of the toxic dose to the antiinflammatory dose) compared favorably with that of other antiinflammatory drugs (Phelps *et al.*, 1968). This finding was confirmed in other laboratories (Hitchens *et al.*, 1967; Lorenzetti, 1970). It was therefore deemed feasible to proceed cautiously with clinical trial.

The early trials of indomethacin confirmed its antiinflammatory activity in man, but undesirable reactions, most frequently headache or gastrointestinal disturbances, were seen in some individuals, and several of the early clinical papers expressed the hope that an analog might be found with somewhat different physical and chemical properties so that some of the undesired effects might be avoided (Hart and Boardman, 1964; Katz *et al.*, 1965). These considerations led to the development and clinical trial of three additional compounds.

The first of these was the 5-dimethylamino analog of indomethacin (Compound **46**, Table 3), MK-825. Though it was slightly less potent than indomethacin in the animal tests, it was postulated that perhaps greater polarity, different ionization characteristics, and increased water solubility could be reflected in a different metabolic fate than indomethacin in man, with subsequent minimizing of undesirable reactions (see section 6.2). Actual trials, however, soon established that the side effects of MK-825 were not substantially different from those of indomethacin, and the compound was not more effective in therapy.

The indene isostere of indomethacin, MK-715 (sections 3.4.4 and 6.3.1), was the next compound judged to be worthy of clinical trial. In the animal tests, its potency was comparable to that of indomethacin, but it required much higher doses to produce gastrointestinal damage. Cautious clinical trial indicated that a considerable degree of separation of antiinflammatory and ulcerogenic activities had indeed been achieved. The headache side effect of indomethacin was also not seen with MK-715 patients. However, a major urinary metabolite, the glucuronide conjugate of MK-715, proved to be relatively insoluble in urine. After crystalluria had been detected in human subjects at 3–400 mg daily doses, the trials were discontinued.

The findings with MK-715 were sufficiently encouraging that exploration of the indene-3-acetic acid series was continued. The compound of choice received the designation MK-231, sulindac (sections 3.4.5, 3.5.4, 5, and 6.3). This compound appeared to retain the activity and favorable anti-inflammatory/ulcerogenic ratio of MK-715, and yielded no insoluble metabolites. In addition, it offered the unique advantage (for systemic use) of being a "pro-drug"; that is, a compound nearly pharmacologically inert *per se*, but metabolized to an active compound after absorption (Duggan *et al.*, 1976). Hence, the gastrointestinal tract would not be exposed to the possible irritating effect which is a common action of potent antiinflammatory agents. Only a small portion of the active metabolite, the sulfide of sulindac, reaches the g.i. tract through enterohepatic recycling and conversion by the intestinal flora (see section 6.3.2) but the concentration is much less than would be expected if the active compound had itself been administered.

Results of clinical trials of sulindac available to date seem to bear out the prediction of the experimental findings. For example, in two double-blind multi-clinic studies, one in ankylosing spondylitis (Liebling *et al.*, 1975) and the other in osteoarthritis of the hip (Calabro *et al.*, 1975), sulindac was found to be effective, and the incidence of adverse reactions did not differ significantly in drug-treated and placebo-treated groups. Likewise, a multi-clinic open study in acute gout (Calabro *et al.*, 1974) reported the compound to produce "dramatic improvement" in all patients tested (series of 15), with no adverse reactions. Other clinical experiences were presented at a recent symposium (Huskisson and Franchimont, 1976).

9.2 CLINICAL REPORTS ON INDOMETHACIN IN RHEUMATIC DISORDERS

Not all of the numerous clinical reports on indomethacin are in full agreement. The majority of the clinical authors have considered indomethacin to be a useful drug, especially in the treatment of acute gout, ankylosing spondylitis, and osteoarthritis of the hip, and to a somewhat lesser degree in rheumatoid arthritis. A number of other conditions have been treated, though the documentation may be less complete (Calabro, 1975).

The present authors are not clinicians, but this review would not be complete without a few comments on the clinical literature. It is more difficult to apply the principles of good experimental design in clinical studies than in laboratory experiments, and there is some disagreement on what constitutes a proper clinical evaluation of a compound. One large study on indomethacin in rheumatoid arthritis (Mainland and A.R.A. Committee, 1967) was highly critical of previous studies on the compound, and referred to "the poor quality of much of the previous research". But the committee study has itself been criticized. All the patients in the committee investigation were permitted unlimited salicylate intake. This aspect of the investigation has given rise to controversy, especially since some experimental evidence suggests a possible antagonism between indomethacin and salicylates (see section 6.5.4). In this respect, neither the committee study nor that of Donnelly and co-workers (1967) can be considered to be truly controlled studies of the basic activity of indomethacin. In spite of this, the committee study showed "a much higher frequency of deterioration" in patients after discontinuance of the drug than after discontinuance of placebo, with aspirin continued in both groups. The committee, however, seemed not to consider this finding as evidence of activity of the compound.

Objective evidence of effectiveness of a drug in rheumatoid arthritis seems to be difficult to obtain with any kind of therapy, nor have efforts of large committees been notably more successful than those of smaller groups or of individual investigators. For example, a well-known committee study, that of the Empire Rheumatism Council (1955) was unable to distinguish between cortisone acetate and aspirin.

In a double blind study comparing aspirin and indomethacin, Pinals and Frank (1967) found 12·5 mg of indomethacin to be about as effective as 400 mg of aspirin. This potency ratio is similar to that found in animal experiments (see section 3). Somewhat higher ratios were obtained in a single blind study by Pitkeathly et al. (1966) in which 50 to 100 mg of indomethacin daily gave results comparable to 4 g of aspirin.

Many of the reported clinical trials of indomethacin have been of relatively short duration, and the drug has been administered in fixed dosage. In this respect, such trials do not mimic the conditions under which a drug is often used in the treatment of rheumatoid arthritis, in which both dosage and duration can be individualized. Long-term studies such as those reported by Rothermich (1966) and Calabro (1975) more nearly approach practical conditions. Such studies were not "controlled" in the conventional sense, but in some of them treatments were interrupted for placebo trials, and reduction of steroid was practiced in patients previously on steroid. It is generally agreed that in certain stages of the investigation of a new drug, single blind and double blind techniques are desirable or even necessary. However, several authors (for example, Ballabio and Caruso, 1964; Rothermich, 1966) have remarked that patients soon learn to recognize when a placebo has replaced indomethacin. Such sophistication on the part of patients has not always been recognized by clinical investigators.

In spite of these difficulties, many double blind studies of indomethacin have been completed; some of these have been reported in the literature. A few were mentioned in the Mainland committee report, and by O'Brien (1968). Others include publications by Ward (1965), Coste et al. (1964), and Catoggio (1964). According to Smyth (1970) most of the controlled studies were of too short a duration to demonstrate effectiveness of the medication. In a study by

Brocklehurst and Humphreys (1965) indomethacin appeared to be better when compared with placebo in a double blind trial than when used in open trial.

Although it is often stated that only about one-third of patients with rheumatoid arthritis improve significantly with indomethacin, Mezey (1966) made a survey of world-wide clinical trials in a wide variety of disorders, and estimated that 66·5 per cent of 2300 patients responded with "good" or "excellent" results. Such terms are imprecise, and the clinic population surveyed by Mezey embraced a wide variety of degrees of statistical control, but his figure is surprisingly close to the 61 per cent reported by Bunim (1955) after a similar survey of early results with cortical steroids and adrenocorticotropic hormone. Any designation of a clinical result that does not involve a mathematical measurement is open to the criticism of non-objectivity, but after all, pain and discomfort (and to some extent mobility) are subjective phenomena. This adds to the difficulty of objective evaluation of patients' responses. In the absence of a "cure", the object of therapy is to improve the patient's well being, a parameter not always amenable to "objective" measurement in the usual sense but which nevertheless should not be ignored.

The majority of side effects of indomethacin fall into one of two categories: "central nervous system" or "cerebral" symptoms (Rothermich, 1966) or gastrointestinal effects. The first category includes headache (the most common single symptom), vertigo, light-headedness, and disturbed sensorium. These symptoms subside when the drug is withdrawn (Healey, 1967) or often even if continued (Calabro, 1975), or they sometimes may be avoided altogether if the daily dosage is started low and increased gradually (Smyth, 1970). The second category is sometimes more serious; it includes epigastric pain, cramping, and peptic ulceration. Boardman and Hart (1967) reviewed the literature on side effects of indomethacin, and added a few cases that did not fit either category. They also found evidence that the incidence of side reactions decrease with increasing age, but others have suggested that the opposite may be true (Brocklehurst and Humphreys, 1965; Emmerson, 1967).

The medical literature is replete with examples of initial exaggerated enthusiasm for a new drug, followed by an over-reaction in the opposite direction, before the final status has been attained. Healey (1967) and Calabro (1975) have commented on this aspect of the clinical history of indomethacin. Overall, it seems fair to conclude that the compound has an acceptable degree of usefulness for those conditions for which other antiinflammatory drugs have been used, that it is reasonably safe if properly employed, and that it is sometimes useful in cases where other remedies have failed (the opposite is also sometimes true). It is not equally effective in all types of rheumatic disorders. The search for better compounds, exemplified by the development of sulindac, is fully justified.

Some of the alleged side effects of indomethacin are somewhat controversial. The often repeated statement that indomethacin increases the effect of coumarin anticoagulants by displacement from binding sites has been discussed in detail above (see section 6.5.2). Suffice it to say at this point that the evidence clearly shows that indomethacin has no clinically significant effect upon the action of coumarin anticoagulants. There has also been much discussion of a possible ocular toxicity. Burns (1966, 1968) described decreased retinal sensitivity as well as corneal and ophthalmoscopic changes in patients receiving indomethacin, but some observers failed to confirm Burns' findings. Davidorf (1972) compared 170 patients receiving daily doses of 50 to 150 mg of indomethacin for 1 to 5 years with 160 patients not taking the drug. Complete ophthalmologic examinations were made at 18 to 24 month intervals. No sign of ocular toxicity was detected in their series. In a smaller group of patients, Carr and Siegel (1973) also found no drug effects as determined by electroretinography and retinal sensitivity profiles; a few abnormalities, present equally in treated and control groups, were consistent with aging changes and were regarded as not related to drug intake. Subsequently, Burns (1973) in a somewhat modified stand, suggested that if a toxic ocular effect of indomethacin does indeed exist, it must be a subtle one, and called for a controlled prospective study.

9.3 MISCELLANEOUS CLINICAL REPORTS

In contrast to these suggestions of possible ocular toxicity, several reports indicate beneficial effects of indomethacin in certain ophthalmological conditions. Experimental background for the use of the compound in treatment of ocular inflammation was supplied by such reports as those of Hanna and Keatts (1967), Baldwin and Borgmann (1970), Hanna (1970), and Conquet et al. (1975). In a double blind trial, Perkins and Macfaul (1965) reported orally administered indomethacin to be useful in the treatment of uveitis. Tuovinen et al. (1966) also thought indomethacin helpful in uveitis, while Obayashi and Kozaki (1968) reported the drug to be especially useful against pain, edema, and congestion following ophthalmic surgery. Novak and Soumarova (1971) compared indomethacin with several other antiinflammatory compounds in patients with episcleritis and scleritis, and found indomethacin to have the most pronounced antiphlogistic effect.

For the most part these results, though encouraging, would be more impressive if they were repeated under more thoroughly controlled conditions. The oral administration was accompanied by the usual side effects, and Gordon (1970) could not confirm the reports of beneficial actions in uveitis. Eakins (1974) suggested that the ocular antiinflammatory actions are due to the inhibition of PG biosynthesis—in line with the prevailing hypothesis seeking to explain antiinflammatory action in other tissues—and he called for the development of new agents with greater selectivity for the eye and with topical activity. There is, however, evidence that indomethacin has topical activity in the eye. Hanna and Sharp (1972) showed that the drug is absorbed when applied topically to the rabbit's cornea, and that absorption is enhanced by inflammation. Evidence of topical activity was also seen in animal experiments by Ku et al. (1975) and by Conquet and co-workers (1975). Thus, a trial of topical indomethacin in human eyes may be indicated, and such tests are in progress.

Attention on the use of indomethacin has been largely concentrated on the treatment of rheumatic disorders, leaving certain other possible clinical uses incompletely explored. One area that has received some notice is in the realm of kidney disorders. Several of the early reports on indomethacin claimed suppression of proteinuria and hematuria in acute and chronic glomerulonephritis, and even (in some reports) improvement of histological lesions as seen on biopsy (Conte et al., 1967; Murisasco et al., 1967; Michielsen and Verberckmoes, 1968; Michielsen et al., 1969). More recent investigators have in general confirmed the value of indomethacin in symptomatic therapy and reduction of proteinuria; for example, Clarkson et al., 1972; Vihert et al., 1973. The latter started their clinical trial after obtaining evidence of the effectiveness of the drug in rats with experimentally induced glomerulonephritis. Patients with renal insufficiency receiving indomethacin for antirheumatic therapy require no alterations in size or frequency of doses, according to Traeger et al. (1972) and Kunze et al. (1974).

Natriuresis induced by furosemide is antagonized by indomethacin, and despite reduction of protein excretion in nephrotic patients receiving indomethacin and furosemide concurrently, edema may not be controlled (Tiggeler et al., 1973). Conversely, administration of furosemide reduces plasma level of indomethacin, and Brooks et al. (1974b) suggested that the two drugs should not be given at the same time. On the other hand, the same group of workers thought that probenecid given with indomethacin increased the effectiveness of the latter, and possibly decreased the side effects (Brooks et al., 1974b); this has been discussed in a previous section of this review (section 6.5.3).

Daha et al. (1973) obtained beneficial results in rats with glomerular nephritis, as well as improved synthesis of glomerular basement membrane in in vitro studies of isolated glomeruli in the presence of $[^{14}C]$-L-proline. The mechanism by which these effects are produced is not clear. Indomethacin inhibits PG biosynthesis in kidneys as well as in other tissues, but the significance of this action in the kidney has been studied primarily with respect to the role of PGs in the regulation of renal blood flow (McGiff et al., 1974). Whether there is any relation between effects on PG synthesis and the relief of symptoms in glomerular nephritis remains to be explored. Barnett and co-workers (1975) reasoned that PG biosynthesis inhibition might account for the antagonism by indomethacin of the diuretic response to calcitonin in man, but their data gave no direct evidence of it.

It has been postulated that PGs synthesized in the kidneys of the blood vessels are important in the regulation of blood pressure, and that a deficiency of PGs may initiate or exaggerate hypertension (Vane and McGiff, 1975). An inhibitor of PG biosynthesis might therefore raise blood pressure. Most observers have not seen hypertension as a side effect of indomethacin, but Lee (1975) noted a rise in blood pressure after initiating treatment with indomethacin in patients with mild essential hypertension, while Wennmalm (1974) described increased aortic pressure in human volunteers receiving indomethacin intravenously.

In a small series of patients, Kerber et al. (1971) observed a favorable action of indomethacin in pericardial effusion of various etiologies. This has been confirmed by several other groups of investigators (references in Minuth et al., 1975). Minuth treated the pericarditis which sometimes occurs during chronic hemodialysis in uremia, and noted prompt defervescence, abatement of pain, disappearance of pericardial friction rub, decrease in cardiac size, resolution of the fusion, and avoidance of the need for surgical intervention. Dramatic relief of pain in pleurisy and pericarditis was also described by Baron (1968).

Pain relief in pleurisy was also noted by Sacks and Kanarek (1973) in a double blind study of single 100 mg suppositories of indomethacin. Relief of bone pain in patients with various hematological conditions was described as "dramatic" by Brodie (1974) in a series of patients whose pain had not responded to aspirin, codeine, or morphine. Pain in dysmenorrhea caused by irregular or excessive uterine contractions responds well to treatment with indomethacin (editorial, British Medical Journal, 31 May, 1975). Decrease in uterine tone and complete alleviation of pain was claimed by Lundström et al. (1976) in a small series of dysmenorrheal patients treated with indomethacin beginning the day before the expected menstrual period.

Sacks and Kanarek speculated that the analgesic effect of indomethacin in pleuritic pain might be due to an interference with the production of chemical mediators of pain. If so, the mediator most likely involved would be one or more of the prostaglandins. PG-synthetase activity in pulmonary vessels is altered in pathological states, and indomethacin blocks the effect of arachidonic acid on circulation in the lung (Hyman et al., 1976). Inhibition of PG biosynthesis is the most likely explanation for analgesia in dysmenorrhea, since PGs are known to be stimulants of uterine contractions. The inhibitory action of indomethacin on uterine contractions has also been utilized in the control of premature labor (Zuckerman et al., 1974).

Inhibition of PG biosynthesis also probably accounts for the suppression of growth of certain experimental tumors by indomethacin in mice as observed by

Humes and co-workers (1974). The tumors studied by Humes were said to be a mixture of inflammatory cells and granulation tissue containing elevated amounts of PGs. Sykes and Maddox (1972) also noted increased PG production in experimental tumors and its inhibition by indomethacin. Some tumors in human patients are accompanied by hypercalcemia not explained by bone metastases, and it has been suggested that such hypercalcemia may be related to enhanced PG production by the tumor. On this basis, Brereton *et al.* (1974) tried indomethacin in a patient with hypercalcemia associated with renal cell adenocarcinoma which was refractory to more traditional modes of therapy. Their success in this case led them to suggest a further trial of the drug in similar situations. Other patients with hypercalcemia were treated by Blum (1975).

A possible use of indomethacin in peridontal disease was suggested by Goldhaber *et al.* (1973) on the basis of results obtained in *in vitro* studies of bone resorption in cultures of human gingival fragments. Inflamed gingival tissues were said to produce significant amounts of PGE_2, which may be responsible for bone resorption in chronic destructive peridontal disease. The authors suggested that long-term studies should be undertaken to determine the efficacy of indomethacin and other PG synthetase inhibitors in the treatment of such disease. To our knowledge, there have been no reports of actual trials in patients, but in a related condition, Harris *et al.* (1973) presented evidence that bone resorption by dental cysts is caused by PGs, and that indomethacin inhibited this action *in vitro*.

In sections 3.1.2 and 7.9.5 we made brief reference to the effectiveness of indomethacin in sunburn. In a double blind study in human volunteers Gruber *et al.* (1972) showed that orally administered indomethacin, aspirin, or fenoprofen delayed the erythemic response to ultraviolet irradiation. Snyder and Eaglstein (1974a, b) observed that indomethacin effectively reduced ultraviolet induced erythema whether injected intradermally or applied topically. A solution containing 2·5 per cent of indomethacin applied externally to the skin after redness had appeared proved to be more effective than a cream containing fluorinated steroid. In these and other publications by the same group of investigators (Snyder, 1975; Greenberg *et al.*, 1975) it was suggested that the erythema might be due to release of PGs in the skin and that inhibition of PG biosynthesis, especially of PGE, is probably the mechanism of action of indomethacin.

Reports such as those described in the last few paragraphs above are somewhat fragmentary, and do not firmly establish new clinical uses for the compounds discussed in this review. They may be indicative, however, of potentialities for further exploration. Whether or not inhibition of PG synthesis is the sole explanation for therapeutic activity of indomethacin and similar compounds, the ubiquitous nature of PGs is well established, and the inhibition of either their synthesis or their pharmacological activities may have therapeutic implications that are as yet undreamed of.

Acknowledgements and final comment

The compilation of information for use in this review, as well as the original research performed in the Merck laboratories, some of which is reported herein for the first time, was made possible by the wholehearted cooperation of many individuals in the Merck Sharp & Dohme Research Laboratories and the Merck Institute for Therapeutic Research. At all stages of the investigations, we were encouraged and advised by Drs Max Tishler, L. H. Sarett, Karl H. Beyer, Jr and C. A. Stone.

The multidisciplinary effort during the development of indomethacin and of sulindac involved several teams of biologists, chemists, physicians and others, whose collaboration it is a pleasure to acknowledge. Among these were Dr John M. Chemerda, responsible for the process development, Dr Louis Schroeter, who supervised most of the pharmaceutical development, and Dr N. H. R. Cantwell, who piloted indomethacin through its initial clinical trials.

Of the scientists, assistants and technicians who devoted their skills to the laboratories under direct supervision of the present authors, special mention should be made of P. Tormo, S. L. Lucas, W. J. Holtz, R. L. Ellis, R. L. Bugianesi, E. A. Risley and G. W. Nuss.

Several colleagues in the Merck laboratories have generously permitted us to use data obtained in their laboratories and never before published. For this material, we are grateful to Drs and Messrs H. M. Peck, R. E. Zwickey, S. E. McKinney, D. A. Brodie, H. B. Hucker, D. E. Duggan, H. M. Hanson, K. C. Kwan, and E. M. Cohen. Dr C. G. Van Arman was involved in much of this research, especially in the elucidation of the pharmacological properties of sulindac. Others contributing importantly during key stages of the development included Drs and Messrs T. B. Windholz, A. Rosegay, B. E. Witzel, Howard Jones, B. O. Linn, A. R. Matzuk, C. H. Shunk, R. Greenwald, M. Fordice, J. McPherson, A. N. Wilson, C. H. Stammer and F. W. Holly. We are indebted to Mrs Carol Babish for her able assistance in assembling the manuscript.

All of these efforts have resulted in useful compounds, but more importantly, they have contributed to scientific knowledge. Our satisfaction comes not only from having been involved in the development of a compound of therapeutic value, but also in proven usefulness as a scientific tool, and in the stimulus these investigations have given to research in many other laboratories.

References

Ackerman, N. R. and Beebe, J. R. (1975). *Journal of Pharmacology and Experimental Therapeutics,* **193**, 603.

Adams, S. S. and Cobb, R. (1958). *Nature,* **181**, 773.

Allais, A., Meier, J., Mathieu, J., Nomine, G., Peterfalvi, M., Deraedt, R., Chifflot, L., Bezoni, J. and Fournex, R. (1975). *European Journal of Medicinal Chemistry,* **10**, 187.

Alvan, G., Orme, M., Bertilsson, L., Ekstrand, R. and Palmer, L. (1975). *Clinical Pharmacology and Therapeutics,* **18**, 364.

Anderson, G. G. and Speroff, L. (1973). *In* "The Prostaglandins" (Ed. P. W. Ramwell), p. 365. Plenum Press, New York, London.

Anderson, K. W. (1965). *In* "Non-steroidal Anti-inflammatory Drugs" (Eds S. Garattini and M. N. G. Dukes). *International Congress Series*, **82**, 245. Excerpta Medica, Amsterdam.

Anton, A. H. and Solomon, H. M. (eds) (1973). "Drug-Protein Binding". *Annals of the New York Academy of Sciences*, **226**.

Arrigoni-Martelli, E. and Conti, I. (1964a). *Farmaco, Editione Practicale*, **19**, 134.

Arrigoni-Martelli, E. and Conti, I. (1964b). *Medicina Experimentalis*, **10**, 164.

Arth, G. E., Fried, J., Johnston, D. B. R., Hoff, D. R., Sarett, L. H., Silber, R. H., Stoerk, H. C. and Winter, C. A. (1958). *Journal of the American Chemical Society*, **80**, 3161.

Asp, K. (1974). *Journal of International Medical Research*, **2**, 203.

Aspinall, R. L. (1970). *Proceedings of the Society for Experimental Biology and Medicine*, **135**, 561.

Aspinall, R. L., Cammarata, P. S., Makao, A., Jiu, J., Miyano, M., Baker, D. E. and Pautsch, W. F. (1973). *In* "Advances in the Biosciences" (Eds S. Bergström and S. Bernhard), vol. 9, p. 419. Pergamon Press, New York.

Atwater, E. C., Mongan, E. S., Wieche, D. R. and Jacox, R. F. (1965). *Archives of Internal Medicine*, **115**, 184.

Baer, J. E. (1972). *Journal of Pharmaceutical Sciences*, **611**, 1674.

Baldwin, H. A. and Borgmann, A. R. (1970). *Proceedings of the Society for Experimental Biology and Medicine*, **133**, 1326.

Ballabio, C. B. (1965). *In* "Non-steroidal Anti-inflammatory Drugs" (Eds S. Garattini and M. N. G. Dukes). *International Congress Series*, **82**, 342. Excerpta Medica, Amsterdam.

Ballabio, C. B. and Caruso, I. (1964). *Rhumatologie*, **16**, 431.

Barnett, D. B., Edwards, I. R. and Smith, A. J. (1975). *British Medical Journal*, **3**, 686.

Baron, B. R. (1968). *New England Journal of Medicine*, **278**, 1291.

Bartelheimer, H. K. and Senft, G. (1968). *Arzneimittel-Forschung*, **18**, 567.

Beatty, C. H., Bocek, R. M., Yong, M. K. and Novy, M. J. (1976). *Prostaglandins*, **11**, 713.

Behrman, H. R. and Anderson, G. G. (1974). *Archives of Internal Medicine*, **133**, 77.

Behrman, H. R. and Caldwell, B. V. (1974). *In* "Physiology Series One, Reproductive Physiology" (Ed. R. O. Greep), p. 63. Butterworths, London, and U. Park Press, Baltimore.

Bennett, A., Stamford, I. F. and Unger, W. G. (1973). *In* "Advances in the Biosciences" (Eds S. Bergström and S. Bernhard), vol. 9, p. 265. Pergamon Press, New York.

Benzi, G. and Frigo, G. M. (1964). *Farmaco, Editione Pratica*, **19**, 498.

Bergström, S. and Bernhard, S. (eds) (1973). "Advances in the Biosciences", vol. 9. Pergamon Press, New York.

Berman, L. (1965). *In* "Non-steroidal Anti-inflammatory Drugs" (Eds S. Garattini and M. N. G. Dukes). *International Congress Series*, **82**, 383. Excerpta Medica, Amsterdam.

Bett, I. M. (1962a). *Annals of the Rheumatic Diseases*, **21**, 63.

Bett, I. M. (1962b). *Annals of the Rheumatic Diseases*, **21**, 388.

Beyer, K. B., Jr. (1960). *Clinical Pharmacology and Therapeutics*, **1**, 274.

Bhattacherjee, P. and Eakins, K. E. (1974). *British Journal of Pharmacology*, **50**, 227.

Bianchi, C., Lumachi, B. and Pegrassi, L. (1967). *Arzneimittel-Forschung*, **17**, 246.

Blackham, A. and Owen, R. T. (1975). *Journal of Pharmacy and Pharmacology*, **27**, 201.

Blackwell, G. J., Flower, R. J. and Vane, J. R. (1975). *Biochemica et Biophysica Acta*, **398**, 178.

Bluestone, R., Kippen, I. and Klinenberg, J. R. (1969). *British Medical Journal*, **4**, 590.

Bluestone, R., Kippen, I., Klinenberg, J. R. and Whitehouse, M. W. (1970). *Journal of Laboratory and Clinical Medicine*, **76**, 85.

Boardman, P. L. and Hart, F. D. (1964). *Rhumatologie*, **16**, 425.

Boardman, P. L. and Hart, F. D. (1967). *Annals of the Rheumatic Diseases*, **26**, 127.

Bogden, A. E., Glenn, E. M., Koslowske, T. and Rigiero, C. S. (1967). *Life Sciences*, **6**, 965.

Bollet, A. J. (1961). *Arthritis and Rheumatism*, **4**, 624.

Botting, J. H. and Salzmann, R. (1973). *British Journal of Pharmacology*, **50**, 119.

Bowery, B. and Lewis, G. P. (1973). *British Journal of Pharmacology*, **47**, 305.

Brereton, H. D., Halushka, P. V., Alexander, R. W., Mason, D. M., Keiser, H. R. and DeVita, V. T., Jr. (1974). *New England Journal of Medicine*, **291**, 83.

Briseid, K., Arntzen, F. C. and Dyrud, O. K. (1971). *Acta Pharmacologica et Toxicologica*, **29**, 265.

Brocklehurst, J. C. and Humphreys, G. S. (1965). *Gerontologia Clinica*, **7**, 270.

Brodie, B. B. (1965). *Proceedings of the Royal Society of Medicine*, **58**, 946.

Brodie, D. A. and Hanson, H. M. (1960). *Gastroenterology*, **38**, 353.

Brodie, D. A., Cokk, P. A., Chase, B. J., Bauer, B. J. and Dagle, G. R. (1970). *Toxicology and Applied Pharmacology*, **17**, 615.

Brodie, G. N. (1974). *Lancet*, **i**, 1160.

Brody, T. M. (1955). *Pharmacological Reviews*, **7**, 335.

Brody, T. M. (1956). *Journal of Pharmacology and Experimental Therapeutics*, **117**, 39.

Brooks, P. M., Bell, M. A., Lee, P., Rooney, P. J. and Dick, W. C. (1974b). *British Journal of Clinical Pharmacology*, **1**, 485.

Brooks, P. M., Bell, M. A., Sturrock, R. D., Famaey, J. P. and Dick, W. C. (1974a). *British Journal of Clinical Pharmacology*, **1**, 287.

Brooks, P. M., Walker, J. J., Bell, M. A., Buchanan, W. W. and Rhymer, A. R. (1975). *British Medical Journal*, **3**, 69.

Brown, J. H., Taylor, J. L. and Waters, I. W. (1971). *Proceedings of the Society for Experimental Biology and Medicine*, **136**, 137.

Bugianesi, R. L. and Shen, T. Y. (1971). *Carbohydrate Research*, **19**, 179.

Bunim, J. J., Sokoloff, L., Williams, R. R. and Black, R. L. (1955). *Journal of Chronic Diseases*, **1**, 168.

Burns, C. A. (1966). *Investigations in Ophthalmology*, **5**, 325.

Burns, C. A. (1968). *American Journal of Ophthalmology*, **66**, 825.

Burns, C. A. (1973). *American Journal of Ophthalmology*, **76**, 312.

Burns, J. J., Rose, R. K., Chenkin, T., Goldman, A., Schulert, A. and Brodie, B. B. (1953). *Journal of Pharmacology and Experimental Therapeutics*, **109**, 346.

Butler, M., Giannina, T., Cargill, D. I., Popick, F. and Steinitz, B. G. (1969). *Proceedings of the Society for Experimental Biology and Medicine*, **132**, 484.

Calabro, J. J. (1975). *Drug Therapy*, **5**, No. 2, 46.

Calabro, J. J., Andelman, S., Bower, R., Caldwell, J., Hamaty, D., Kaplan, H., Maltz, B., Saville, P. and Umbenhauer, E. (1975). *American Society of Clinical Pharmacology and Therapeutics*, Washington, D.C., Mar. 20–22.

Calabro, J. J., Khoury, M. I. and Smyth, C. J. (1974). *Acta Rheumatologia, Portuguesa II*, 163.

Carlson, J. C., Barcikowski, B., Cargill, V. and McCracken, J. A. (1974). *Journal of Clinical Endocrinology and Metabolism*, **39**, 399.

Carr, R. E. and Siegel, I. M. (1973). *American Journal of Ophthalmology*, **75**, 302.

Carson, J. R., McKinstry, D. N. and Wong, S. (1971). *Journal Medicinal Chemistry*, **14**, 646.

Caruso, I. (1971). *Arzneimittel-Forschung*, **21**, 1824.

Caruso, I., Forcella, E. and Marczzan, E. (1964). *Reumatismo*, **16**, 393.

Casagrande, C., Invernizzi, A., Ferrini, R. and Miragoli, G. (1971). *Farmaco Editione Scienza*, **26**, 1059.

Cashin, C. H. and Heading, C. E. (1968). *British Journal of Pharmacology*, **34**, 148.

Casolo, G., Fontana, G., Mentasi, G. and Greco, V. (1965). *In* "Non-steroidal Anti-inflammatory Drugs" (Eds S. Garattini and M. N. G. Dukes). *International Congress Series*, **82**, 373. Excerpta Medica, Amsterdam.

Catoggio, P. (1964). *Rhumatologie*, **16**, 441.

Champion, G. D., Paulus, H. E., Mongan, E., Okun, R., Pearson, C. M. and Sarkissian, E. (1972). *Clinical Pharmacology and Therapeutics*, **13**, 239.

Chanh, P. H., Junstad, M. and Wennmahn, A. (1972). *Acta Physiologica Scandinavica*, **86**, 563.

Chang, Y. H. (1968). *Arthritis and Rheumatism*, **11**, 473.

Chang, Y. H. (1972). *Journal of Pharmacology and Experimental Therapeutics*, **183**, 235.

Chaplin, M. D., Roszkowski, A. P. and Richards, R. K. (1973). *Proceedings of the Society for Experimental Biology and Medicine*, **143**, 667.

Chiavarelli, N., Griseta, V. and Schena, P. (1974). *Circulation*, **50**, Supplement III, 291.

Chignell, C. F. and Starkweather, D. K. (1971). *Molecular Pharmacology*, **7**, 299.

Chivasta, T. E. and Cooke, A. R. (1972). *Journal of Laboratory and Clinical Medicine*, **79**, 302.

Christ, E. J. and Van Dorp, D. A. (1973). *In* "Advances in the Biosciences" (Eds S. Bergström and S. Bernhard), vol. 9, p. 35. Pergamon Press, New York.

Ciosek, C. P., Ortel, R. W., Thanassi, N. M. and Newcombe, D. S. (1974). *Nature*, **251**, 148.

Clark, R. L., Pessalano, A. A., Rogers, E. F., Sarett, L. H. and Stone, C. A. (1957). 132nd American Chemical Society Meeting, New York, Abstract 180.

Clarke, E. H. (1972). *Journal of Pharmaceutical Sciences*, **61**, 1678.

Clarkson, A. R., MacDonald, M. K., Cash, J. D. and Robson, J. S. (1972). *British Medical Journal*, **3**, 255.

Cohen, M., Sztokalo, J. and Hinsch, E. (1973). *Life Sciences*, **13**, 317.

Collier, H. O. J. (1971). *Nature*, **232**, 17.

Collier, H. O. J., Saeed, S. A., Schneider, C. and Warren, B. T. (1973). *In* "Advances in the Biosciences" (Eds S. Bergström and S. Bernhard), vol. 9, p. 413. Pergamon Press, New York.

Conquet, P., Plazonnet, B. and LeDouarec, J. C. (1975). *Investigations in Ophthalmology*, **14**, 772.

Conte, J., Suc, J. M. and Mignon-Conte, M. (1967). *Journal of Urology and Nephrology*, **73**, 850.

Coste, F., Delbarre, F., Braun, S. and Nastorg, G. (1964). *Rhumatologie*, **16**, 415.

Daha, M. R., Blok, A. P. R. and DeGraeff, J. (1973). *Netherlands Journal of Medicine,* **16**, 276.

D'Amour, F. E. and Smith, D. L. (1941). *Journal of Pharmacology and Experimental Therapeutics,* **72**, 74.

Davidorf, F. H. (1972). *Ohio State Medical Journal,* **68**, 1022.

Davies, G. E., Holman, G., Johnston, T. P. and Lowe, J. S. (1966). *British Journal of Pharmacology,* **28**, 212.

Davis, H. A. and Horton, E. W. (1972). *British Journal of Pharmacology,* **46**, 658.

Deby, C., Descamps, M., Binon, F. and Bacq, Z. M. (1975). *Biochemical Pharmacology,* **24**, 1092.

DeGaetano, G., Vermylen, J., Donati, M. B., Dotremont, G. and Michielsen, P. (1974). *British Medical Journal,* **2**, 301.

Denko, C. W. (1974a). *Journal of Rheumatology,* **1**, 222.

Denko, C. W. (1974b). *Pharmacology,* **12**, 331.

Dieppe, P. A., Huskisson, E. C., Crocker, P. and Willoughby, D. A. (1976). *Lancet,* **i**, 266.

DiPasquale, G. and Welaj, P. (1973). *Journal of Pharmacy and Pharmacology,* **25**, 831.

DiRosa, M., Giroud, J. P. and Willoughby, D. A. (1971a). *Journal of Pathology,* **104**, 15.

DiRosa, M., Papadimitriou, J. M. and Willoughby, D. A. (1971b). *Journal of Pathology,* **105**, 239.

DiRosa, M. and Sorrentino, L. (1970). *British Journal of Pharmacology,* **38**, 214.

DiRosa, M. and Willoughby, D. A. (1971). *Journal of Pharmacy and Pharmacology,* **23**, 297.

DiRosa, M., Sorrentino, L. and Parente, L. (1972). *Journal of Pharmacy and Pharmacology,* **24**, 576.

Dodge, P. W., Brodie, D. A., Young, P. R., Krause, R. A. and Tekeli, S. (1974). *Digestive Diseases,* **19**, 449.

Doebel, K. J. and Wasley, J. W. F. (1972). *Journal of Medicinal Chemistry,* **15**, 1081.

Domenjoz, R. (1952). *International Record of Medical and General Practice Clinics,* **165**, 467.

Domenjoz, R. (1966). *Advances in Pharmacology,* **4**, 143.

Domenjoz, R. and Mörsdorf, K. (1965). *In* "Non-steroidal Anti-inflammatory Drugs" (Eds S. Garattini and M. N. G. Dukes). *International Congress Series,* **82**, 162. Excerpta Medica, Amsterdam.

Donnelly, P., Lloyd, K. and Campbell, H. (1967). *British Medical Journal,* **1**, 69.

Dorrego, F., Sunkel, C. and Armijo, M. (1976). *Archivos de Farmacologia y Toxicologia,* **11**, 1.

Dougherty, T. F., Brown, H. E. and Berliner, D. L. (1958). *Endocrinology,* **62**, 455.

Douwes, F. R. (1974). *International Journal of Clinical Pharmacology, Therapeutics and Toxicology,* **9**, 243.

Drees, D. T., Robbins, T. L. and Crago, F. L. (1974). *Toxicology and Applied Pharmacology,* **27**, 194.

Duggan, D. E., Hogans, A. F., Kwan, K. C. and McMahon, F. G. (1972). *Journal of Pharmacology and Experimental Therapeutics,* **181**, 563.

Duggan, D. E., Hooke, K. F., Noll, R. M. and Kwan, K. C. (1975). *Biochemical Pharmacology,* **24**, 1749.

Duggan, D. E., Hooke, K. F., Carlson, R. and Van Arman, C. G. (1976). *Pharmacologist,* **18**, 164.

Duggan, D. E., Hare, L. E., Ditzler, B. A., Lei, B. W. and Kwan, K. C. (1977a). *Clinical Pharmacology and Therapeutics* (in press).

Duggan, D. E., Hooke, K. F., White, S. D., Noll, R. M. and Stevenson, C. R. (1977b). *Journal of Pharmacology and Experimental Therapeutics*, **201**, 463.

Duggan, D. E., Hooke, K. F., Risley, E. A., Shen, T. Y. and Van Arman, C. G. (1977c). *Journal of Pharmacology and Experimental Therapeutics*, **201**, 8.

Eakins, K. E. (1974). *In* "Prostaglandin Synthetase Inhibitors" (Eds H. J. Robinson and J. R. Vane), p. 343. Raven Press, New York.

Eakins, K. E., Whitelocke, R. A., Bennett, A. and Martenet, A. C. (1972). *British Medical Journal*, **3**, 452.

Eakins, K. E., Whitelocke, R. A. F., Perkins, E. S., Bennett, A. and Unger, W. G. (1973). *In* "Advances in the Biosciences" (Eds S. Bergström and S. Bernhard), vol 9, p. 427. Pergamon Press, New York.

Ellis, E. F., Oelz, O., Nies, A. S., Wilkinson, G. R. and Oates, J. A. (1976). *Federation Proceedings*, **35**, 297.

Emmerson, B. T. (1967). *British Medical Journal*, **2**, 272.

Emori, H. W., Champion, G. D., Bluestone, R. and Paulus, H. E. (1973). *Annals of the Rheumatic Diseases*, **32**, 433.

Emori, H. W., Champion, G. D., Paulus, H. E., Bluestone, R. and Pearson, C. M. (1974). *Australian and New Zealand Journal of Medicine*, **4**, 212.

Empire Rheumatism Council (1955). *Annals of the Rheumatic Diseases*, **14**, 353.

Erspamer, V. (1961). *In* "Progress in Drug Research" (Ed. E. Jucker), vol. 3, p. 151. Birkhäuser, Basel and Stuttgart, Interscience, New York.

Ezer, E., Palosi, E., Hajos, G. and Szporny, L. (1976). *Journal of Pharmacy and Pharmacology*, **28**, 655.

Feldberg, W. (1974). *In* Prostaglandin Synthetase Inhibitors" (Eds H. J. Robinson and J. R. Vane), p. 197. Raven Press, New York.

Ferreira, S. H., Moncada, S. and Vane, J. R. (1971). *Nature New Biology*, **231**, 237.

Ferreira, S. H., Moncada, S. and Vane, J. R. (1973). *British Journal of Pharmacology*, **49**, 86.

Ferreira, S. H., Moncada, S. and Vane, J. R. (1974). *In* "Prostaglandin Synthetase Inhibitors" (Eds H. J. Robinson and J. R. Vane), p. 175. Raven Press, New York.

Ferreira, S. H. and Vane, J. R. (1974). *Annual Review of Pharmacology*, **14**, 57.

Fitch, K. D. and Gray, S. D. (1974). *Medical Journal of Australia*, **1**, 260.

Fleming, J. S., Bierwagen, M. E., Pircio, A. W. and Pindell, M. H. (1969). *Archives Internationales de Pharmacodynamie et de Thérapie*, **199**, 164.

Floman, Y. and Zor, U. (1976). *Prostaglandins*, **12**, 403.

Flower, R. J. (1974). *Pharmacological Reviews*, **26**, 33.

Flower, R. J., Gryglewski, R., Herbaczynska-Cedro, K. and Vane, J. R. (1972). *Nature New Biology*, **238**, 104.

Fontaine, L., Grand, M., Quentin, Y. and Merle, S. (1965). *Medicina et Pharmacologia Experimentalis*, **13**, 137.

Formiller, M. and Cohon, M. S. (1969). *American Journal of Hospital Pharmacy*, **26**, 574.

Frost, H. and Hess, H. (1966). *In* "Die Entzündung" (Eds R. Heitz and H. F. Hofmann), p. 374. Urban and Schwartzenberg, Munich, Berlin, Vienna.

Gander, G. W. and Goodale, F. (1969). *Federation Proceedings*, **28**, 357.

Garnham, J. C., Raymond, K., Shotton, E. and Turner, P. (1975). *European Journal of Clinical Pharmacology*, **8**, 107.

Gáspárdy, G., Balint, G. and Gáspárdy, G., Jr. (1967). *Zeitschrift für Rheumaforschung*, **26**, 332.

Gerber, D. A. (1965). *Clinical Research*, **13**, 543.

Gerber, D. A., Giustra, R. and Cohen, N. (1966). *Arthritis and Rheumatism*, **9**, 507.

Gerber, D. A., Cohen, N. and Giustra, R. (1967). *Biochemical Pharmacology*, **16**, 115.

Giordano, M., Cappelli, L. and Chianese, U. (1975). *Arzneimittel-Forschung*, **25**, 435.

Glamkowski, E. J., Gal, G. and Sletzinger, M. (1973). *Journal of Medicinal Chemistry*, **16**, 176.

Glenn, E. M. and Bowman, B. J. (1969). *Proceedings of the Society for Experimental Biology and Medicine*, **130**, 1327.

Glenn, E. M., Bowman, B. J., Koozers, W., Koslowske, T. and Meyers, M. L. (1967). *Journal of Pharmacology and Experimental Therapeutics*, **155**, 157.

Glenn, E. M., Bowman, B. J., Lyster, S. C. and Rohloff, N. A. (1971). *Proceedings of the Society for Experimental Biology and Medicine*, **138**, 235.

Glenn, E. M., Bowman, B. J. and Rohloff, N. A. (1972). *In* "Prostaglandins in Cellular Biology" (Eds P. W. Ramwell and B. P. Pharriss), p. 239. Plenum Press, New York.

Glenn, E. M. and Sekhar, N. C. (1971). *In* "Immunopathology of Inflammation", (Eds J. Houck and B. Forscher), p. 13. Excerpta Medica, Amsterdam.

Glynn, L. E. (1963). *International Archives of Allergy and Applied Immunology*, **22**, 236.

Goldhaber, P., Rabadjija, L., Beyer, W. R. and Kornhauser, A. (1973). *Journal of the American Dental Association*, **87**, 1027.

Gordon, D. M. (1970). *In* "Ocular Anti-inflammatory Therapy" (Ed. H. E. Kaufman), p. 146. Charles C. Thomas, Springfield.

Görög, P. and Kovacs, I. B. (1970). *Journal of Pharmacy and Pharmacology*, **22**, 86.

Greaves, M. W. and McDonald-Gibson, W. (1973). *Journal of Investigative Dermatology*, **61**, 127.

Green, A. F., Young, P. A. and Godfrey, T. A. (1951). *British Journal of Pharmacology*, **6**, 572.

Greenberg, R. A., Eaglstein, W. H., Turnier, H. and Houdek, P. V. (1975). *Archives of Dermatology*, **111**, 328.

Greenwald, R. B. and Shen, T. Y. (1970). *Journal of Heterocyclic Chemistry*, **7**, 683.

Grennan, D. M., Zeitlin, I. J., Mitchell, W. S., Buchanan, W. W. and Dick, W. C. (1975). *Prostaglandins*, **9**, 800.

Gruber, C. M., Jr., Ridolfo, A. S., Nickander, R. and Mikulaschek, W. M. (1972). *Clinical Pharmacology and Therapeutics*, **13**, 109.

Grunnet, I. and Bojesen, E. (1976). *Biochemica et Biophysica Acta*, **419**, 365.

Gryglewski, R. J. (1974). *In* "Prostaglandin Synthetase Inhibitors" (Eds H. J. Robinson and J. R. Vane), p. 33. Raven Press, New York.

Gryglewski, R. J. (1976). *Pharmacology Research Communications*, **8**, 337.

Gryglewski, R. J. and Gryglewski, T. A. (1966). *Biochemical Pharmacology*, **15**, 1171.

Gund, P. and Shen, T. Y. (1977). *Journal of Medicinal Chemistry*, **20**, 1146.

Gupta, M. B., Gupta, G. P., Tangri, K. K. and Bhargava, K. P. (1969). *Biochemical Pharmacology*, **18**, 531.

Guzman, F., Braun, C., Lim, R. K. S., Potter, G. D. and Rodgers, D. W. (1964). *Archives Internationales de Pharmacodynamie et de Thérapie*, **149**, 571.

Hagenfeldt, L. and Wennmalm, A. (1975). *European Journal of Clinical Investigation*, **5**, 235.

Hamberg, M. and Samuelsson, B. (1971). *Journal of Biological Chemistry*, **246**, 6713.

Hamberg, M. and Samuelsson, B. (1973). *Proceedings of the National Academy of Sciences, USA*, **70**, 899.

Hamberg, M. and Samuelsson, B. (1974). *Proceedings of the National Academy of Sciences, USA*, **71**, 3400.

Hamberg, M., Svensson, J. and Samuelsson, B. (1974). *Proceedings of the National Academy of Sciences, USA*, **71**, 3824.

Hamberg, M., Svensson, J. and Samuelsson, B. (1975). *Proceedings of the National Academy of Sciences, USA*, **72**, 2994.

Hamberg, M., Svensson, J., Wakabayashi, T. and Samuelsson, B. (1974). *Proceedings of the National Academy of Sciences, USA*, **71**, 345.

Hanna, C. and Keatts, H. C. (1967). *Archives of Ophthalmology*, **77**, 554.

Hanna, C. and Sharp, J. D. (1972). *Archives of Ophthalmology*, **88**, 196.

Hansen, H. S. (1974). *Prostaglandins*, **8**, 95.

Hansen, H. S. (1976). *Prostaglandins*, **12**, 647.

Hare, L. E., Ditzler, D. A., Hichens, M. and Duggan, D. E. (1974). *Pharmacologist*, **16**, 221.

Harman, R. E., Meisinger, M. A. P., Davis, G. E. and Kuehl, F. A., Jr. (1964). *Journal of Pharmacology and Experimental Therapeutics*, **143**, 215.

Harris, M., Jenkins, M. V., Bennett, A. and Wills, M. R. (1973). *Nature*, **245**, 213.

Hart, F. D. and Boardman, P. L. (1964). *Practitioner*, **192**, 828.

Healey, L. A. (1967). *Bulletin of Rheumatic Diseases*, **18**, 483.

Hedqvist, P. (1973). *In* "Advances in the Biosciences" (Eds S. Bergström and S. Bernhard), vol. 9, p. 461. Pergamon Press, New York.

Heimlich, K. R. (1972). *Journal of Pharmaceutical Sciences*, **61**, 1686.

Heller, J. and Tata, P. S. (1968). *Physiologica Bohemoslovenica*, **17**, 1.

Hench, P. S., Kendall, E. C., Slocumb, C. H. and Polley, H. F. (1949). *Proceedings of the Staff Meetings of the Mayo Clinic*, **24**, 181.

Herzog, H. L., Nobile, A., Tolksdorf, S., Charney, W., Hershberg, E. B., Perlman, P. L. and Pechet, M. M. (1955). *Science*, **121**, 176.

Heymann, M. A., Rudolph, A. M. and Silverman, N. H. (1976). *New England Journal of Medicine*, **295**, 530.

Hichens, M. (1974). *In* "Medicinal Chemistry, 13-II, Antiinflammatory Agents (Eds R. A. Scherrer and M. W. Whitehouse), p. 264. Academic Press, New York.

Higgs, G. A., Vane, J. R., Hart, F. D. and Wojtulewski, J. A. (1974). *In* "Prostaglandin Synthetase Inhibitors" (Eds H. J. Robinson and J. R. Vane), p. 165. Raven Press, New York.

Hinman, J. W. (1972). *Annual Review of Biochemistry*, **41**, 161.

Hitchens, J. T., Goldstein, S., Sambuca, A. and Shemano, I. (1967). *Pharmacologist*, **9**, 326.

Hoffbrand, B. I. and Kininmonth, D. A. (1967). *British Medical Journal*, **2**, 838.

Hogans, A. F., Hooke, K. F. and Duggan, D. E. (1971). *Pharmacologist*, **13**, 237.

Hoogsteen, K. and Trenner, N. R. (1970). *Journal of Organic Chemistry*, **35**, 521.

Hucker, H. B. and Hoffman, E. (1971). *Journal of Pharmaceutical Sciences*, **60**, 1049.

Hucker, H. B., Stauffer, S. C., Bower, R. J., Umbenhauer, E. R. and McMahon, F. G. (1972). *Federation Proceedings*, **31**, 577.

Hucker, H. B., Stauffer, S. C., White, S. D., Rhodes, R. E., Arison, B. H., Umbenhauer, E. R., Bower, R. J. and McMahon, F. G. (1973). *Drug Metabolism and Disposition*, **1**, 721.

Hucker, H. B., Zacchei, A. G., Cox, S. V., Brodie, D. A. and Cantwell, N. H. R. (1966). *Journal of Pharmacology and Experimental Therapeutics*, **153**, 237.

Humes, J. L., Cupo, J. J., Jr. and Strausser, H. R. (1974). *Prostaglandins*, **6**, 463.

Huskinsson, E. C. and Franchimont, P. (eds) (1976). "Clinoril in the Treatment of Rheumatic Diseases". Raven Press, New York.

Hussar, D. A. (1967). *American Journal of Pharmacy*, **139**, 215.

Hussar, D. A. (1969). *American Journal of Pharmacy*, **141**, 107.

Hyman, A. L., Mathe, A. S., Spannhake, E. W. and Kadowitz, P. J. (1976). *Physiologist*, **19**, 236.

Ignarro, L. J. (1971). *Biochemical Pharmacology*, **20**, 2847, 2861.

Ignarro, L. J. (1972). *Journal of Pharmacology and Experimental Therapeutics*, **182**, 179.

Ignarro, L. J. and Colombo, C. (1972). *Nature New Biology*, **239**, 155.

Inglot, A. D. and Wolna, E. (1968). *Biochemical Pharmacology*, **17**, 269.

Janoff, A. (1972). *Annual Review of Medicine*, **23**, 177.

Jansen, J. A., Hvidberg, E. and Lausen, H. H. (1970). *Acta Pharmacologica et Toxicologica*, **28**, Supp. 1, 54.

Jansen, J. A. and Schou, J. (1971). *Acta Pharmacologica et Toxicologica*, **30**, 153.

Jansen, J. A. and Schou, J. (1972). *Acta Pharmacologica et Toxicologica*, **31**, 209.

Jeremy, R. and Towson, J. (1970). *Medical Journal of Australia*, **2**, 127.

Jones, H., Bugianesi, R. L. and Shen, T. Y. (1976). *Journal of Carbohydrates, Nucleosides and Nucleotides*, **3**, 369.

Juby, P. F. and Hudyma, T. W. (1969). *Journal of Medicinal Chemistry*, **12**, 396.

Kaiser, D. G., Glenn, E. M., Johnson, R. H. and Johnston, R. L. (1967). *Journal of Pharmacology and Experimental Therapeutics*, **155**, 174.

Kalbhen, D. A., Gelderblom, P. and Domenjoz, R. (1970). *Pharmacology*, **3**, 353.

Kamiya, K., Wada, Y. and Nichkawa, M. (1975). *Chemical and Pharmaceutical Bulletin*, **23**, 1589.

Kantrowitz, F., Robinson, D. R., McGuire, M. B. and Levine, L. (1975). *Nature*, **258**, 737.

Katz, A. M., Pearson, C. M. and Kennedy, J. M. (1965). *Clinical Pharmacology and Therapeutics*, **6**, 25.

Kent, T. H., Cardelli, R. M. and Stamler, F. W. (1969). *American Journal of Pathology*, **54**, 237.

Kerber, R. E., Spivack, A. P. and Harrison, D. C. (1971). *Circulation*, **44**, Supplement 1, 185.

Kistenmacher, T. J. and Marsh, R. E. (1972). *Journal of American Chemical Society*, **94**, 1340.

Kobayashi, S. and Takagi, H. (1968). *Arzneimittel-Forschung*, **18**, 939.

Komatsu, T., Saito, C., Awata, H., Sakai, Y., Inukai, T., Kurokawa, H. and Yamamoto, H. (1973). *Arzneimittel-Forschung*, **23**, 1690.

Ku, E. C., Eakins, K. E. and Signor, C. (1975). International Conference on Prostaglandins, Florence, Abstract 94.

Kuehl, F. A., Jr., Cirillo, V. J., Ham, E. A. and Humes, J. L. (1973). *In* "Advances in the Biosciences" (Eds S. Bergström and S. Bernhard), vol. 9, p. 155. Pergamon Press, New York.

Kuehl, F. A., Jr., Oien, H. G. and Ham, E. A. (1974). *In* "Prostaglandin Synthetase Inhibitors" (Eds H. J. Robinson and J. R. Vane), p. 53. Raven Press, New York.

Kunze, M., Stein, G., Kunze, E. and Traeger, A. (1974). *Deutsche Gesundheitswesen*, **29**, 351.

Kwan, K. C., Breault, G. O., Umbenhauer, E. R., McMahon, F. G. and Duggan, D. E. (1976). *Journal of Pharmacokinetics and Biopharmacy*, **4**, 255.

Lange, O. (1966). *In* "Die Entzündung" (Eds R. Heister and H. F. Hofmann), p. 337. Urban and Schwarzenberg, Munich, Berlin, Vienna.

Langkilde, M. (1965). Indomethacin Symposium, Amsterdam, 69.
Lee, J. B. (1975). *Medical Clinics of North America*, **59**, 713.
Lee, R. E. (1974). *Prostaglandins*, **5**, 63.
Lee, Y. H., Mollison, K. W. and Cheng, W. D. (1971). *Archives Internationales de Pharmacodynamie et de Thérapie*, **191**, 370.
Lemberger, L. (1972). *Journal of Pharmaceutical Sciences*, **61**, 1690.
Levy, L. (1974). *In* "Antiinflammatory Agents" (Eds R. A. Scherrer and M. W. Whitehouse), p. 193. Academic Press, New York.
Lewis, A. J., Cottney, J. and Sugrue, M. F. (1975). *Journal of Pharmacy and Pharmacology*, **27**, 375.
Liebling, M. R., Altman, R. D., Benedek, T. G., Bennahum, D. A., Blaschke, J. A., Bower, R. J., Calabro, J. J., Caldwell, J. R., Collins, R. L., Felt, J., Hamaty, D., Jimenea, C. V., Umbenhauer, E. R. and Wilkins, R. (1975). Proceedings of 39th Annual Meeting, American Rheumatism Foundation, Section Arthritis, New Orleans, June 5, p. 30.
Lim, R. K. S. (1960). *Annals of the New York Academy of Sciences*, **86**, 73.
Lim, R. K. S. (1967). *Anesthesiology*, **28**, 106.
Lim, R. K. S., Miller, D. G., Guzman, F., Rodgers, D. W., Rogers, R. W., Wang, S. K., Chao, P. Y. and Shih, T. Y. (1967). *Clinical Pharmacology and Therapeutics*, **8**, 521.
Linquist, B., Jensen, K. M., Johansson, H. and Hansen, T. (1974). *Clinical Pharmacology and Therapeutics*, **15**, 247.
Lippman, W. (1974). *Prostaglandins*, **7**, 1, 231.
Lorber, A. (1966). *Clinical Research*, **14**, 334.
Lorenzetti, O. J. (1970). *Pharmacologist*, **12**, 334.
Lövgren, O. and Allander, E. (1965). *British Medical Journal*, **1**, 996.
Lowry, P. J., McMartin, C. and Peters, J. (1973). *Journal of Endocrinology*, **59**, 43.
Lundström, V., Green, K. and Wiqvist, N. (1976). *Prostaglandins*, **11**, 893.
Mafii, G. and Schiatti, P. (1966). *Toxicology and Applied Pharmacology*, **8**, 138.
Maickel, R. P., Bush, M. T., Jondorf, W. R., Miller, F. P. and Gillette, J. R. (1966). *Molecular Pharmacology*, **2**, 491.
Maickel, R. P., Miller, F. P. and Brodie, B. B. (1965). *Pharmacologist*, **7**, 182.
Maickel, R. P., Miller, F. P. and Brodie, B. B. (1969). *Arzneimittel-Forschung*, **19**, 1803.
Main, I. H. M. and Whittle, B. J. R. (1973). *British Journal of Pharmacology*, **47**, 666P.
Mainland, D. and Cooperating Clinics of the American Rheumatism Association (1967). *Clinical Pharmacology and Therapeutics*, **8**, 11.
Majerus, P. W. and Stanford, N. (1977). *British Journal of Clinical Pharmacology*, **4**, 15S.
Martyak, S. N. (1974). *Drug Therapy*, **4/5**, 19.
Mason, R. W. and McQueen, E. G. (1974). *Pharmacology* **12**, 12.
Mattila, M. J. and Saarnivaara, L. (1967a). *Scandinavian Journal of Clinical and Laboratory Investigation*, **19**, Supplement **95**, 63.
Mattila, M. J. and Saarnivaara, L. (1967b). *Annales Medicinae Experimentales et Biologiae Fenniae*, **45**, 360.
McCall, E. and Youlten, L. J. F. (1974). *British Journal of Pharmacology*, **52**, 452P.
McDonough, J. and Levine, L. (1975). *Nature*, **258**, 739.
McGiff, J. C., Terragno, N. A. and Irskovitz, H. D. (1974). *In* "Prostaglandin Synthetase Inhibitors" (Eds H. J. Robinson and J. R. Vane), p. 259. Raven Press, New York.

McMillan, M. (1960). *Journal of Clinical Pathology,* **13,** 140.

McQueen, E. G. (1973). *Drugs,* **6,** 104.

Meier, R., Schuler, W. and Desaulles, P. (1950). *Experientia,* **6,** 469.

Menasse-Gdynia, R. and Krupp, P. (1974). *Toxicology and Applied Pharmacology,* **29,** 389.

Menguy, R. and Desbaillets, L. (1967). *American Journal of Digestive Diseases,* **12,** 862.

Menguy, R. and Desbaillets, L. (1968). *Annals of Surgery,* **168,** 475.

Mezey, K. C. (1966). *In* "Die Entzündung" (Eds R. Heister and H. F. Hofmann), p. 294. Urban and Schwarzenberg, Munich, Berlin, Vienna.

Michielsen, P. and Verberckmoes, R. (1968). *Medicinae Scientia Donat,* **1,** 45.

Michielsen, P., Verberckmoes, R., Desmet, V. and Hemerijckx, W. (1969). *Journal of Urology and Nephrology,* **75,** 315.

Michotte, L. J. and Wanters, M. (1964). *Acta Rheumatologica Scandinavia,* **10,** 273.

Mielens, Z. E., Drobeck, H. P., Rozitis, J. and Sansone, V. J. (1968). *Journal of Pharmacy and Pharmacology,* **20,** 567.

Mills, J. A. (1974). *New England Journal of Medicine,* **290,** 1002.

Milton, A. S. (1973). *In* "Advances in the Biosciences" (Eds S. Bergström and S. Bernhard), p. 495. Pergamon Press, New York.

Minuth, A. N. W., Nottebohm, G. A., Eknoyan, G. and Suki, W. N. (1975). *Archives of Internal Medicine,* **135,** 807.

Mizushima, Y., Sakai, S. and Yamaura, M. (1970). *Biochemical Pharmacology,* **19,** 227.

Moncada, S., Ferreira, S. H. and Vane, J. R. (1974). *In* "Prostaglandin Synthetase Inhibitors" (Eds H. J. Robinson and J. R. Vane), p. 189. Raven Press, New York.

Moncada, S., Needleman, P., Bunting, S. and Vane, J. R. (1976). *Prostaglandins,* **12,** 323.

Morrelli, H. F. and Melmon, K. L. (1968). *California Medicine,* **109,** 280.

Mörsdorf, K. (1965). *In* "Non-steroidal Anti-inflammatory Drugs" (Eds S. Garattini and M. N. G. Dukes), *International Congress Series,* **82,** 85. Excerpta Medica, Amsterdam.

Müller, K. H. and Herrman, K. (1966). *Medizinische Welt,* **17,** 1553.

Müller, K. H. and Zollinger, W. (1966). *In* "Die Entzündung" (Eds R. Heister and H. F. Hofmann), p. 376. Urban and Schwarzenberg, Munich, Berlin, Vienna.

Murisasco, A., Picon, G., Hebreard, J., Sansot, M., Aubert, L., Taramasco, J., Martin, J. and Manassero, L. (1967). *Marseille Médical,* **104,** 787.

Nakanishi, M. and Goto, K. (1975). *Biochemical Pharmacology,* **24,** 421.

Neufeld, A. H. and Sears, M. L. (1973). *Prostaglandins,* **4,** 157.

Newcombe, D. S., Thanassi, N. M. and Ciosek, C. P. (1974). *Life Sciences,* **14,** 505.

Niemegeers, C. J. E., Verbruggen, F. J. and Janssen, P. A. J. (1964). *Journal of Pharmacy and Pharmacology,* **16,** 810.

Novak, V. and Soumarova, H. (1971). *Ceskoslovenska Oftalmologie,* **27,** 352.

Novy, M. J., Cook, M. J. and Manaugh, L. (1974). *American Journal of Obstetrics and Gynecology,* **118,** 412.

Nucifera, T. L. and Malone, M. H. (1971). *Archives Internationales de Pharmacodynamie et de Thérapie,* **191,** 345.

Obayashi, K. and Kozaki, M. (1968). *Japanese Review of Clinical Ophthalmology,* **62,** 479.

O'Brien, W. M. (1968). *Clinical Pharmacology and Therapeutics,* **9,** 94.

Odegaard, A. E. (1974). *Tidsskrift for den Norske Laegeforening*, **94**, 2313, 2330.

Oliw, E., Kover, G., Larsson, C. and Anggard, E. (1976). *European Journal of Pharmacology*, **38**, 95.

Olson, D. R., Wheeler, W. J. and Wells, J. N. (1974). *Journal of Medicinal Chemistry*, **17**, 167.

Oronsky, A. L., Triner, L., Steinsland, O. S. and Nahas, G. G. (1969). *Nature*, **223**, 619.

Palmer, L., Bertilsson, L., Alvan, G., Orme, M., Sjöqvist, F. and Holmstedt, B. (1974). *In* "Prostaglandin Synthetase Inhibitors" (Eds H. J. Robinson and J. R. Vane), p. 91. Raven Press, New York.

Pantuck, E. J., Hsiao, K. C., Kuntzman, R. and Conney, A. H. (1975). *Science*, **187**, 744.

Patrono, C., Ciabattoni, G., Greco, F. and Grossi-Belloni, D. (1976). *In* "Advances in Prostaglandins and Thromboxane Research" (Eds B. Samuelsson and R. Paoletti), vol. 1, p. 125. Raven Press, New York.

Paul, W. D., Strottmann, M. P., Routh, J. I. and Mergner, W. (1964). *Rheumatologie*, **16**, 411, 413.

Paulus, H. E. and Whitehouse (1973). *Annual Review of Pharmacology*, **13**, 107.

Pearson, C. M. (1966). *Clinical Pharmacology and Therapeutics*, **7**, 416.

Peck, H. M. (1964a). *Journal of the American Medical Association*, **187**, 341.

Peck, H. M. (1964b). *Annals of the New York Academy of Sciences*, **111**, 689.

Peck, H. M. (1966). *Bioscience*, **16**, 696.

Peck, H. M. (1968). *In* "Importance of Fundamental Principles in Drug Evaluation" (Eds D. H. Tedeschi and R. E. Tedeschi), p. 449. Raven Press, New York.

Peck, H. M., Mattis, P. A., Stonier, P. F. and Zwickey, R. E. (1967). *Drug Information Bulletin*, January/March, 32.

Pelczarska, A. and Gieldanowski, J. (1970). *Journal of Pharmacy and Pharmacology*, **22**, 617.

Perkins, E. S. and MacFaul, P. A. (1965). *Transactions of the Ophthalmology Society, UK*, **85**, 53.

Phelps, A. H., Bagdon, W. J., Mattis, P. A., Winter, C. A. and Zwickey, R. E. (1968). *Federation Proceedings*, **27**, 598.

Phelps, P. and McCarty, D. J., Jr. (1966). *Arthritis and Rheumatism*, **9**, 532.

Phelps, P. and McCarty, D. J. Jr., (1967). *Journal of Pharmacy and Pharmacology*, **22**, 617.

Piliero, S. J., Graeme, M. L., Sigg, E. B., Chinea, G. and Colombo, C. (1966). *Life Sciences*, **5**, 1057.

Pinals, R. S. and Frank, S. (1967). *New England Journal of Medicine*, **276**, 512.

Pitkeathly, D. A., Banerjee, N. R., Harris, R. and Sharp, J. (1966). *Annals of the Rheumatic Diseases*, **25**, 334.

Podos, S. H., Becker, B. and Kass, M. A. (1973). *Investigative Ophthalmology*, **12**, 426.

Pollock, S. H. and Brown, J. H. (1971). *Journal of Pharmacology and Experimental Therapeutics*, **178**, 609.

Prema, K. and Gopinathan, K. P. (1974). *Biochemical Journal*, **143**, 613.

Prema, K. and Gopinathan, K. P. (1976). *Biochemical Pharmacology*, **25**, 1299.

Ramunni, M. (1966). *Gazzetta Medica Italiana*, **125**, 131.

Ramwell, P. W. (ed.) (1973). "The Prostaglandins I". Plenum Press, New York.

Randall, L. O. and Selitto, J. J. (1957). *Archives Internationales de Pharmacodynamie et de Thérapie*, **111**, 409.

Rao, C. V. (1974). *Prostaglandins,* **6,** 313.

Riesterer, L. and Jaques, R. (1967). *Helvetica Physiologica et Pharmacologica Acta,* **25,** 156.

Robert, A. (1974a). *Prostaglandins,* **6,** 523.

Robert, A. (1974b). *Gastroenterology,* **66,** 765.

Robinson, D. R. and McGuire, M. B. (1974). Abstract 23, New York Academy of Sciences Conference on Mechanisms of Tissue Injury with Reference to Rheumatoid Arthritis, Nov. 20–22.

Robinson, H. J. and Vane, J. R. (eds) (1974). "Prostaglandin Synthetase Inhibitors". Raven Press, New York.

Robinson, H. J., Phares, H. F. and Graessle, O. E. (1974). *In* "Prostaglandin Synthetase Inhibitors" (Eds H. J. Robinson and J. R. Vane), p. 327. Raven Press, New York.

Rome, L. H., Lands, W. E. M., Roth, G. J. and Majerus, P. W. (1976). *Prostaglandins,* **11,** 23.

Rosenthale, M. E., Dervinas, A., Kassarich, J. and Singer, S. (1972). *Journal of Pharmacy and Pharmacology,* **24,** 149.

Roth, G. J., Stanford, N. and Majerus, P. W. (1975). *Proceedings of the National Academy of Sciences, USA,* **72,** 3073.

Roth, S. H. and Englund, D. W. (1969). *Arthritis and Rheumatism,* **12,** 328.

Rothermich, N. O. (1966). *Journal of the American Medical Association,* **195,** 531; 1102.

Roubal, Z. and Nemecek, O. (1966). *Journal of Medicinal Chemistry,* **9,** 840.

Rubegni, M., Provvedi, D., Bellini, P. G., Bandinelli, C. and Demauro, G. (1975). *Minerva Medica,* **66,** 1689.

Rubin, A., Rodda, B. E., Warrick, P., Gruber, C. M., Jr. and Ridolfo, A. S. (1973). *Arthritis and Rheumatism,* **16,** 635.

Sacks, P. V. and Kanarek, D. (1973). *American Review of the Respiratory Diseases,* **108,** 666.

Samuelsson, B., Granstrom, E., Green, K., Hamberg, M. and Hammarstrom, S. (1975). *Annual Review of Biochemistry,* **44,** 669.

Sarett, L. H. (1971). *Arzneimittel-Forschung,* **21,** 1759.

Schayer, R. W. (1963). *In* "Progress in Allergy" (Eds P. Kallos and B. H. Waksman), vol. 7, p. 187. Karger, Basel.

Scheidt, S., Alonso, D. R., Wilner, G. and Killip, T. (1974). *Bulletin of the New York Academy of Sciences,* **50,** 247.

Schölkens, B. A. and Steinbach, R. (1975). *Archives Internationales de Pharmacodynamie et Thérapie,* **214,** 328.

Segre, E. J., Chaplin, M., Forchielli, E., Runkel, R. and Sevelius, H. (1974). *Clinical Pharmacology and Therapeutics,* **15,** 374.

Selye, H. (1970a). *Münchener Medizinische Wochenschrift,* **112,** 1401.

Selye, H. (1970b). *Review of Canadian Biology,* **29,** 49.

Selye, H. (1971). *Experientia,* **27,** 1445.

Shanahan, R. W. (1968). *Archives Internationales de Pharmacodynamie et de Thérapie,* **175,** 186.

Sharkawi, M. (1972). *British Journal of Pharmacology,* **44,** 544.

Shaw, D. and Wischmeier, C. (1973). *Journal of Dental Research,* **52,** 180.

Shaw, E. (1955). *Journal of the American Chemical Society,* **77,** 4319.

Shaw, E. and Wooley, D. W. (1954). *Journal of Pharmacology and Experimental Therapeutics,* **111,** 43.

Shen, T. Y. (1965). *In* "Non-steroidal Anti-inflammatory Drugs" (Eds S. Garattini and M. N. G. Dukes), p. 13. Excerpta Medica Foundation, Amsterdam.

Shen, T. Y. (1967). *In* "Topics in Medicinal Chemistry" (Eds J. L. Rabinowitz and R. M. Myerson), vol. 1, p. 29. Interscience Publishers, New York.

Shen, T. Y. (1972). *Angewandte Chemie International Edition*, **11**, 460.

Shen, T. Y. (1976). *In* "Clinoril in the Treatment of Rheumatic Disorders" (Eds E. C. Huskisson and P. Franchimont), p. 1. Raven Press, New York.

Shen, T. Y. (1977). *In* "Prostaglandins and Thromboxanes" (Eds F. Berti, B. Samuelson and G. P. Velo), p. 111. Plenum Publishing Corporation, New York.

Shen, T. Y., Holtz, W. J., Witzel, B. E., Lucas, S. and Sarett, L. H. (1962). Abstracts Papers 142nd Meeting, American Chemical Society, Atlantic City, New Jersey, 910.

Shen, T. Y., Windholz, T. B., Rosegay, A., Witzel, B. E., Wilson, A. N., Willett, J. D., Holtz, W. J., Ellis, R. L., Matzuk, A. R., Lucas, S., Stammer, C. H., Holly, F. W., Sarett, L. H., Risley, E. A., Nuss, G. W. and Winter, C. A. (1963). *Journal of the American Chemical Society*, **85**, 488.

Shen, T. Y., Witzel, B. E., Jones, H., Linn, B. O., McPherson, J., Greenwald, R., Fordice, M. and Jacob, A. (1972). *Federation Proceedings*, **31**, 577.

Shen, T. Y., Ham, E. A., Cirillo, V. J. and Zanetti, M. (1974). *In* "Prostaglandin Synthetase Inhibitors" (Eds H. J. Robinson and J. R. Vane), p. 19. Raven Press, New York.

Sherrer, R. A. and Whitehouse, M. W. (eds) (1974). "Antiinflammatory Agents", Medicinal Chemistry Monographs, Academic Press, New York, San Francisco, London.

Shuman, R. F., Pines, S. H., Shearin, W. E., Czaja, R. F., Abramson, N. L. and Tull, R. (1977). *Journal of Organic Chemistry*, **42**, 1914.

Sih, C. J. and Takeguchi, C. A. (1973). *In* "The Prostaglandins I" (Ed. P. W. Ramwell), p. 83. Plenum Press, New York.

Silver, M. J. and Smith, J. B. (1975). *Life Sciences*, **16**, 1635.

Sim, M. F. (1965). *In* "Non-steroidal Anti-inflammatory Agents" (Eds S. Garattini and M. N. G. Dukes). *International Congress Series*, **82**, 207. Excerpta Medica, Amsterdam.

Sjaastad, O. (1975). *Danish Medical Bulletin*, **22**, 109.

Skeith, M. D., Simkin, P. A. and Healey, L. A. (1968). *Clinical Pharmacology and Therapeutics*, **9**, 89.

Skidmore, I. F. and Whitehouse, M. W. (1966a). *Biochemical Pharmacology*, **15**, 1965.

Skidmore, I. F. and Whitehouse, M. W. (1966b). *Journal of Pharmacy and Pharmacology*, **18**, 558.

Smith, J. B. and Willis, A. L. (1971). *Nature New Biology*, **231**, 235.

Smith, J. B., Ingerman, C. M., Kocsis, J. J. and Silver, M. J. (1974). *In* "Prostaglandin Synthetase Inhibitors" (Eds H. J. Robinson and J. R. Vane), p. 229. Raven Press, New York.

Smith, M. J. H. (1966). *In* "The Salicylates" (Eds M. J. H. Smith and P. K. Smith), chap. 3. Interscience, New York.

Smyth, C. J. (1965). *Arthritis and Rheumatism*, **8**, 921.

Smyth, C. J. (1968). *Postgraduate Medicine*, **44**, 77.

Smyth, C. J. (1970). *Annals of Internal Medicine*, **72**, 430.

Snyder, D. S. (1975). *Journal of Investigative Dermatology*, **64**, 322.

Snyder, D. S. and Eaglstein, W. H. (1973). *Clinical Research*, **21**, 742.

Snyder, D. S. and Eaglstein, W. H. (1974a). *Journal of Investigative Dermatology*, **62**, 47.

Snyder, D. S. and Eaglstein, W. H. (1974b). *British Journal of Dermatology*, **90**, 91.

Sofia, R. D., Knobloch, L. C. and Vassar, H. B. (1975). *Journal of Pharmacology and Experimental Therapeutics*, **193**, 918.

Solez, K., Fox, J. A., Miller, M. and Heptinstall, R. H. (1974). *Prostaglandins*, **7**, 91.

Solomon, H. M., Schrogie, J. J. and Williams, D. (1968). *Biochemical Pharmacology*, **17**, 143.

Solymoss, D., Toth, S., Varga, S. and Selye, H. (1971). *Toxicology and Applied Pharmacology*, **18**, 586.

Somogyi, A., Kovacs, K. and Selye, H. (1969). *Journal of Pharmacy and Pharmacology*, **21**, 122.

Spector, W. G. (ed.) (1964). The Acute Inflammatory Response. *Annal of the New York Academy of Sciences*, **116**, 747.

Spiera, H. (1963). *Arthritis and Rheumatism*, **6**, 364.

Splawinski, J. A., Nies, A. S., Sweetman, B. and Oates, J. A. (1973). *Journal of Pharmacology and Experimental Therapeutics*, **187**, 501.

Standish, J., Maiorana, K. and Graeme, M. L. (1972). *Federation Proceedings*, **31**, 577.

Stanford, N., Roth, G. J., Shen, T. Y. and Majerus, P. W. (1977). *Prostaglandins*, **13**, 669.

Steele, A. D. and Phelps, P. (1971). *Arthritis and Rheumatism*, **14**, 415.

Stenlake, J. B., Williams, W. D., Davidson, A. G. and Downie, W. W. (1971). *Journal of Pharmacy and Pharmacology*, **23**, 146.

Stone, C. A., Van Arman, C. G., Peck, H. M., Minsker, D. H. and Ham, E. A. (1974). *In* "Prostaglandin Synthetase Inhibitors" (Eds H. J. Robinson and J. R. Vane), p. 79. Raven Press, New York.

Stripp, B. and Gillette, J. R. (1972). *Journal of Pharmaceutical Sciences*, **61**, 1682.

Sundberg, D. K., Fawcett, C. P., Illner, P. and McCann, S. M. (1975). *Proceedings of the Society for Experimental Biology and Medicine*, **148**, 54.

Suzuki, T. (1966). Abstract of Symposium on Vaso-active Peptides, Ribeirão Prêto.

Svensson, J., Hamberg, M. and Samuelsson, B. (1976). *Acta Physiologica Scandinavia*, **98**, 285.

Swingle, K. F. (1974). *In* "Medicinal Chemistry", 13-II, Antiinflammatory Agents, (Eds R. A. Scherrer and M. W. Whitehouse), p. 33. Academic Press, New York.

Swingle, K. F., Grant, T. J., Jaques, L. W. and Kvam, D. C. (1970). *Journal of Pharmacology and Experimental Therapeutics*, **172**, 423.

Swingle, K. F., Grant, T. J. and Kvam, D. C. (1971a). *Proceedings of the Society for Experimental Biology and Medicine*, **137**, 536.

Swingle, K. F., Hamilton, R. R., Harrington, J. K. and Kvam, D. C. (1971b). *Archives Internationales de Pharmacodynamie et de Thérapie*, **189**, 129.

Sykes, J. A. C. and Maddox, I. S. (1972). *Nature New Biology*, **237**, 59.

Thomas, G. and West, G. B. (1973). *Journal of Pharmacy and Pharmacology*, **25**, 747.

Thompson, M. M. (1964). *Rheumatologie*, **16**, 439.

Tiggeler, R. G. W. L., Van Leusen, R., Koene, R. and Wijdeveld, P. (1973). *Netherlands Journal of Medicine*, **16**, 61.

Tolman, E. L. and Partridge, R. (1975). *Prostaglandins*, **9**, 349.

Tomlinson, R. V., Ringold, H. J., Qureshi, M. C. and Forchielli, E. (1972). *Biochemical and Biophysical Research Communications*, **46**, 552.

Topliss, J. G. (1972). *Journal of Medicinal Chemistry*, **15**, 1006.

Traeger, A., Stein, G., Kunze, M. and Zaumseil, J. (1972). *International Journal of Clinical Pharmacology*, **6**, 237.

Tuovinen, E., Esila, R. and Liesmaa, M. (1966). *Acta Ophthalmologica*, **44**, 585.

Ubatuba, F. B., Harvey, E. A. and Ferreira, S. H. (1975). *Agents and Actions*, **5**, 31.

Van Arman, C. G. (1974). *Clinical Pharmacology and Therapeutics*, **16**, 900.

Van Arman, C. G. and Nuss, G. W. (1969). *Journal of Pathology*, **99**, 245.

Van Arman, C. G. and Carlson, R. P. (1970). *In* "Bradykinin and Related Kinins", p. 525. Plenum Press, New York.

Van Arman, C. G., Nuss, G. W., Winter, C. A. and Flataker, L. (1968). Proceedings of the 3rd International Pharmacology Meeting, vol. 9, p. 25. Pergamon Press, New York, London.

Van Arman, C. G., Carlson, R. P., Risley, E. A., Thomas, R. H. and Nuss, G. W. (1970a). *Journal of Pharmacology and Experimental Therapeutics*, **175**, 459.

Van Arman, C. G., Carlson, R. P., Brown, W. R. and Itkin, A. (1970b). *Proceedings of the Society for Experimental Biology and Medicine*, **134**, 163.

Van Arman, C. G., Carlson, R. P. and Kling, P. J. (1971). *Ciencia e Cultura*, **23**, 555.

Van Arman, C. G., Noss, G. W. and Risley, E. A. (1973). *Journal of Pharmacology and Experimental Therapeutics*, **187**, 400.

Van Arman, C. G., Risley, E. A. and Nuss, G. W. (1972). *Federation Proceedings*, **31**, 577.

Van Arman, C. G., Carlson, R. P., Kling, P. J., Allen, D. J. and Bondi, J. V. (1974). *Arthritis and Rheumatism*, **17**, 439.

Van Arman, C. G., Risley, E. A., Nuss, G. W., Hucker, H. B. and Duggan, D. E. (1976). *In* "Clinoril in the Treatment of Rheumatic Disorders" (Eds E. C. Huskisson and P. Franchimont), p. 9. Raven Press, New York.

Van den Berg, G., Bultsma, T. and Nauta, W. T. (1975). *Biochemical Pharmacology*, **24**, 1115.

Van den Berg, G. and Nauta, W. T. (1975). *Biochemical Pharmacology*, **24**, 815.

Vane, J. R. (1971). *Nature New Biology*, **231**, 232.

Vane, J. R. (1973). *In* "Advances in the Biosciences" (Eds S. Bergström and S. Bernhard), vol. 9, p. 395. Pergamon Press, New York.

Vane, J. R. (1974). *In* "Prostaglandin Synthetase Inhibitors" (Eds H. J. Robinson and J. R. Vane), p. 155. Raven Press, New York.

Vane, J. R. and McGiff, J. C. (1975). *Circulation Research*, **36**, Supplement 1, 168.

Vecchio, C., Fontana, A. and Tavazzi, L. (1964). *Archivic "E. Maragliano" di Patologia e Clinica Genova*, **20**, 275; *Reumatismo*, **16**, 404.

Venuto, R. C., O'Dorisio, T., Ferris, T. F. and Stein, J. H. (1975). *Prostaglandins*, **9**, 817.

Vesell, E. S., Passananti, G. T. and Johnson, A. O. (1975). *Journal of Clinical Pharmacology*, **15**, 486.

Vihert, A. M., Glezer, G. A., Megrelishvili, R. I. and Ryff, I. M. (1973). *Arzneimittel-Forschung*, **23**, 991.

Vinegar, R., Schreiber, W. and Hugo, R. (1969). *Journal of Pharmacology and Experimental Therapeutics*, **166**, 96.

Vinegar, R., Truax, J. F. and Selph, J. L. (1976). *Federation Proceedings*, **35**, 2447.

Vischer, T. L., Bretz, U. and Baggiolini, M. (1976). *Journal of Experimental Medicine*, **14**, 863.

Volterra, G., Pisanti, N. and Meli, A. (1974). *Proceedings of the Society for Experimental Biology and Medicine*, **146**, 146.

Von Kaulla, K. N. (1967). *Federation Proceedings,* **26,** 759.
Wallach, E. E., Del la Cruz, A., Hunt, J., Wright, K. H. and Stevens, V. C. (1975). *Prostaglandins,* **9,** 645.
Walter, J. E. and Diener, R. M. (1971). Abstract, 10th Annual Meeting, Society for Toxicology, Washington, Mar. 7–11.
Walters, M. N. and Willoughby, D. A. (1965). *Journal of Pathology,* **90,** 641.
Walton, E., Stammer, C. H., Nutt, R. F., Jenkins, S. R. and Holly, F. W. (1965). *Journal of Medicinal Chemistry,* **8,** 204.
Wanka, J. and Dixon, A. S. (1964). *Annals of the Rheumatic Diseases,* **23,** 288.
Wanka, J., Jones, L. I., Wood, P. H. N. and Dixon, A. S. (1964). *Annals of the Rheumatic Diseases,* **23,** 218.
Ward, J. R. (1965). *In* "Non-steroid Anti-inflammatory Drugs" (Eds S. Garattini and M. N. G. Dukes). *International Congress Series,* **82,** 353. Excerpta Medica, Amsterdam.
Ward, J. R. and Cloud, R. S. (1966). *Journal of Pharmacology and Experimental Therapeutics,* **152,** 116.
Ward, P. A. and Zwaifler, N. J. (1971). *Journal of Clinical Investigation,* **50,** 606.
Wax, J., Winder, C. V., Tessman, D. K. and Stephens, M. D. (1975). *Journal of Pharmacology and Experimental Therapeutics,* **192,** 172.
Weil, C. S. (1952). *Biometrics,* **8,** 249.
Weiner, M. and Piliero, S. J. (1970). *Annual Review of Pharmacology,* **10,** 171.
Weinshenker, N. M. and Andersen, N. H. (1973). *In* "Prostaglandins I" (Ed. P. W. Ramwell), p. 5. Plenum Press, New York.
Welstead, W. J., Stauffer, H. F. and Sancilio, L. F. (1974). *Journal of Medicinal Chemistry,* **17,** 544.
Wennmalm, A. (1974). *Research in Clinical Pharmacology and Therapeutics,* **2,** 1099.
Whitehouse, M. W. (1965). *In* "Progress in Drug Research" (Ed. E. Jucker), vol. 8, p. 321. Birkhäuser, Basel and Stuttgart, Interscience, New York.
Whitehouse, M. W. and Boström, H. (1965). *Biochemical Pharmacology,* **14,** 1173.
Whitehouse, M. W. and Skidmore, I. F. (1965). *Journal of Pharmacy and Pharmacology,* **17,** 688.
Wilhelmi, G. (1974). *Pharmacology,* **11,** 220.
Wilhelmi, G., Herrman, B. and Tedeschi, G. (1959). *Arzniemittel-Forschung,* **9,** 241.
Williamson, H. E., Bourland, W. A. and Marchand, G. R. (1974). *Prostaglandins,* **8,** 297.
Williamson, H. E., Bourland, W. A. and Marchand, G. R. (1975). *Proceedings of the Society for Experimental Biology and Medicine,* **148,** 164.
Williamson, N. and Holt, P. J. L. (1968). *Annals of the Rheumatic Diseases,* **27,** 477.
Willis, A. L. (1969). *In* "Prostaglandins, Peptides and Amines" (Eds P. Mantegazza and E. W. Horton), p. 31. Academic Press, New York.
Willis, A. L. (1974). *Science,* **183,** 325.
Willis, A. L., Davison, P., Ramwell, P. W., Brocklehurst, W. E. and Smith, B. (1972). *In* "Prostaglandins in Cellular Biology" (Eds P. W. Ramwell and B. P. Pharriss), p. 227. Plenum Press, New York.
Willis, A. L., Kuhn, D. C. and Weiss, H. J. (1974). *Science,* **183,** 327.
Willoughby, D. A. and DiRosa, M. (1972). *Annals of the Rheumatic Diseases,* **31,** 540.
Winder, C. V. (1959). *Nature,* **184,** 494.
Winder, C. V. (1966). *Annals of Physical Medicine,* Supplement 7.
Winship, D. H. and Bernhard, G. C. (1970). *Gastroenterology,* **58,** 762.

Winter, C. A. (1965). *In* "Non-steroidal Anti-inflammatory Drugs" (Eds S. Garattini and M. N. G. Dukes). *International Congress Series*, **82**, 190. Excerpta Medica, Amsterdam.

Winter, C. A. (1966a). *In* "Progress in Drug Research" (Ed. E. Jucker), vol. 10, p. 139. Birkhäuser, Basel and Stuttgart, Interscience, New York.

Winter, C. A. (1966b). *Annual Review of Pharmacology*, **6**, 157.

Winter, C. A. (1969). *California Medicine*, **110**, 175.

Winter, C. A. (1971). *Arzneimittel-Forschung*, **21**, 1805.

Winter, C. A. and Flataker, L. (1965a). *Journal of Pharmacology and Experimental Therapeutics*, **148**, 373.

Winter, C. A. and Flataker, L. (1965b). *Journal of Pharmacology and Experimental Therapeutics*, **150**, 165.

Winter, C. A. and Nuss, G. W. (1963). *Toxicology and Applied Pharmacology*, **5**, 247.

Winter, C. A. and Nuss, G. W. (1966). *Arthritis and Rheumatism*, **9**, 394.

Winter, C. A. and Porter, C. C. (1957). *Journal of the American Pharmaceutical Association, Scientific Edition*, **46**, 515.

Winter, C. A. and Risley, E. A. (1965). *Arzniemittel-Forschung*, **15**, 427.

Winter, C. A., Risley, E. A. and Nuss, G. W. (1962). *Proceedings of the Society for Experimental Biology and Medicine*, **111**, 544.

Winter, C. A., Risley, E. A. and Nuss, G. W. (1963). *Journal of Pharmacology and Experimental Therapeutics*, **141**, 369.

Winter, C. A., Risley, E. A. and Silber, R. H. (1968). *Journal of Pharmacology and Experimental Therapeutics*, **162**, 196.

Winter, J. C. and Gessner, P. K. (1968). *Journal of Pharmacology and Experimental Therapeutics*, **162**, 286.

Wong, S., Gardocki, J. F. and Pruss, T. P. (1973). *Journal of Pharmacology and Experimental Therapeutics*, **185**, 127.

Yamamoto, H., Hirohashi, A., Izumi, T. and Koshiba, M. (1971). U.S.P. 3 798 235.

Yamamoto, H. and Nakao, M. (1968). U.S. Patent 3 629 284.

Yamamoto, H. and Nakao, M. (1969). *Journal of Medicinal Chemistry*, **12**, 176.

Yamamoto, H., Nakao, M. and Kobayashi, A. (1968). *Chemical and Pharmaceutical Bulletin, Japan*, **16**, 647.

Yamamoto, H., Saito, C., Okamoto, T., Awata, H., Inukai, T., Hirohashi, A. and Yukawa, Y. (1969b). *Arzneimittel-Forschung*, **19**, 981.

Yaron, M., Yaron, I. and Allalouf, D. (1971). *Annals of the Rheumatic Diseases*, **30**, 613.

Yesair, D. W., Callahan, M., Remington, L. and Kenslar, C. J. (1970a). *Biochemical Pharmacology*, **19**, 1579.

Yesair, D. W., Remington, L., Callahan, M. and Kenslar, C. J. (1970b). *Biochemical Pharmacology*, **19**, 1591.

Ziboh, V. A., McElligott, T. and Hsia, S. L. (1973). *In* "Advances in the Biosciences" (Eds S. Bergström and S. Bernhard), vol. 9, p. 457. Pergamon Press, New York.

Zuckerman, H., Reiss, U. and Rubinstein, I. (1974). *Obstetrics and Gynecology*, **44**, 787.

Zurier, R. B. and Ballas, M. (1973). *Arthritis and Rheumatism*, **16**, 251.

Bromocriptine

DAVID PARKES, MD, FRCP

University Department of Neurology, Institute of Psychiatry and King's College Hospital, London, England

Abbreviations

CA, catecholamine; DA, dopamine (1); NA, noradrenaline, epinephrine; GABA, gamma-aminobutyric acid; 5-HT, 5-hydroxytryptamine, serotonin; 5-HTP, 5-hydroxytryptophan; HVA, homovanillic acid; 5-HIAA, 5-hydroxyindole acetic acid; 6-OH-DA, 6-hydroxydopamine; NPA, norpropylaporphine; TIDA, tubero-infundi-bular dopamine; CNS, central nervous system; GH, growth hormone; GHRF, growth hormone releasing factor; GHRIF, growth hormone release-inhibiting factor, somato-statin; TRF, thyrotropin releasing factor; ACTH, adrenocorticotropic hormone; PIF, prolactin inhibitory factor; MSH, melanocyte stimulating hormone; MIF, MSH-release inhibiting factor; FSH, follicle stimulating hormone; LH, luteinizing hormone; GRF, gonadotropin releasing factor; LRF, luteinizing hormone releasing factor; HPr, human prolactin.

1 Introduction

Ergot alkaloids have made a formidable contribution to the relief of human suffering. Professor Chassair Moir wrote in 1932 that ergot was of the nature of a treasure chest. He was referring to the number and the variety of the chemical substances isolated from the parasitic fungus, *Claviceps purpurea*, that grows on rye and grain, and also to the immense amount of pharma-cological work devoted to these compounds (Saameli, 1976). Dale's work on adrenaline remains the corner stone of the pharmacology of ergot (Dale, 1906). Dale showed that ergot alkaloids selectively block what we now describe as α-adrenoceptors, whilst β-adrenoceptors are relatively unaffected. Certain ergot alkaloids may stimulate as well as block α-adrenoceptors. In addition to these actions on the adrenergic system, ergot alkaloids have powerful effects on the DA nervous system.

Today, a number of naturally occurring ergot alkaloids are recognized, and hundreds of chemically related compounds have been produced by partial synthesis. One of the most interesting of these compounds is bromocriptine, a powerful DA stimulant drug.

The inhibition of lactation by ergot was described by Dodart in 1676, and from mediaeval times it has been recognized that women with St Anthony's fire, due to eating ergot-contaminated grain, failed to lactate. However, it was not until 1954 that the possible mechanism of this was elucidated, when Shelesnyak found that ergotoxine prevented implantation in the rat by suppressing prolactin secretion. Shelesnyak suggested that ergotoxine inhibited the release of prolactin from the pituitary. With the observation that levodopa increases the content of a prolactin-inhibiting factor (PIF) in the pituitary portal blood, a possible relationship between ergot derivatives and dopamine was shown (Kamberi *et al.*, 1971). This work led to the concept that tubero-infundibular dopaminergic activity modulated the secretion of inhibiting factors which were carried by the portal circulation to control secretion of prolactin by the anterior pituitary. In a search for ergot derivatives that would inhibit prolactin secretion, Flückiger found that bromocriptine was highly active, well tolerated, and without the oxytocic or cardiovascular effects of the parent compound. Flückiger believed such a compound would have great therapeutic importance (Flückiger and Wagner, 1968). Hyperprolactinaemia often causes impotence in the male, and failure of menstruation and ovulation in the female. Bromocriptine, as well as suppressing prolactin levels, restores normal gonadal function and fertility in these subjects.

In 1973, Corrodi and his colleagues showed that bromocriptine was a dopamine stimulant, which altered the motor behaviour of animals in a similar fashion to levodopa. Because of this similarity, it was suggested that bromocriptine would be a potent antiparkinsonism drug.

In addition to the effect of bromocriptine on lactation and in parkinsonism, it is also effective in acromegaly. This is also due to the DA stimulant effect of bromocriptine. Dopamine causes a rise in plasma growth hormone (GH) levels in normal subjects, but for reasons still not completely understood, a fall in acromegalics. However, levodopa does not cause a prolonged suppression of elevated GH levels in acromegaly nor reversal of soft tissue swelling or the other consequences of excess circulating GH. Bromocriptine, in contrast, causes a sustained fall of plasma GH levels with reversal of many of the clinical features of acromegaly.

The antiparkinsonism and hormonal effects of bromocriptine are likely to result from the stimulation of DA receptors in different regions of the brain and pituitary. There are, however, many differences in the action of bromocriptine and the classic DA agonist drug, apomorphine. These differences indicate that the mode of receptor agonism due to the two drugs is different, and suggests there may be two or more DA receptor types, both inside and outside the CNS.

The relationship of catecholamines and peptide hormones poses a challenge undreamt of by conventional 19th century concepts of neuronal organization. The brain itself is a target organ for hormones or local chemical messengers, and some of the behavioural consequences of bromocriptine treatment result from the release of peptides from neurosecretory neurones. These peptides have local and distant effects via the circulation, but also modify neuronal excitability, may act as neurotransmitters, and alter the metabolism and central effects of catecholamines.

2 Dopamine systems

2.1 DOPAMINE SYSTEMS IN THE BRAIN

In the rat brain, there are three well-defined DA systems (Ungerstedt, 1971):

   i. In the substantia nigra compact zones, neurones project to the neostriatum and central portion of the amygdaloid nuclei.

  ii. In the mesolimbic system, cell bodies are located dorsal to the inter-peduncular nuclei in the ventral tegmental area, and innervate the nucleus accumbens and olfactory tubercles.

  iii. In the tubero-infundibular dopamine (TIDA) system, cell bodies are largely central to the arcuate nuclei of the hypothalamus, and innervate the median eminence.

In addition, the results of human and animal experiments suggest the presence of at least two further dopamine systems:

  iv. A system with nerve terminals within the cerebral cortex, demonstrated by fluorescence microscopy studies in animals (Thierry *et al.*, 1973).

  v. A medullary DA system, with neurones possibly sited in the medullary emetic area.

There are important differences between these systems in animals. The TIDA system is relatively insensitive to the normal destructive action of 6-OH-DA, and when activated for any length of time the terminals become markedly depleted of transmitter (Cooper *et al.*, 1974). In contrast, nigrostriatal and limbic DA systems are readily destroyed by 6-OH-DA. Some ergolene derivatives preferentially stimulate the mesolimbic DA system.

In the human brain the extremely complicated CA neuronal system (Nobin and Björklund, 1973) appears to correspond well to that in animals. The function of different DA systems in man can be deduced from animal studies and the effects of disease and drugs. Destruction of the nigrostriatal and possibly the mesolimbic DA systems results in parkinsonism, and destruction of the TIDA system causes abnormal prolactin and GH secretion. A cortical DA system may malfunction in schizophrenia. The medullary DA system is involved in the control of vomiting and blood pressure. In man, DA agonists cause a rise in plasma GH levels, a fall in prolactin levels, hypotension, emesis, and when used in the treatment of parkinsonism (in which there is pre-existing brain damage), involuntary movements and neuropsychiatric changes. They also cause metabolic changes and sometimes loss of weight. Dopamine antagonists have, on the whole, opposite effects. In animals, DA agonists have a number of actions whose exact counterpart in man is uncertain. In addition to stimulating motor behaviour and blocking ovulation in rodents, they produce hypothermia, and antagonize different aspects of sexual behaviour (Fuxe *et al.*, 1975). Thus, bromocriptine blocks ovulation in immature rats treated with pregnant mare serum. Dopaminergic agonists may possibly alter sexual receptivity of castrated female rats.

2.2 DOPAMINE RECEPTOR TYPES IN THE CNS

There may be two distinct types of DA receptor in the nervous system (Cools and van Rossum, 1976). The evidence for the possible existence of two receptor types is based on the finding of two histochemically different types of DA terminal structure in the brain (Fuxe *et al.*, 1974b) and the fact that DA causes inhibitory postsynaptic potentials at most caudate neurones, but excitatory potentials at a minority (Connor, 1970; York, 1970). Some of the many discrepancies between the behavioural and biochemical properties of different DA stimulants may be due to stimulation of different DA receptor types.

Levodopa, apomorphine and a number of other dopaminergic and anti-dopaminergic agents sometimes affect motor behaviour in unexpected ways. In Huntington's chorea and parkinsonism, levodopa causes or increases chorea whilst apomorphine may alleviate chorea. Dopamine stimulants and DA-blocking drugs given separately are occasionally effective in the treatment of torsion dystonia, and the combination of amantadine and haloperidol may be of value in a number of patients with spasmodic torticollis. The long-term treatment of parkinsonism with levodopa and psychotic patients with neuro-leptics produces dyskinesias in both cases. In contrast to levodopa and apomorphine, the DA stimulant piribedil (2) is not therapeutically effective in most subjects with parkinsonism. Levodopa does not apparently influence the motor behaviour of healthy subjects (Cools and van Rossum, 1976).

None of this evidence forms a satisfactory basis for establishing the existence of two distinct DA receptor types in the human brain. Some of the above inconsistencies do not bear close scrutiny. The agonist–antagonist effects of apomorphine and piribedil result from complex metabolic transfor-mations in the body. The effects of pre-existing brain damage will influence the motor response to drugs. A dopaminergic defect has not been convincingly demonstrated in torsion dystonia. The clinical observation of dyskinesias is often misleading and patterns of involuntary movement may change dramatically over a short time period for no apparent cause. Cools and van Rossum (1976) proposed that levodopa dyskinesias were produced because of an imbalance between the degree of stimulation of two hypothetical DA receptor types. However, it seems more probable that the presence or absence, and possibly the type, of dyskinesias in parkinsonism subjects treated with DA stimulants depends on the relative degree of damage to nigrostriatal and mesolimbic systems (Parkes *et al.*, 1976c).

There is no definite evidence for the occurrence of two or more distinct DA receptor types in the brain of man or animals, although Cools *et al.* (1975) demonstrated behavioural differences following electrical stimulation of different DA receptor areas in the monkey brain, stimulation of one region causing choreic movements, and of a different area, torticollis.

2.3 DOPAMINE SYSTEMS OUTSIDE THE BRAIN

The peripheral effects of DA on the vascular system cannot be exactly mimicked by NA or adrenaline, and vasodilator effects of DA can be prevented by the DA-blocking drugs, pimozide and metoclopramide, but not by adrenergic blocking drugs, phentolamine or propranolol. Thus, DA appears to be involved in the control of the mesenteric, coronary and cerebral circulation (Goldberg, 1972; Thorner, 1975).

Dopamine is synthesized in the kidney, and levodopa causes a considerable increase in renal blood flow in man. The urinary excretion of free DA is much greater than that of NA and adrenaline. The excretion of DA is proportional to the sodium excretion (Wayne *et al.*, 1974). Thus, when salt intake is restricted, urinary sodium and free DA excretion fall whilst after saline infusion, urinary sodium and free DA content rise. Dopamine may have an important physiological role in the control of sodium excretion and renal blood flow in man.

The evidence that DA has a physiological role in other systems is less well defined, although DA has been identified in the autonomic nervous system, thyroid, pancreas, salivary glands, gastrointestinal mucosa, and stomach (Falck and Hellman, 1964; Cegrell, 1967; Hakanson and Owman, 1967; Hakanson *et al.*, 1970; Hakanson, 1970). Levodopa causes minor changes in plasma renin and glucagon levels, but the physiological significance of these remains to be established. The evidence for existence of pituitary DA receptors is reviewed in section 7.3.

2.4   STRUCTURE OF DOPAMINE RECEPTORS

The DA receptor in the central and autonomic nervous systems appears to be a DA-binding component of the DA-sensitive enzyme, adenylate cyclase. In the autonomic nervous system, stimulation of pre-ganglionic fibres in superior cervical ganglia results in DA release from interneurones, followed by stimulation of a specific adenylate cyclase mechanism in postganglionic neurones, with accumulation of cAMP. The intracellular accumulation of cAMP results in hyperpolarization of postganglionic neural membranes with inhibitory postsynaptic potentials (Greengard and Kebabian, 1974; Jacobowitz and Greene, 1974; Libet and Owman, 1974; Kebabian *et al.*, 1975). Thus changes in DA transmission within the ganglia will modulate nicotinic cholinergic transmission (Greengard *et al.*, 1972).

In the brain, the presence of dopaminergic innervation at various regions correlates well with the occurrence of DA-sensitive adenylate cyclase (Horn *et al.*, 1974) which is found in the following structures: (i) caudate nucleus (Kebabian *et al.*, 1972); (ii) olfactory tubercle (Clement-Cormier *et al.*, 1974; Horn *et al.*, 1974); (iii) nucleus accumbens (Clement-Cormier *et al.*, 1974; Horn *et al.*, 1974); (iv) amygdala (Clement-Cormier *et al.*, 1974); (v) cerebral cortex (McCune *et al.*, 1971); (vi) retina (Brown and Makman, 1972).

Dopamine receptors are also present on pituitary lactotrophs (see MacLeod, 1976). The prolactin cell is remarkable in that whilst increase in cAMP leads to increased secretion, dopaminergic stimulation does not lead to an increase in cAMP, and produces *inhibition* of prolactin secretion. Bromocriptine appears to have a direct DA-receptor effect on the lactotroph (Flückiger, 1976). The effect of bromocriptine in causing prolactin inhibition is completely reversed by chlorpromazine. Chlorpromazine causes DA-receptor blockade and an increase in plasma prolactin concentration in a dose-dependent fashion (MacLeod and Lehmayer, 1974).

2.5 DOPAMINE AUTORECEPTORS

There appear to be specific DA receptor sites, termed autoreceptors by Carlsson (1975a), on the neuronal cell body. The soma of DA neurones is responsive to the direct micro-iontophoretic application of either DA or the DA agonist, apomorphine. If the terminals of DA neurones also have DA receptors, these may be involved in receptor-mediated feedback control of striatal tyrosine hydroxylase activity at DA synapses (Kehr *et al.*, 1972; Aghajanian and Bunney, 1973), resulting in the control of biosynthesis of DA from tyrosine. A different feedback mechanism is probably involved in the case of the DA-responsive lactotroph and the TIDA neurone, which are separated by the portal circulation, and prolactin will alter DA turnover in TIDA neurones. The physiological reason for the presence of DA receptors on the soma of DA neurones is problematical, although certain presynaptic receptors may conceivably respond to hormones such as prolactin and somatostatin, and form the mechanism whereby these peptides depress neuronal excitability.

The ability of a drug to modify striatal DA synthesis after impulse flow is inhibited in the DA neurones can be considered an index of the drug's direct effect on dopaminergic nerve terminals. Gamma-butyrolactone has the property of blocking impulse flow in the nigro-neostriatal pathway. When this pathway is blocked, the affinity of pre- and postsynaptic receptors for DA antagonists may be different (Walters and Roth, 1976). Presynaptic receptors may have little functional significance under physiological conditions, although it is possible that they mediate some of the actions of DA agonists, such as apomorphine, and also DA stimulants, such as bromocriptine. Clinical studies may answer the question as to whether drugs with less presynaptic effects and greater postsynaptic effects can be developed.

2.6 SUPERSENSITIVITY

The stimulation or interruption of synaptic transmission can result in a state of increased or decreased sensitivity to the subsequent administration of a neuro-transmitter or to its antagonist (Trendelenberg, 1963). With the chronic administration of neuroleptics, the sensitivity of DA receptors may alter so that when the drug is stopped, there is an increased sensitivity to very low doses of DA agonists (Tarsy and Baldessarini, 1973). It is several weeks before normal responses are re-established. The mechanism of supersensitivity in the DA nervous system is uncertain. On the whole, there is no change in the activity of DA-sensitive adenylate cyclase in the basal ganglia following 6-OH-DA or surgical denervation (Voigtlander *et al.*, 1973), although Mishra *et al.* (1974) apparently demonstrated that following denervation the adenylate cyclase response to DA was considerably increased in homogenates of striatal tissue. An increased number of DA-sensitive adenylate cyclase sites may be present in denervated tissues or, alternatively, other membrane characteristics may be altered.

In contrast to the effects of neuroleptics such as chlorpromazine, the feeding of large quantities of levodopa to animals for several months does not alter behavioural responses to dopamine (Pycock and Marsden, 1977). If this finding is relevant to humans, long-term levodopa treatment of parkinsonism is unlikely to cause a change in DA-receptor sensitivity. If progressive receptor denervation is a factor involved in disease progression in parkinsonism, levodopa or bromocriptine treatment is unlikely to arrest this.

3   Dopamine receptor stimulants

A high degree of structural specificity is required for CNS DA-receptor agonists. Phenethylamines lacking the catecholamine hydroxy groups, or substances in which the side chain contains one or three carbon atoms instead of the two in catecholamines, have no dopamine-agonist activity. A number of compounds in which the side chain is held in a second ring system are dopamine agonists. Those having the dopamine side chain locked in a tetra-hydroisoquinoline nucleus are weaker DA agonists than those in which the side chain is in an extended form as in apomorphine (3) from which it is concluded that the most active conformation of DA at CNS receptors may be that in which the side chain is in the fully extended *trans* form (Miller *et al.*, 1974; Iversen, 1975).

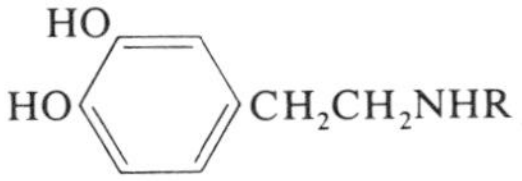

HO
HO⟨ ⟩CH₂CH₂NHR

R = H, dopamine (DA)
R = CH₃, epinine

(1)

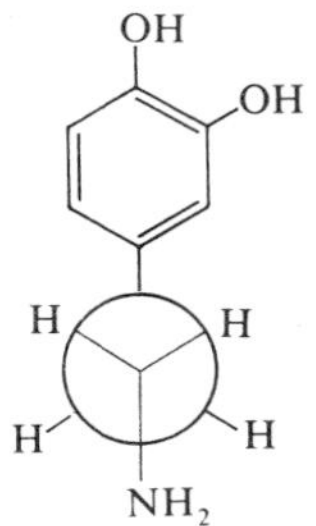

OH
OH
H   H
H   H
NH₂

trans-conformation of DA

Dopamine agonists cause a reduction of DA turnover in the brain and in rodents with unilateral 6-OH-DA nigral lesions, turning towards the intact side.

Piperonylpyrimidyl piperazines. The best known of the piperonylpyrimidyl amines which cause DA-receptor stimulation, is piribedil (ET 495) (2), which probably acts by formation of an active phenolic metabolite (Corrodi *et al.*, 1971). Piribedil causes long-lasting circling behaviour in animals with unilateral nigral lesions and reduces DA turnover in the brain.

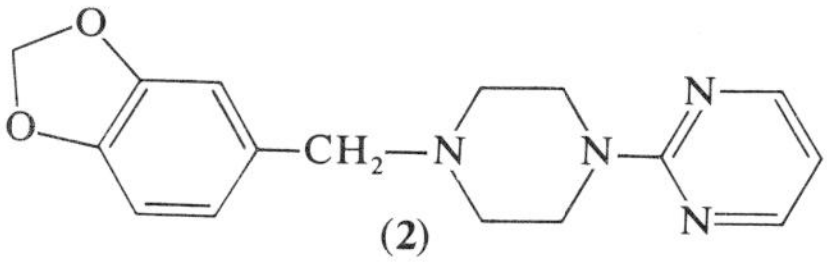

(2)

Apomorphine derivatives. Apomorphine (3) and its derivatives have been largely investigated in animals and used in man as DA-receptor stimulants.

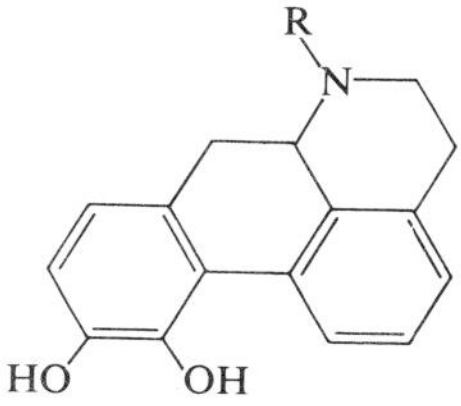

	R
Apomorphine	$-CH_3$
Norapomorphine	$-H$
N-Ethylnorapomorphine	$-CH_2CH_3$
N-n-Propylnorapomorphine	$-CH_2CH_2CH_3$
N-Cyclopropylmethylnorapomorphine	$-CH_2-\triangleleft$ 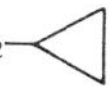

(3)

The behavioural effects of these apomorphine analogues are qualitatively similar to that of apomorphine (Menon *et al.*, 1976). The n-propyl derivative is more potent than apomorphine in a number of respects. Like piribedil (2), these apomorphine derivatives cause circling behaviour in animals with uni-lateral nigrostriatal lesions, and reduce DA turnover in the brain.

Ergot alkaloids and their derivatives

These belong to a class of indole alkaloids, the majority having a condensed four-ring structure known as ergoline (4). Two main types may be differentiated: the lysergic acid derivatives (5) and the clavines (6). The

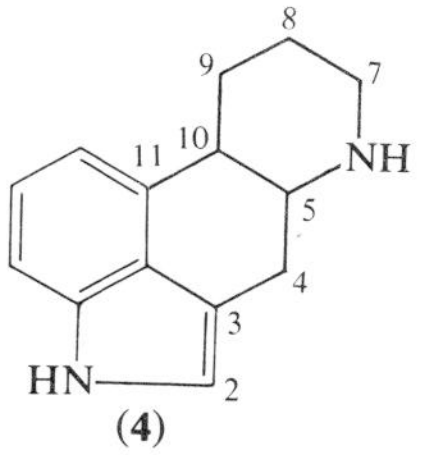

(4)

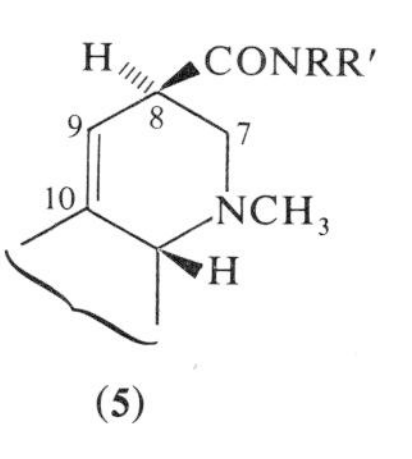

(5)

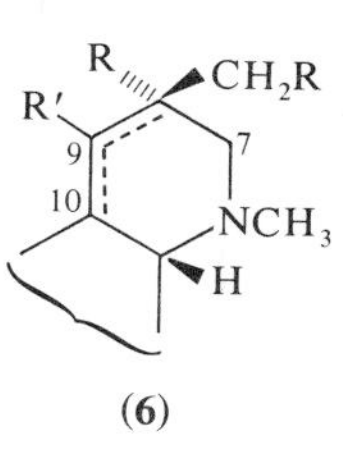

(6)

clavines are 6,8-dimethyl substituted ergolines and may have a double bond at C-8 or C-9. The lysergic acid derivatives are either simple amides or cyclic peptides.

Ergoline (**4**) has the phenethylamine moiety of DA, fixed in a rigid extended structure but lacks the phenolic groups of catecholamines. However, dopamine-receptor agonists have been found in all three classes.

Among the lysergic acid derivatives, ergometrine (also known as ergonovine) (**5**: R = H; R′ = CH(CH$_3$)CH$_2$OH) and methylergometrine (**5**: R = H; R′ = CH(CH$_2$CH$_3$)CH$_2$OH) are potent DA-receptor agonists.

TABLE 1

The ovum implantation inhibitory potencies of the natural peptide ergot alkaloids

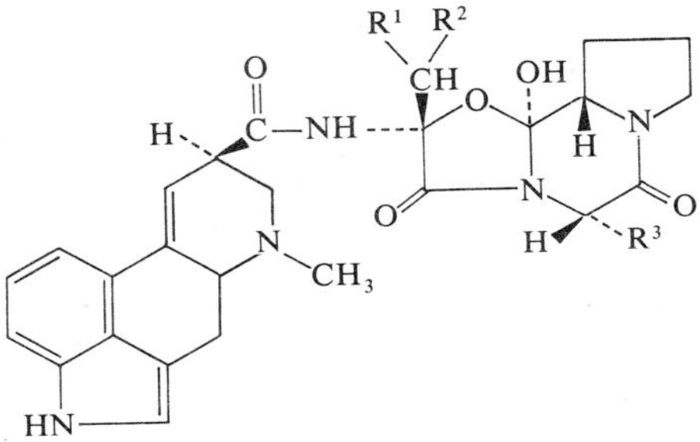

| R^1 | R^2 | | R^3 | |
		−CH$_2$C$_6$H$_5$	−CH$_2$CH(CH$_3$)$_2$	−CH(CH$_3$)$_2$
H	H	ergotamine >20[a]	ergosine 5·7	ergovaline 9·0
CH$_3$	CH$_3$	ergocristine 4·2	α-ergocryptine 1·1	ergocornine 2·7
H	CH$_3$	ergostine >20	ergoptine 4	ergonine 4·6

[a] ED$_{50}$ (mg kg^{-1}) after sc injection of inseminated rats (Flückiger and Wagner, 1968). This ED$_{50}$ is a measure of the prolactin secretion inhibitory activity (from Flückiger et al., 1976).

The ergot alkaloids shown in Table 1 are cyclic peptide derivatives of lysergic acid and of these ergocornine, α-ergocryptine and its 2-bromo derivative bromocriptine (**7**) are potent DA agonists as shown by their effect on animal behaviour (see section 6). Bromocriptine has little vasoconstrictor or oxytocic activity and in this respect it resembles the 9,10-dihydro ergot alkaloids rather than its parent α-ergocryptine.

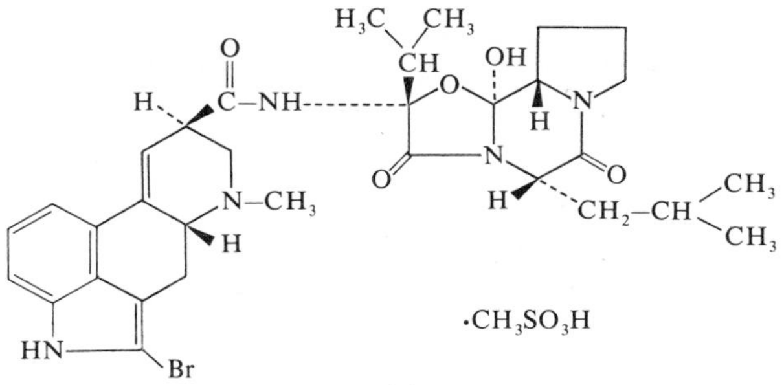

(7)

Bromocriptine is also more active in the rat as an implantation inhibitor (ED_{50} 0·7 mg kg^{-1}) than α-ergocryptine (ED_{50} 1·1 mg kg^{-1}; see Table 1); and it is less potent as an ovulation inhibitor in the rat (ED_{50} 20) than α-ergocryptine (ED_{50} 1·7 mg kg^{-1}) (Flückiger et al., 1976) (see Tables 1 and 2).

The clavine derivatives lergotrile (**8**; 2-chloro-8β-cyanomethyl-6-methylergoline) and PTR 17402 (**9**; (5R, 8R)-8-(4-p-methoxyphenyl-1-piperazinyl-

TABLE 2

The ovum implantation inhibitory potencies of the 9,10-dihydro derivatives of the natural peptide ergot alkaloids

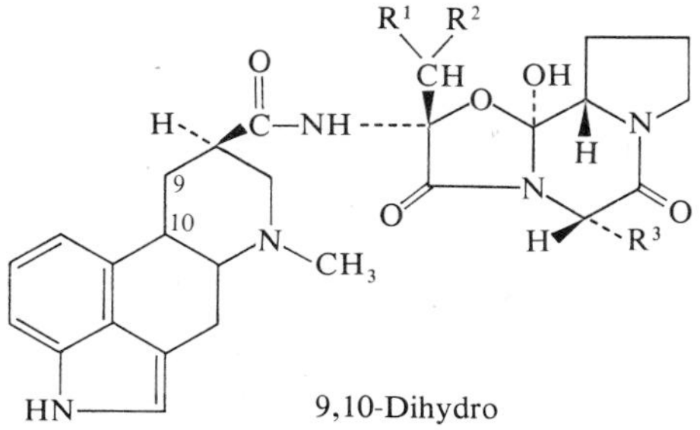

9,10-Dihydro

		R³		
R¹	R²	$-CH_2C_6H_5$	$-CH_2CH(CH_3)_2$	$-CH(CH_3)_2$
H	H	-ergotamine >20[a]	-ergosine 20	-ergovaline >20
CH₃	CH₃	-ergocristine >3	-α-ergocryptine 4·8	-ergocornine >3
H	CH₃	-ergostine >3	-ergoptine >3	-ergonine >3

[a] See footnote of Table 1.

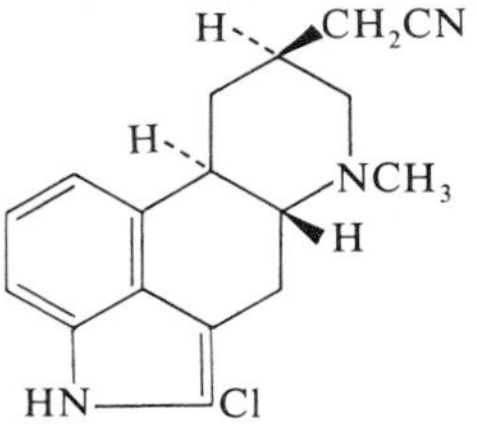

H··₂ CH₂CN

H··₂

NCH₃

H

HN——Cl

(8)

H··₂ CH₂N

NCH₃

H

HN——

OCH₃

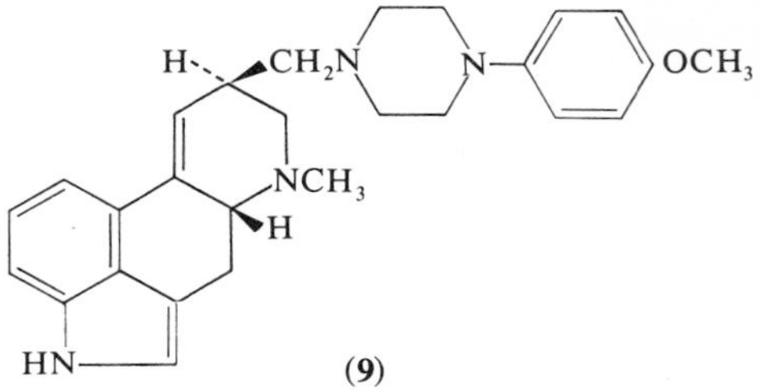

(9)

methyl)-6-methylergolene) are dopamine-receptor agonists and there is evidence that PTR 17402 may act preferentially at DA receptors in the limbic forebrain (Fuxe *et al.*, 1975).

4   Pharmacokinetic studies

2-Bromo-α-ergocryptine (bromocriptine, **7**) like all ergot alkaloids is a weak base insoluble in water-forming salts which have an acid reaction in water. It is available as the methanesulphonate (mesylate) (Parlodel®, Sandoz) in the form of tablets or capsules.

4.1   BROMOCRIPTINE METABOLISM AND PHARMACOKINETICS

The absorption of bromocriptine from the g.i. tract, plasma levels urinary and faecal excretion have been determined following ³H or ¹⁴C-labelled bromocriptine in different species.[1] Although virtually insoluble in water, the central effects indicate that bromocriptine does penetrate most areas of the brain.

Bromocriptine is rapidly and fairly completely absorbed from the gastro-intestinal tract in man. Following oral dosage, absorption amounts to around 40–90 per cent in the rat, rabbit and monkey. Higher blood bromocriptine levels are achieved after intravenous than after oral administration. Very low levels persist for at least 4 days after oral administration. In the rat, low levels of bromocriptine can be determined in all organs except the liver, stomach and intestines, 2 hours after oral dosage, and small traces persist in a few organs for up to 24 hours.

The major route of elimination of bromocriptine in the investigated species is biliary. The metabolic pattern of drug excretion in the bile is extremely complex, with at least 30 partially or completely characterized metabolites in the rat and monkey. Three processes appear to be going on in the body:

i.   isomerization at C-8 of the bromolysergic acid moiety;
ii. hydrolysis of the lysergic acid amide group;
iii. oxidative attack on the proline fragment of the peptide moiety, the major pathway.

[1] Data in this section is unpublished, and reproduced by kind permission of Sandoz Ltd.

At least 10 different metabolites of bromocriptine have been identified in human urine, whilst only a very small portion of unchanged bromocriptine is present. Bromolysergic acid is the main metabolite, accounting for approximately half the excreted radioactivity. In the rat and rhesus monkey, as well as in man, 2-bromolysergic acid and 2-bromo-isolysergic acid are the main urinary metabolites. The cumulative excretion of ^{3}H-labelled material in the urine of man is approximately 6 per cent of the dose after oral administration and 7 per cent after intravenous administration, whereas 70 per cent appears in the faeces over 120 hours following a single oral dose of bromocriptine 2·5 mg.

A technique for the estimation of bromocriptine levels in human plasma has been developed using radioimmuno assay techniques. Following high single oral bromocriptine dosages (50 mg) in man, peak levels occur 2–3 hours after drug administration, at approximately the same time as the peak antiparkinsonism action, maximum severity of dyskinesias, and shortly after peak GH levels are achieved.

5 Toxicology

5.1 ACUTE AND CHRONIC TOXICITY IN MAN AND ANIMALS

The acute toxicity of bromocriptine has been determined in mice, rats and rabbits. In oral tests, no deaths occurred at the highest possible dose in rats and rabbits, and the mortality was only 80 per cent in mice (Grauwiler and Griffith, 1974). Following intravenous dosage, the mean LD_{50} was 190, 72, and 12·5 mg kg^{-1} in mice, rats and rabbits respectively.

No specific toxic effects of chronic bromocriptine treatment on any body organ in rats, rhesus monkeys or dogs have been determined (Griffith, 1974; Griffith and Richardson, 1975).

Bromocriptine has no effect on foetal development. In reproductive studies in rats and rabbits, bromocriptine has no teratogenic effect and also has no effect on animal fertility, embryonic development or postnatal viability.

The acute toxicity of bromocriptine in man is largely confined to the consequences of postural hypotension causing sudden acute collapse accompanied by yawning, sweating, pallor, and great prostration (Thorner, 1975). This occurs in approximately 1–2 per cent of parkinsonism and normal subjects given a single oral bromocriptine dosage of 2·5 mg. These symptoms rapidly recover. Haloperidol would be a logical treatment for bromocriptine poisoning.

Chronic oral treatment with bromocriptine 10–60 mg daily po results in digital vasospasm in a small number of subjects (Duvoisin, 1976; Wass et al., 1976). This condition, unlike Raynaud's disease, is sometimes painless. However, other ergot drugs, although relatively safe compounds, may cause endothelial damage.

The possibility that bromocriptine may be associated with gastric ulceration was discussed by Wass *et al.* (1976). There is no direct evidence that this is so. No consistent haematological or biochemical changes due to bromocriptine treatment in low or high dosage (2·5–300 mg daily) have been reported.

Bromocriptine, unlike the DA-releasing drugs amphetamine and amantadine, has little or no CNS stimulant effect, but may cause mild sedation. In contrast to anticholinergic drugs used in parkinsonism, bromocriptine does not commonly cause dryness of the mouth, urinary retention, difficulty in focusing or constipation. Nasal stuffiness occurs in a few subjects treated with bromocriptine; this side effect is also caused by reserpine, although the mechanism is uncertain. Side effects reported during clinical trials of bromocriptine are shown in Table 3 (from data obtained by Sandoz Ltd and reprinted by kind permission).

6   Pharmacodynamic studies

6.1   GENERAL PHARMACOLOGY OF BROMOCRIPTINE

Most of the pharmacological effects of bromocriptine can be attributed to DA receptor stimulation. Otherwise, bromocriptine is remarkably pharmacologically inert, although it does have a mild stimulant effect on 5-HT receptors in the brain, and like several other DA stimulants, bromocriptine has a weak antagonist effect on α-adrenoceptors. Bromocriptine differs from other ergot alkaloids such as ergometrine and ergotamine in many ways, and in particular has no major actions on the uterus or cardiovascular system of animals and man.

The DA stimulant effect of bromocriptine is likely to account for the potent action of this drug on animal mobility, plasma GH and prolactin levels. Other actions of bromocriptine on the gut, cardiovascular system and kidney are also likely to be due to a DA-receptor stimulant effect.

The action of bromocriptine on the heart and cardiovascular system is slightly different in different species, possibly partly owing to a different distribution of renal and mesenteric vessel DA receptors (Yeh *et al.*, 1969). Bromocriptine lowers blood pressure and decreases resistance in the superior mesenteric vascular bed in the dog and this action is prevented by haloperidol pretreatment (Flückiger, 1976). When vascular beds which possibly contain DA-receptors are excluded from the circulation by ligating the coeliac, mesenteric and renal arteries, bromocriptine does not affect the blood pressure. In the cat, the injection iv of extremely low concentrations of bromocriptine causes a fall in blood pressure and heart rate. Since such low concentrations given intravenously have no direct effect on the cardiovascular system, these changes are likely to be due to a central action of the drug. In a pithed rat, bromocriptine causes a dose-dependent increase in blood pressure, although it is much less potent that the parent compound, ergocryptine. Bromocriptine has little or no stimulant effect upon isolated blood vessels of dogs, but does inhibit the venous response to NA and the arterial response to 5-HT (Flückiger, 1976).

In man bromocriptine causes vasospasm, symptomatic postural hypotension and cardiac irregularities in approximately 1 per cent of all subjects. These changes are not necessarily dose dependent and have been reported following bromocriptine dosages as low as 2·5 mg po. Similar changes may follow levodopa or DA infusion in man.

The effects of DA upon the kidney, water and salt excretion are complex and may result from changes in prolactin secretion as well as changes in renal blood flow and tubular water and electrolyte reabsorption (Edwards and Jeffcoate, 1976). Dopamine, levodopa and DA-receptor stimulants cause an increase in renal plasma flow, glomerular filtration rate, and Na^+ excretion (Meyer et al., 1976). Thus bromocriptine causes an increase in urine volume which is accompanied by a fall in osmolarity, and a rise in Ca^{++}, Na^+ and K^+ excretion (Mahajan et al., 1976).

Dopamine, apomorphine and other DA stimulants will antagonize the antinocioceptive action of morphine (Vigouret et al., 1973). Bromocriptine iv reduces the antinocioceptive action of morphine in a dose-dependent manner (Loew et al., 1976). It has been assumed that in this test system bromocriptine acts as a DA-receptor stimulant on the striate nuclei, possibly resulting in a decreased inhibitory input to the afferent sensory system. The injection of pimozide into the third but not into the fourth ventricle prevents this action of bromocriptine.

Bromocriptine reduces gastrointestinal propulsion in animals, but only in large doses, considerably higher than those which are necessary to inhibit prolactin secretion. Normal animals quickly develop tolerance to this inhibitory effect on the gut. Inhibition may result from stimulation of a DA-sensitive mechanism in gut smooth muscle, counteracting the actions of acetylcholine.

Bromocriptine has no oxytocic activity although it does inhibit the uterine response to methylergometrine (Flückiger, 1976).

6.2   EFFECTS OF BROMOCRIPTINE ON BRAIN AMINES

6.2.1   Bromocriptine and catecholamines

Bromocriptine, in common with DA agonists such as apomorphine, and in contrast to DA antagonists, causes a reduction in DA turnover in the CNS, in the same dose range as causes behavioural changes in rats. Decrease of DA turnover due to bromocriptine is accompanied by a fall in brain homovanillic

TABLE 3

Side effects during bromocriptine treatment for inhibition or suppression of puerperal lactation, hypogonadism, premenstrual syndrome, acromegaly and Parkinson's disease (by courtesy of Sandoz Limited)

Side effect	Inhibition or suppression of puerperal lactation ($n = 793$)	Hypogonadism/galactorrhoea Average dosage 5–7.5 mg day⁻¹ ($n = 835$)	Premenstrual syndrome Average dosage 5 mg day⁻¹ ($n = 125$)	Acromegaly[a] Average dosage 10–40 mg day⁻¹ ($n = 338$)	Parkinson's disease Dosage variable Average 30–80 mg day⁻¹ ($n = 293$)
Gastrointestinal symptoms (not specified)	—	—	—	—	16 (8.00%)
Nausea	5 (0.73%)	51 (8.5%)	10 (8.93%)	35 (23.17%)	22 (11.00%)
Vomiting	6 (0.89%)	2 (0.33%)	—	4 (2.65%)	6 (3.00%)
Constipation	—	—	1 (0.89%)	27 (17.88%)	19 (9.5%)
Diarrhoea	—	1 (0.17%)	2 (1.79%)	—	—
Dyspepsia/heartburn	—	1.00%	—	3 (1.99%)	—
Stomach ache	—	1 (0.17%)	2 (1.79%)	—	—
Anorexia/weight loss	—	6 (1.00%)	—	—	—
Flatus	—	—	1 (0.89%)	—	—
Dizziness/giddiness/light headedness/vertigo	8 (1.18%)	11 (1.83%)	9 (8.04%)	1 (0.66%)	14 (7%)
Postural hypotension with or without fainting	2 (0.30%)	15 (2.5%)	—	—	16 (8%)
Fall in blood pressure	—	—	—	4 (2.65%)	—
Headache	4 (0.59%)	5 (0.83%)	5 (4.46%)	2 (1.32%)	1 (0.5%)
Salivary duct obstruction	—	—	—	2 (1.32%)	—
Dry mouth	—	—	—	7 (4.64%)	6 (3.0%)
Nasal stuffiness	—	—	1 (0.89%)	3 (1.99%)	1 (0.5%)
Mild sedation (drowsiness, fatigue, lassitude, lethargy, somnolence)	1 (0.15%)	1 (0.17%)	—	—	21 (10.5%)

Sleep disturbance	—	—	—	—	2 (1·0%)
Insomnia on drug withdrawal	—	—	—	—	4 (2·0%)
Hallucinations	—	—	—	—	14 (7%)
Confusion	—	—	—	—	3 (1·5%)
Affective disorders	—	—	—	—	2 (1·0%)
Psychosis on drug withdrawal	—	—	—	—	—
Restlessness	—	—	—	—	3 (1·5%)
Visual defects	1 (0·13%)	1 (0·12%)	—	—	3 (1·5%)
Hearing defects	1 (0·13%)	—	—	—	—
Cramp	—	—	2 (1·79%)	6 (1·78%)	—
Digital vasospasm[a]	—	—	—	24 (7·1%)	1 (0·34%)
Exacerbation of existing Raynaud's phenomenon	—	—	—	5 (1·48%)	1 (0·34%)
Dyskinesia	—	—	—	—	41 (13·99%)
Hyperkinesia	—	—	—	3 (0·89%)	4 (1·37%)
Bradykinesia	—	—	—	—	1 (0·34%)
Abnormal involuntary movements	—	—	—	—	10 (3·41%)
Dystonic posture	—	—	—	—	3 (1·02%)
Limb chorea	—	—	—	—	1 (0·34%)
Palpitations	—	—	—	—	3 (1·02%)
Ventricular premature contractions	—	—	—	—	1 (0·34%)
Metrorrhagia	1 (0·1%)	3 (0·36%)	—	—	—
Rash	—	1 (0·12%)	—	—	—
Numbness	—	—	—	—	—
Decreased tolerance to alcohol	—	—	—	5 (1·48%)	—
Flushes	—	—	—	—	1 (0·34%)

[a] In a study of articular and limb changes in 26 acromegalics, 14 subjects suffered from Raynaud's phenomenon (53-85%). *Quarterly Journal of Medicine* (NS) 1952, **21**, 405.

acid (HVA) synthesis. Ergocornine also causes a fall in DA turnover, but other amino acid alkaloids such as ergotamine and dihydrogenated ergotoxine alkaloids are less potent (Johnson *et al.*, 1973).

Bromocriptine and ergocornine cause a reduction in DA turnover in all brain areas containing DA. However, PTR 17402 (**9**), preferentially reduces DA turnover in limbic and certain nigrostriatal DA nerve terminals (Fuxe *et al.*, 1975a).

Bromocriptine, although reducing DA turnover, has little effect on endogenous DA levels in the CNS, and total levels of DA in rat brain are not altered by bromocriptine or ergocornine at doses up to 5 mg kg^{-1} (Corrodi *et al.*, 1973; Snider *et al.*, 1976). However, the effect of bromocriptine on DA turnover is revealed following the inhibition of endogenous DA synthesis, when the disappearance of DA is retarded by bromocriptine. The decrease in DA turnover can be visualized by histochemical studies of limbic and neostriatal DA terminals, which show a dose-dependent deceleration of disappearance of DA fluorescence.

In contrast to the effect on DA levels in the brain, bromocriptine and ergocornine cause a partial depletion of endogenous NA stores, possibly owing to a weak reserpine-like action on NA neurones (Corrodi *et al.*, 1973). Bromocriptine, in common with many other DA stimulants, has a weak NA antagonist action.

Bromocriptine in low dosage (0·1–2·5 mg kg^{-1}) causes motor inhibition and in high dosage (5 mg kg^{-1}), excitation. Both inhibition and stimulation are associated with decreased DA turnover in the brain. Inhibition is also associated with a decreased release of NA, but stimulation is accompanied by increased NA release, both in the brain and adrenals (Snider *et al.*, 1976).

The fall in brain DA turnover following bromocriptine is likely to be largely due to the reflex consequences of DA receptor stimulation. However, hormonal changes may also be involved, particularly in TIDA neurones. Suppression of prolactin release by bromocriptine will result in changes in uptake, storage and release of DA (Hökfelt and Fuxe, 1972). Both prolactin and GH in high dosages increase DA turnover in the TIDA system in normal rats, and especially after hypophysectomy (see section 7.3.1).

6.2.2   *Bromocriptine and serotonin*

Bromocriptine, like certain other ergot alkaloids, has a weak stimulant effect on 5-HT receptors (Corrodi *et al.*, 1975; Snider *et al.*, 1975, 1976). Bromocriptine may reduce 5-HT turnover in rats, since brain 5-HIAA is decreased 30–40 per cent. 5-HIAA concentration is reduced in the cerebrospinal fluid of bromocriptine-treated subjects with parkinsonism (Curzon, 1975).

6.3 EFFECTS OF BROMOCRIPTINE ON ANIMAL BEHAVIOUR

Bromocriptine, in common with other DA stimulants, causes stereotyped behaviour in rodents, turning behaviour in animals with electrolytic or 6-OH-DA lesions in nigrostriatal or related pathways, enhanced locomotor activity, and antagonism of reserpine-induced catalepsy. These effects are prevented by pretreatment with DA-receptor blocking drugs. Motor responses due to bromocriptine are delayed in onset, prolonged in duration, and a period of inhibition may precede stimulation.

6.3.1 Bromocriptine and locomotor hyperactivity

Increased spontaneous motor activity in rodents results from changes in both DA and NA systems (van Rossum, 1970; Andén et al., 1973). Dopamine stimulant drugs cause an increase in animal mobility in a dose-dependent manner, but low doses of bromocriptine, apomorphine and amantadine, will inhibit rather than stimulate normal motor activity (Stromberg, 1970; Stromberg and Svensson, 1971; Thornberg and Moore, 1972; Carlsson, 1975a; Johnson et al., 1976; Snider et al., 1976). Extremely high dosages of some of these drugs may also inhibit, rather than enhance movement. Thus, in animals, amantadine in a dosage of 160 mg kg^{-1} sc inhibits movement, possibly owing to a toxic effect (Abuzzahab, 1971; Thornberg and Moore, 1972), and high levodopa and bromocriptine dosages are occasionally less effective than lower dosages in the treatment of parkinsonism (Calne et al., 1970; Debono et al., 1976). High dosages may cause receptor depolarization, and result in postsynaptic receptor antagonism, rather than agonism.

In rats, bromocriptine 2·5–10 mg kg^{-1} sc causes an initial reduction in movement for approximately 1–2 hours, and as the dosage of bromocriptine is increased, the period of inhibition is shorter (Snider et al., 1976; Johnson et al., 1976). A prolonged period of motor excitation follows with peak activity at 3–4 hours (Fig. 1). After bromocriptine 10 mg kg^{-1} sc hyperactivity persists for at least 7 hours, a considerably longer period than following levodopa, apomorphine, amphetamine, or amantadine.

The reason why a period of motor inhibition precedes motor excitation with bromocriptine and other DA stimulant drugs has not been definitely established. Low concentrations of these drugs may cause presynaptic DA autoreceptor stimulation without causing postsynaptic stimulation, resulting in a reduction of presynaptic DA release. In contrast, high dosages may stimulate both pre- and postsynaptic receptors, but the postsynaptic effect is dominant. In favour of this concept is the finding that low bromocriptine dosages occasionally increase rather than decrease disability in parkinsonism (Carlsson, 1975b). Alternatively, inhibition-stimulation may result from mixed antagonist–agonist effects of certain DA stimulant drugs and their metabolites.

Bromocriptine-stimulated motor activity in rodents is partially or completely prevented when DA synthesis is blocked by α-methyl-*p*-tyrosine. This also prevents locomotor hyperactivity due to levodopa, amphetamines, amantadine and piribedil, but has no effect on apomorphine-stimulated locomotor hyperactivity. In contrast, previous DA-receptor blockade by haloperidol or pimozide blocks motor hyperactivity due to all these drugs, although large doses are required to antagonize the effect of apomorphine.

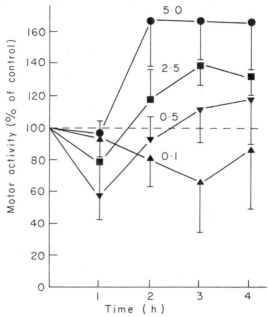

Fig. 1. Biphasic motor response to bromocriptine. Motor activity after bromocriptine. 0·1 (▲), and 0·5 (▼), 2·5 (■) or 5·0 (●) mg kg^{-1}, was given to groups of 4 rats and activity measurements were made on single rats for 4 min 1, 2, 3 and 4 h after bromocriptine. Control rats were measured in parallel. Each point represents the mean ±1 SEM of 4 values expressed as percentages of respective control. (After Snider *et al.*, 1976).

Atropine and other anticholinergic drugs potentiate motor hyperactivity in animals due to levodopa and other DA stimulants (Arnfred and Randrup, 1968; Costall and Olley, 1971). This illustrates the interrelationship of cholinergic and dopaminergic systems in the striatum. In man, anticholinergic drugs have an additive effect with levodopa and probably also with bromocriptine in parkinsonism.

6.3.2 *Bromocriptine and stereotyped behaviour*

Bromocriptine, apomorphine and levodopa all cause sniffing, gnawing and rearing in rats, although the dosages required are 10–100 times greater than those required to produce turning behaviour (Ernst, 1967; Voigtlander and Moore, 1973). Stereotyped behaviour is dependent upon NA activity as well as DA-receptor activity in an intact striatum (Amsler, 1923; Corrodi *et al.*, 1970; Fuxe and Ungerstedt, 1970).

Bromocriptine 1–10 mg kg^{-1} sc causes dose-dependent stereotyped behaviour (mainly sniffing) in rats. This is slow in onset, but maintained much longer than following levodopa or apomorphine. Apomorphine 0·3–10 mg kg^{-1} sc, causes more intense stereotopies than does bromocriptine 1–10 mg kg^{-1} sc, and biting is more marked. Stereotyped behaviour caused by bromo-criptine and apomorphine is completely prevented by previous DA-receptor blockade with pimozide 1 mg kg^{-1} sc. The inhibition of DA storage or synthesis by α-methyl-*p*-tyrosine 200 mg kg^{-1} sc, or reserpine 5 mg kg^{-1} sc prevents stereotopies due to bromocriptine but not due to apomorphine (Johnson *et al.*, 1976).

6.3.3   *Bromocriptine antagonism of catalepsy*

The production of catalepsy by neuroleptics in mice is believed to be due to antagonism of DA mechanisms. The tranquillizing action of reserpine which depletes 5-HT as well as CA stores in the brain, is reversed by levodopa, but not by the 5-HT precursor 5-hydroxytryptophan (Carlsson *et al.*, 1957). Neuroleptic-induced catalepsy in animals is also antagonized by anti-cholinergic drugs (Morpurgo, 1962).

Although the motor stimulant effects of bromocriptine are, to some extent, prevented by reserpine, bromocriptine will antagonize reserpine-induced catalepsy in mice, with an ED$_{50}$ of 1·8 mg kg^{-1} sc, as compared with (+)-amphetamine which is more potent in this respect (ED$_{50}$ 0·1 mg kg^{-1} sc); apomorphine (0·75 mg kg^{-1} sc) and levodopa (38 mg kg^{-1} sc without decarboxylase inhibitor, 3·7 mg kg^{-1} sc with inhibitor). Reversal of catalepsy by bromocriptine is slow in onset and well maintained (Johnson *et al.*, 1976).

6.3.4   *Bromocriptine and animal circling behaviour*

In animals in which the basal ganglia or pathways leading to them have been destroyed or interrupted unilaterally, drugs which act on DA neurone systems cause both postural asymmetries and turning behaviour. Injection of 6-OH-DA (which causes destruction of DA neurones, but not receptors), electrolytic or other lesions in the caudate nucleus, lesions which do not destroy the nigrostriatal tract but alter its activity (e.g. in the zona reticulata, Dray *et al.*, 1975), or lesions in the nucleus accumbens; all cause animals to circle in the presence of DA stimulants. The most intense circling is caused by lesions in the medial forebrain bundle in the lateral hypothalamus (Costall *et al.*, 1975). Circling results from interactions between the nigrostriatal and mesolimbic DA systems (Kelly and Moore, 1976). Mesolimbic dopaminergic activity has no directional influence, for rats with unilateral 6-OH-DA-induced destruction of mesolimbic DA neurons do not rotate in response to amphetamine or apomorphine (Kelly, 1975) and unilateral injections of DA agonists into the nucleus accumbens do not cause rotation (Elkhawad and Woodruff, 1975). However, the nigrostriatal and mesolimbic DA systems seem to interact physiologically and there are connections between the accumbens and the caudate nuclei (Powell and Leman, 1976) and substantia nigra (Smith, 1930; Rioch, 1931) which might provide the anatomical basis for this relationship. Mesolimbic as well as nigrostriatal DA neurones are damaged in certain motor disorders in man (Hornykiewicz, 1976).

In animals with 6-OH-DA lesions of the substantia nigra or ascending DA pathways, apomorphine causes turning to the intact side whilst DA-releasing drugs such as amantadine and amphetamine cause turning to the denervated side. The direction of turning behaviour may depend on the development of DA receptor supersensitivity on the denervated side (Ungerstedt, 1971). Thus, DA receptor stimulants increase the DA receptor activity preferentially on the denervated side, and the rat rotates to the intact side (Andén et al., 1967a). In contrast, DA-releasing agents (Carlsson et al., 1966) increase DA receptor activity only on the intact side, and the rat rotates to the denervated side.

In animals with 6-OH DA nigral lesions, bromocriptine 0.5 to 5.0 mg kg^{-1} sc cause dose-dependent rotation to the intact side (Corrodi et al., 1973; Johnson et al., 1973; Fuxe et al., 1974a). Bromocriptine rotation is late in onset and with high dosages, as intense as that due to apomorphine, the animal making about 20 turns min^{-1} (Fig. 2). Ergocornine-rotation is rapid in onset.

The circling effect of bromocriptine is prevented by pretreatment with DA receptor blocking drugs and potentiated by caffeine and theophylline (Fuxe and Ungerstedt, 1974; Fuxe et al., 1975). These drugs inhibit cAMP phosphodiesterases in the neostriatum (Butcher and Sutherland, 1962), and higher amounts of cAMP may be formed on stimulation at the supersensitive denervated CA receptors than at the intact receptor. However, in man the anti-parkinsonism effects of bromocriptine are not potentiated by theophylline or caffeine (Calne et al., 1976).

The rotatory effects of apomorphine in 6-OH-DA-lesioned mice are not altered when CA synthesis is prevented by α-methyl-p-tyrosine or when brain amine stores are depleted by reserpine. In contrast, the effects of bromocriptine (and also those of piribedil) are partially or completely prevented (Corrodi et al., 1973; Fuxe et al., 1974a; Johnson et al., 1976).

In rats with electrolytic lesions in the zona reticulata, bromocriptine 5–25 mg kg^{-1} ip, apomorphine 2–6 mg kg^{-1} and (+)-amphetamine 2–6 mg kg^{-1} cause dose-related rotation towards and not away from the denervated site. Lesions in the zona reticulata do not destroy the nigrostriatal DA pathway, but alter its activity. In these animals high bromocriptine dosages (50 mg kg^{-1}) cause sedation rather than turning. Apomorphine-induced turning is rapid in onset, whilst that due to bromocriptine is delayed. During this latency, bromocriptine will reduce apomorphine-induced rotation, but enhance amphetamine-induced rotation (Dray and Oakley, 1976).

The injection of DA stimulants into the mesolimbic and into the nigrostriatal DA system results in different kinds of behaviour, and the direct injection of apomorphine into the nucleus accumbens may antagonize the effects of ip levodopa in animals with bilateral 6-OH-DA lesions. Apomorphine

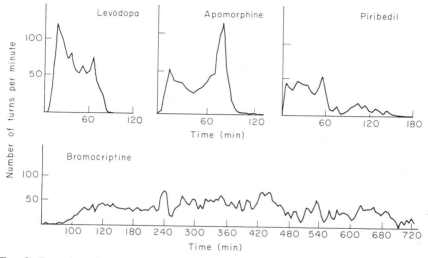

FIG. 2. Duration of turning in rodents with unilateral 6-OH-DA nigrostriatal lesions in response to bromocriptine and other DA stimulants. (After Fuxe *et al.*, 1975.)

will anatagonize the DA response in small doses that do not cause stereotopies (0·065–0·25 mg kg^{-1} sc), whilst bromocriptine antagonizes the hyperactivity response only in large doses (50 mg kg^{-1} ip). Apomorphine and bromocriptine thus have important differences in their effects on DA systems that determine circling behaviour (Costall and Naylor, 1976).

6.4   MODE OF ACTION OF BROMOCRIPTINE

6.4.1   *Differences in response to bromocriptine and apomorphine*

Bromocriptine shares many of the DA stimulant properties of the classic DA agonist, apomorphine, and other stimulant drugs, such as piribedil. However, there are substantial differences in response, which can be conveniently summarized here. Bromocriptine and other ergot drugs differ from apomorphine as follows (Pijneburg *et al.*, 1973; Struyker-Boudier *et al.*, 1974):

(i) There are species differences in response to bromocriptine and apomorphine. Unlike apomorphine, bromocriptine does not cause behavioural excitation in baboons (Anlezark *et al.*, 1975), does not greatly increase motility in mice (Puech *et al.*, 1975), or cause prominent stereotopies in rats (Snider *et al.*, 1976). These inconsistencies may depend upon species differences in bromocriptine metabolism, or be dose dependent.

(ii) Motor activation due to bromocriptine is delayed in onset and of longer duration than that due to apomorphine or levodopa in rodents with 6-OH-DA lesions (Fuxe *et al.*, 1974a; Johnson *et al.*, 1976; Snider *et al.*, 1976; see section 6.3).

(iii) The effect of bromocriptine (and also that of piribedil) but not that of apomorphine, on locomotor hyperactivity, is prevented when DA synthesis is prevented by α-methyl-p-tyrosine, or when CA stores are depleted by reserpine (Andén *et al.*, 1967a, b, c; Fuxe *et al.*, 1975; Johnson *et al.*, 1976; see section 6.3).

(iv) Bromocriptine (and also piribedil) in contrast to apomorphine, do not cause stimulation of DA-sensitive adenylate cyclase in striatal homogenates *in vitro* (see below). However, bromocriptine is a potent stimulator of cAMP formation in the rabbit retina (Schorderet, 1976).

6.4.2 *Effects of bromocriptine on cyclic AMP*

Bromocriptine in the rat causes an increase of striatal cAMP concentration *in vivo* but not *in vitro*. This increase is dose dependent, with a maximal cAMP concentration 10–15 min after bromocriptine 2 mg kg^{-1} ip. Two hours later, cAMP levels return to control values (Trabucchi *et al.*, 1976). These changes in cAMP concentration do not correlate with the onset of motor hyperactivity, which does not occur in the first hour following bromocriptine, but then persists for at least 6 hours.

In striatal homogenates *in vitro* bromocriptine in high concentration (10^{-4} M) does not stimulate cAMP formation and eventually causes a moderate inhibition. In low concentration (10^{-6} M) bromocriptine causes noncompetitive inhibition of accumulation of cAMP in response to DA (Trabucchi *et al.*, 1976) comparable to the activity of some neuroleptic drugs, although these cause a competitive inhibition.

Apomorphine, in contrast to bromocriptine, stimulates the formation of cAMP both *in vitro* and *in vivo* (Kebabian *et al.*, 1972). The differences in the effects of bromocriptine on cAMP production *in vitro* and *in vivo* could be explained by the possibility that *in vivo*, bromocriptine is transformed into an active metabolite, as occurs with piribedil (Miller and Iverson, 1974). However, *in vivo* bromocriptine causes a rapid increase of striatal cAMP levels, which is therefore unlikely to be due to the formation of a metabolite. Bromocriptine may possibly exert its effect on cAMP by a mechanism linked to the release of DA, a mode of action more similar to that of amphetamine than apomorphine, and only detected *in vivo*. Amphetamine stimulates the formation of cAMP *in vivo*, and like bromocriptine, does not stimulate striatal DA-sensitive adenylate cyclase systems *in vitro* (Carenzi *et al.*, 1975). However, many of the actions of bromocriptine are different from those of amphetamines. Bromocriptine decreases DA turnover at doses which cause an increase of spontaneous motor activity, whilst amphetamines increase DA turnover in the striatum (Costa *et al.*, 1972). Bromocriptine causes contralateral turning whereas amphetamines cause ipsilateral turning in rats with unilateral 6-OH-DA lesions (Johnson *et al.*, 1976).

Dopamine receptors can be studied *in vitro* by their ability to bind different drugs (Creese *et al.*, 1975, 1976; Burt *et al.*, 1975). Using this technique, agonist and antagonist states of the DA receptor can be recognized. ^{3}H-Dopamine selectively labels the agonist state of the DA-receptor, while ^{3}H haloperidol, the antagonist state. Dopamine and other DA agonists have about 30 times more affinity for ^{3}H-DA than ^{3}H-haloperidol binding sites, while the reverse occurs with DA antagonists such as the phenothiazines and butyrophenones. Bromocriptine has a similar affinity for the two sites and in this model acts as a mixed agonist–antagonist.

6.4.3   Is bromocriptine a dopamine-receptor agonist?

A DA agonist is a drug that causes direct stimulation of DA-receptors. There are several indirect indications that bromocriptine is a DA-receptor agonist. In animals, bromocriptine causes a fall in DA turnover and apparently direct stimulation of supersensitive denervated DA-receptors. In severely disabled patients with parkinsonism, who are likely to have considerable destruction of DA neurones but intact DA-receptors, bromocriptine often causes considerable improvement. The actions of bromocriptine on prolactin and GH in acromegalics are likely to result from direct stimulation of pituitary DA receptors. Bromocriptine causes a reduction and not an increase in CSF HVA concentration in man, indicating a reduced and not an increased DA turnover. This change in DA turnover is the likely reflex consequence of receptor stimulation (Kehr *et al.*, 1972).

Bromocriptine may be a partial rather than a complete DA agonist, i.e. a drug causing receptor blockade as well as stimulation. If bromocriptine did possess such mixed agonist–antagonist properties, this would explain the finding that high dosages are sometimes less effective than low dosages in parkinsonism, and the fact that in animals bromocriptine will sometimes antagonize the action of other DA stimulants on motor behaviour (Schnieden and Cox, 1976). However, there is no clinical evidence that bromocriptine antagonizes the effect of other antiparkinsonism drugs in man.

Bromocriptine is possibly a slightly less potent DA agonist than dopamine as suggested by the finding that in some, but not all subjects with parkinsonism, levodopa may cause a slightly greater degree of improvement. However, there is probably no great difference in potency between bromocriptine and levodopa, both of which cause a comparable degree of stimulation in hormonal systems, although bromocriptine has a more prolonged effect.

The effects of bromocriptine may depend partly upon the formation of active metabolites. This would explain the initial latency in response and subsequent prolonged period of motor excitation although, as already discussed (see section 6.3.1), initial motor inhibition may result from preferential presynaptic DA-receptor stimulation by low bromocriptine dosages. The apparently contradictory effects of bromocriptine on cAMP *in vivo* and *in vitro* may be explained by the formation of active metabolites *in vivo*. However, bromocriptine causes suppression of prolactin both *in vivo* and *in vitro* (Pasteels *et al.*, 1971), and this indicates that bromocriptine itself has a direct DA stimulant effect.

It is not clear why some of the actions of bromocriptine depend, at least partially, on intact DA stores. The metabolism of bromocriptine may be linked with that of DA and the formation of active bromocriptine metabolites prevented by α-methyl-*p*-tyrosine or reserpine. It seems probable that bromocriptine has dual actions on the DA nervous system, acting like apomorphine in causing direct receptor stimulation, but also acting like amphetamine in requiring intact DA stores. In addition to these pre- and postsynaptic actions, bromocriptine may also, like dihydrogenated ergot alkaloids, cause brain-specific inhibition of cAMP phosphodiesterase, and so enhance DA systems in the brain (Meier-Ruge and Iwangoff, 1976).

6.5   INTERACTIONS   OF   DOPAMINE,   NORADRENALINE   AND   SEROTONIN SYSTEMS IN THE BRAIN

Dopamine, NA and 5-HT systems interact in the control of motor behaviour and also in hormonal control (see sections 7.3 and 8.2) and the action of dopaminergic, cholinergic and other antiparkinsonism drugs is probably the result of complex changes in several neurotransmitter systems. Thus the action of levodopa, which causes a minor increase in NA in the brain, is likely to be different from that of bromocriptine which has a weak NA antagonist effect. The interconnections of DA, NA, and 5-HT neurones is almost certainly different in the DA-hormonal, and the DA-motor, system in the brain.

The noradrenergic system has a major role in influencing motor behaviour.

Lesions of the locus coeruleus, which contains a compact mass of NA neurones, result in circling behaviour (Donaldson *et al.*, 1976). The NA agonist clonidine (which has no effect on DA synthesis or on electrophysiologic activity of DA neurones; Rochette and Bralet, 1975; Svensson *et al.*, 1975), potentiates the locomotor stimulant effect of apomorphine (Andén *et al.*, 1973; Pycock *et al.*, 1976). Clonidine has the same effect as inhibition of 5-HT systems. In contrast to the effect of clonidine, adrenergic blockade will depress motor stimulation due to DA agonists (Andén and Strombom, 1974; Pycock *et al.*, 1975b).

Serotonin systems appear to be less important than NA or DA systems in the control of motor behaviour although reduction of brain 5-HT levels in rodents will potentiate circling (Modigh, 1974; Milson and Pycock, 1976). The influence of serotonin systems on motor behaviour demands an intact DA system (Green and Graheme-Smith, 1974).

In parkinsonism there is a considerable reduction in NA content in many areas of the brain. The enzyme responsible for acetylcholine synthesis, choline acetyltransferase is reduced to about 50 per cent of normal (Lloyd *et al.*, 1975) whilst absolute levels of acetylcholinesterase are also slightly reduced. In addition, striatal glutamic acid decarboxylase (GAD) levels are reduced to 50 per cent of normal (Lloyd *et al.*, 1973).

Drugs affecting the noradrenergic system, such as clonidine and the NA precursor dihydroxyphenylserine (DOPS) apparently do not greatly alter disability in parkinsonism (Birkmayer and Hornykiewicz, 1962; Tarsy *et al.*, 1975). However, anticholinergic drugs which penetrate the brain cause a minor improvement in rigidity and tremor, whilst centrally acting anticholinesterase drugs increase disability (Duvoisin, 1967). In the case of 5-HT, the precursor 5-HTP increases parkinsonism disability although when 5-HT synthesis is blocked by p-chlorphenylalanine, there is no obvious improvement (Chase, 1974). Taking these facts into consideration, the major antiparkinsonism effects of bromocriptine due to DA stimulation, may be slightly reduced by the weak antagonist effect of bromocriptine on NA systems, and the stimulant effect on 5-HT systems.

7   Bromocriptine and prolactin

7.1   INTRODUCTION

In man, prolactin is necessary for milk secretion (McNeilly, 1974, 1975). In animals, prolactin has a multitude of other actions ranging from osmoregulation in fish to hepatic lipogenesis in birds (Nicholl and Bern, 1972). Prolactin secretion from the anterior pituitary is under predominant inhibitory control. Dopamine appears to be one of the major physiologically active prolactin-inhibitory factors. Dopamine stimulants suppress prolactin levels in the blood, whilst DA antagonists or drugs which prevent the synthesis of DA, cause hyperprolactinaemia. Both physiological and nonphysiological lactation (galactorrhoea) are accompanied by hyperprolactinaemia. This has many different causes. Hyperprolactinaemia may be accompanied by hypogonadism, largely due to prolactin-blockade of the effects of gonadotropins on the gonads. Thus, hyperprolactinaemia may be accompanied by infertility in both males and females. Suppression of raised prolactin levels in the blood by bromocriptine will reverse this consequence of hyperprolactinaemia. Thus, bromocriptine, as well as preventing puerperal lactation, will prevent galactorrhoea and restore fertility in infertile subjects with high prolactin levels.

7.1.1 *Structure and synthesis of prolactin*

Prolactin is a hormone synthesized in the anterior pituitary. It contains about 190 amino acid residues with a molecular weight of around 22 000, although prolactin has not been completely characterized in the human. Prolactin is present in both men and women. A substance having similar physiological properties and a closely related structure, placental lactogen, is synthesized in the placenta. High concentrations of prolactin, presumably of foeto-placental origin, occur in the amniotic fluid.

Prolactin is structurally related to GH, and the two hormones may interfere during radioimmunoassay unless precautions are taken to avoid this. Unlike GH, prolactin is not stored in the pituitary to an appreciable extent. Specific pituitary cells manufacture prolactin although GH may also be produced in certain of these cells. During pregnancy, there is a great hypertrophy of the pituitary lactotroph.

Prolactin is transported in the plasma as an unbound molecule and is rapidly inactivated in the liver. Prolactin in the blood has a short half-life, approximately 15–20 minutes. Many tissues as well as the mammary gland take up prolactin, including the ovary, uterus, liver, kidney, and cerebral cortex. Prolactin stimulates milk secretion by binding to specific mammary tissue receptors and inducing formation of specific milk proteins (Turkington, 1971).

7.1.2 *Actions of prolactin*

Prolactin is one of a complex of hormones, including ACTH and insulin, necessary for normal milk secretion and lactation. There are two distinct phases of lactation, the synthesis of milk within the mammary alveolar cells and milk excretion into the alveolar lumen being followed by milk ejection into larger ducts and sinuses, where it is obtainable by suckling. The first phase is dependent upon prolactin, and the second upon oxytocin.

Prolactin has a direct effect upon the ovaries, for high levels inhibit progesterone synthesis *in vitro* (McNatty *et al.*, 1974). Prolactin is present in the fluid of Graafian follicles; follicular fluid prolactin levels are similar to circulating blood levels until just before ovulation when prolactin levels decrease markedly whilst those of LH and progesterone increase.

Under normal circumstances in the rat, prolactin stimulates the corpus luteum to secrete progesterone, and progesterone prepares the endometrium for implantation. Suppression of prolactin in the rat results in failure of implantation, but this is not so in the human, and bromocriptine is not contraceptive in man, as in the rat.

Prolactin may have an action on the hypothalamus, since puerperal women have low FSH levels which rise as prolactin levels fall during treatment with bromocriptine (Nader *et al.*, 1976). The alternative explanation for this phenomenon is that prolactin blocks the effect of gonadotropins on the gonads, and this prevents the normal feedback control of gonadotropin secretion. Under normal circumstances high prolactin levels do not correlate well with low FSH levels, but rather with the occurrence of acyclical FSH production.

The function of prolactin in the male is not known, but as in the female, high circulating prolactin levels may block the effects of the male gonadotropins on the gonads.

In animals prolactin is involved together with oestrogens in the regulation of puberty (Wuttke *et al.*, 1976), but in the human species, mean prolactin levels do not alter at this time.

Prolactin is associated with water and electrolyte metabolism. Oral water loading causes a fall in mean prolactin levels to 7 per cent of their basal levels in normal subjects. However, in subjects with hyperprolactinaemia, this fall is much less marked or may not occur (Perez-Lopez, 1975). The main stimulus to aldosterone secretion is angiotensin II formation following an increase in plasma renin levels. Under normal circumstances the diuretic frusemide causes a rise in plasma aldosterone levels due to an increase in plasma renin activity. Bromocriptine inhibits this rise following frusemide, but this is not apparently due to an action on renin secretion, since plasma renin activity is increased rather than decreased by bromocriptine (Edwards *et al.*, 1975). The action of bromocriptine in inhibiting plasma aldosterone levels may be due to an effect of prolactin on angiotensin II-stimulated aldosterone release. Prolactin is known to have a role in ovarian steroid formation and may also have a physiological role in the formation of the adrenal mineralocorticoid, aldosterone.

7.1.3 *Prolactin and steroid metabolism*

Prolactin appears to have considerable effects upon sex and adrenal steroids. In men and women with hyperprolactinaemia, sex steroid levels on the whole are within the normal range. However, testosterone may stimulate androgen-sensitive target organs mainly following conversion to the more active metabolite, dihydrotestosterone, and in women, the most active oestrogen is the oestrone metabolite, 17β-oestradiol. Patients with hyperprolactinaemia may be deficient in these potent steroids, although total sex steroid concentrations are normal, and reduction in prolactin levels by bromocriptine may cause an increase in 17β-oestradiol and dihydrotestosterone levels (Magrini *et al.*, 1976; Dickey and Stone, 1976). Prolactin may interfere with 5α-reductase activity, thus inhibiting dihydrotestosterone formation.

In respect of adrenal steroids, hyperprolactinaemia may be accompanied by an increase in adrenal androgen production, dihydroepiandosterone (Edwards and Jeffcoate, 1976). The abnormal production of this steroid may possibly play a role in the development of the polycystic ovary syndrome. About a third of such patients have abnormal prolactin levels, and have been treated successfully with bromocriptine.

7.2 PROLACTIN SECRETION

7.2.1 *Normal values*

In normal female subjects, mean day-time plasma prolactin levels are around 12 ng ml^{-1}, rising slightly to around 14 ng ml^{-1} in the evenings. At midnight, these levels increase to nearly double day-time values.

However, in contrast to these mean values, during the day prolactin levels show a wide fluctuation and the release of prolactin into the blood stream is episodic, serum levels showing irregular peaks. Release into the blood stream is probably in the form of a bolus, the mean serum prolactin level being dependent upon the amplitude of release rather than the frequency (Leighton *et al.*, 1976). Changes in prolactin levels during the night may not be related to sleeping or waking, but appear to depend upon chronological time, although this is debated (Sassin *et al.*, 1973).

7.2.2 *Prolactin and menstruation*

Prolactin does not appear to play any part in the regulation of the normal menstrual cycle. On rare occasions, a peak of prolactin occurs coincident with the mid-cycle peak of LH, but on the whole, there is no relationship between prolactin levels and LH, FSH, oestrogen or progesterone levels, or the occurrence of menstruation (McNeilly and Chard, 1974). Despite suppression of normal prolactin levels by bromocriptine in menstruating women, this does not cause any alteration in the biphasic temperature response of ovulating women, or gross alteration in the cyclical sequence of hormonal changes (del Pozo *et al.*, 1975). However, under certain conditions in rodents, bromocriptine influences the phasic secretion of LH, but not FSH and bromocriptine may induce a short luteal phase in normal women. In such subjects, if bromocriptine 7·5 mg daily is given for one complete cycle, there is a reduction in luteal progesterone secretion (Kunzig *et al.*, 1977). Prolactin may possibly exert luteotrophic effects in the human female via follicular maturation.

7.2.3   *Prolactin and luteinizing hormone*

Prolactin does not appear to have any direct effect upon gonadotropin secretion. However, subjects with hyperprolactinaemia often have no LH surge during the menstrual cycle and prolactin may interfere indirectly with LH secretion (Tyson *et al.*, 1975b). This finding does not necessarily preclude the hypothesis that prolactin blocks the effects of the gonadotropins on the gonads. In the normal menstrual cycle, LH peaks occur approximately 2 days following 17β-oestradiol peaks, and the reduction of 17β-oestradiol levels in subjects with hyperprolactinaemia may possibly account for failure of the LH surge (Glass *et al.*, 1976).

7.2.4   *Prolactin and pregnancy*

Prolactin levels in the blood increase progressively during pregnancy from the 8th week of gestation to reach a maximum at term. This rise in prolactin of pituitary origin is paralleled by a rise in human placental lactogen. In the second trimester, mean plasma prolactin levels of around 50 ng ml^{-1} occur, and at term, the mean level is 200 ng ml^{-1}. Much higher prolactin levels (up to 2500 ng ml^{-1}) occur in the amniotic fluid (Berle and Apostolakis, 1971).

Despite rising prolactin levels during pregnancy, lactation does not occur. Why do not women lactate during pregnancy? The effect of pituitary and placental prolactin upon the mammary gland is prevented by the high levels of ovarian and placental steroids occurring during pregnancy (Lyons *et al.*, 1958; Nandi, 1959). The immediate decline in steroid levels at delivery removes this block to prolactin, and milk secretion occurs. In hypophysectomized rodents, proliferation of breast tissue can be induced by a combination of prolactin, oestrogens, progesterone, GH and adrenal steroids. Milk secretion will then occur if prolactin is continued, whilst stopping the ovarian hormones. In lactating women, treatment with oestrogens will inhibit milk production, although prolactin levels remain high. Growth hormone is not essential for milk production in the human, for lactation has occurred despite its total absence.

7.3 CONTROL OF PROLACTIN SECRETION

7.3.1 *Factors affecting prolactin secretion*

Prolactin-releasing factors. Many factors cause a rise in prolactin levels in the blood. A prolactin-releasing factor is present in hypothalamic extracts, distinct from TRF activity (Boyd *et al.*, 1976). Operation, decarboxylase inhibitors (Pontiroli *et al.*, 1976), rapid falls in blood sugar concentration, and the serotonin precursor 5-HTP, cause a modest (5–10-fold) increase in plasma prolactin levels, and running upstairs may double plasma prolactin values (Horrobin, 1973). Various hypothalamic-releasing factors may control more than one hormone, and TRF, as well as causing TSH release, causes an elevation of basal prolactin levels to 5–12 times resting values, with 30 minutes of administration (Bowers and Folkers, 1973). The threshold for TSH and prolactin release by TRF is similar (Bowers *et al.*, 1971), but under normal circumstances TSH release usually does not parallel prolactin release (Meites, 1974). Thyrotropin-releasing factor is unlikely to be involved in the suckling response, for despite rises in plasma prolactin levels, there is no rise in TSH levels during suckling.

Prolactin-inhibiting factors. Prolactin secretion in man is under predominant inhibitory control, mediated by inhibitory factors (PIFs) which are produced in the hypothalamus and travel to the anterior pituitary via the portal vessels. These inhibitory factors can be extracted from the hypothalamus, and cause suppression of prolactin output by the pituitary both *in vitro* and *in vivo*. The most active hypothalamic extract has a high CA but no peptide content, and DA itself appears to be the major physiologically active PIF (Schally *et al.*, 1974; Thorner, 1975). This is shown by the finding that DA will inhibit prolactin production by the isolated pituitary *in vitro*, and also that injection of DA into the portal circulation in intact animals results in prolactin suppression (Takahara *et al.*, 1974; MacLeod and Lehmeyer, 1974). In addition, DA antagonists cause hyperprolactinaemia in man and will antagonize the effect of DA on prolactin in animals (Olson *et al.*, 1971). However, pituitary extracts which lack any CA content may cause prolactin inhibition. The nature of non-CA PIFs has not yet been elucidated (see review by Schally, 1976).

Noradrenaline and prolactin control. Both NA and DA inhibit prolactin release when infused into hypophyseal portal vessels, although probably DA is the more important physiologically. Some highly purified hypothalamic extract fractions which inhibit prolactin in doses smaller than 1 μg ml^{-1} contain a significant amount of NA, but little or no DA, and with such extracts the magnitude of inhibition of prolactin release is related to the NA content. However, the NA precursor dihydroxyphenylserine causes a minor increase rather than a decrease in prolactin output from the pituitary gland. On the whole, the potency of DA in inhibiting prolactin release is greater than that of NA. Attempts to measure either catecholamine in the portal blood have as yet been unsuccessful. The inhibition of prolactin by both NA and DA can be prevented by pretreatment by DA- and α-receptor blocking drugs, although not by the β-receptor blocking drug, propranolol (Schally, 1976).

Noradrenaline systems, unlike DA systems in the brain, are relatively unaffected by lactation, pregnancy or castration. Noradrenaline neurones are, however, clearly sensitive to sex steroids and respond with a clear-cut inactivation on treatment with glucocorticoids (Hökfelt and Fuxe, 1972).

Dopamine and prolactin control. Dopamine may act in two ways to suppress prolactin levels, firstly by stimulation of DA receptors on the pituitary lactotroph, resulting in inhibition of prolactin release; and secondly by stimulating the hypothalamic release of a peptide PIF. There are several physiologically active PIFs. This is shown by the finding that levodopa causes only a 50 per cent suppression of prolactin levels in normal subjects, and levodopa therapy is not as effective as hypophysectomy in suppressing prolactin levels in subjects with pituitary tumours.

7.3.2 Hypothalamic control of prolactin secretion

The physiologic role of hypothalamic control of prolactin secretion in animals is shown by the finding that prolactin production by a transplanted pituitary (into the mammary gland or anterior chamber of the eye) is largely autonomous. The anatomical basis for DA control of prolactin secretion is the presence of TIDA neuronal terminals bordering portal blood vessels (Fuxe and Hökfelt, 1969).

Prolactin may act by a short feedback control loop to modulate PIF-DA secretion, and prolactin causes change in DA turnover in TIDA neurones (see section 6.2.1). During pregnancy and lactation there is an increase in DA turnover in these neurones (Fuxe and Hökfelt, 1967) and, during the ovarian cycle, there is a higher DA turnover during metoestrus and dioestrus than at other times (Fuxe *et al.*, 1967; Ahren *et al.*, 1971). No such cyclical change in DA turnover in TIDA neurones occurs in the male rat. Hypophysectomy leads to a decrease in TIDA turnover in both male and female rats and this is restored by hypophyseal transplant (Olson *et al.*, 1971).

7.3.3 Hypothalamic dopamine systems and gonadotropin control

Tubero-infundibular DA neurones modulate the activity of gonadotropin releasing factors (GRF) in addition to PIF. Thus, gonadal and certain antifertility steroids which cause changes in LH and FSH secretion, cause a dose-dependent activation of the TIDA system. This activation is unlikely to be due primarily to the release of prolactin, since high doses of prolactin do not cause such marked activation of TIDA neurones as do oestrogens or testosterone in castrated rats.

7.3.4   Dopamine and prolactin utilization

Dopamine may have a peripheral effect on prolactin utilization and possibly activates peripheral prolactin receptors to bind the circulating hormone (van der Gugten et al., 1976a). This is suggested by the finding that levodopa, although causing a marked decrease in plasma prolactin levels in rats with pro-lactin-producing pituitary tumours, does not alter pituitary prolactin content. Any blockade of pituitary prolactin secretion is not accompanied by increased storage, and apparently prolactin synthesis is not depressed. However, accompanying the considerable increase in plasma prolactin levels following DA-receptor blockade, there is a marked decrease of pituitary prolactin content (van der Gugten et al., 1976b).

7.4   BROMOCRIPTINE AND PROLACTIN

7.4.1   Introduction

For centuries it had been recognized that milk cows eating grain contaminated with ergot fail to produce milk, but the reason for this was obscure until Shelesnyak in 1954 found that ergotoxine affected endometrial function in the rat and prevented implantation of the ovum in the uteri of pregnant rats. In rats, but not in man, implantation is dependent upon progesterone secretion by the corpus luteum, which is stimulated by prolactin. The suppressive effects of ergot on implantation in the rat can be prevented by progesterone or prolactin and Shelesnyak (1954, 1957) suggested that ergot had a direct effect on either the pituitary or hypothalamus.

   This observation was the starting point in a search by Flückiger for an ergot alkaloid whose main action was suppression of prolactin. This search proved difficult and laborious, largely owing to initial difficulties in prolactin estimation, but culminated in the development of bromocriptine.

7.4.2   Prolactin inhibition by ergot alkaloids

Before the development of a satisfactory radioimmunoassay for prolactin, Flückiger et al. (1968, 1976) used implantation inhibition in the rat to assess the prolactin inhibitory potency of ergot alkaloids. With this technique, great differences in potency of the naturally occurring peptide derivatives of lysergic acid were found. Of the first group of ergot compounds isolated by Barger *et al.* (1906), all of which were 9–10 unsaturated compounds and contained in the mixture known as ergotoxine, ergocryptine was the most active, ergocornine moderately active, and ergovoline the least active in inhibiting implantation.

Ergotoxine alkaloids inhibit both ovulation and implantation in the rat, although these activities are largely independent. Flückiger found that molecular manipulation, with bromine in position 2 of the lysergic acid moiety, resulted in a compound that was a potent implantation inhibitor (and thus causing powerful suppression of prolactin), but that did not inhibit ovulation. Bromocriptine is many times more active in inhibiting implantation, and many times less active in suppressing ovulation, than the parent compound, ergocriptine.

7.4.3   Specificity of bromocriptine action on prolactin

In all animal species tested, bromocriptine causes suppression of prolactin levels and of lactation. Bromocriptine also blocks the prolactin response to TRF. It has little direct effect upon other hormones concerned in the reproductive cycle. In normal female subjects bromocriptine causes a marked suppression of prolactin levels without much change in gonadotropin levels (del Pozo *et al.*, 1975), although in conditions of prolactin dominance accompanied by acyclical gonadotropin secretion, suppression of elevated prolactin levels by bromocriptine is accompanied by a return of normal cyclical gonadotropin levels (Besser *et al.*, 1972; del Pozo *et al.*, 1972). If a state of prolactin dominance is induced in animals by implantation of an ectopic pituitary gland, suppression of high prolactin levels by bromocriptine results in a LH surge.

7.4.4   Mode of action of bromocriptine on prolactin

Bromocriptine, like DA, has a direct inhibitory effect on prolactin secretion by pituitary cells *in vitro* (Pasteels *et al.*, 1971; Tashjian and Hoyt, 1972; Gautvik *et al.*, 1973; Gourdji *et al.*, 1973; Nagasowa *et al.*, 1973; McLeod and Lehmeyer, 1974). Thus Pasteels *et al.* (1971), and del Pozo and Flückiger (1973) showed that bromocriptine reduces elevated serum prolactin levels in rodents with ectopic pituitaries beneath the kidney capsule or implanted into the mammary gland, and Pasteels *et al.* (1971) demonstrated that bromocriptine inhibits the secretion of prolactin from rat and human foetal pituitary glands in culture.

7.5   BROMOCRIPTINE AND PUERPERAL LACTATION

Prolactin and human placental lactogen levels remain elevated for 3 to 6 weeks in the postpartum period in lactating women. Levels are highest immediately following delivery and decline slowly over the subsequent 3 weeks. After this prolactin release is maintained by reflex feedback to the hypothalamus in response to suckling, and prolactin levels fluctuate widely. If the woman fails to breast feed, prolactin levels fall to normal values by 3 weeks postpartum (Bonnar et al., 1975).

Follicular stimulating hormone (FSH) levels are high at delivery and fall postpartum for 2 weeks before returning to normal values. During this two-week period when FSH levels are low, there is also a failure of the normal FSH response to GRF. Episodic prolactic release following suckling may have an inhibitory effect on the hypothalamic–pituitary axis and the ovary, accounting for amenorrhoea in lactating women. The FSH response to GRF is depressed for longer in lactating than nonlactating women.

The concentration of placental sex steroids, oestrogens and progesterone, is high in the last trimester of pregnancy. These steroids disappear from the blood stream in the few days immediately following birth. Plasma levels of oestrogen begin to rise by about 17 days postpartum in women who do not breast feed, and on cessation of milk production in women who do breast feed. However, oestrogen levels do not *greatly* increase in nonlactating women until week 5 postpartum, and then ovulation can occur by about the 6th week, whilst in women who breast feed, ovulation is delayed until about the 10th week. Plasma oestrogen levels do not rise in lactating women despite the rise in FSH levels, probably because of raised plasma prolactin levels (Bonnar et al., 1975).

Human chorionic gonadotropin (HCG) and luteinizing hormone (LH) levels are high at the time of delivery and fall to low levels within 3 weeks, irrespective of whether lactation occurs or not.

7.5.1   *Hormonal changes postpartum and bromocriptine*

Suppression of lactation and lowering of raised plasma prolactin levels postpartum by bromocriptine is accompanied by a return of FSH and LH levels to normal more rapidly than occurs naturally (Besser et al., 1972). Thus, following bromocriptine, FSH levels return to normal by day 12 postpartum (Rolland et al., 1975) whilst LH levels return to the normal cyclic range when human chorionic gonadotropin (HGC) has cleared, approximately 2–3 weeks after delivery. There is no exact correlation between the fall in prolactin level and the rise in FSH level.

The immediate fall in plasma oestradiol level which occurs postpartum is not altered by bromocriptine treatment (Nader et al., 1975) although in bromocriptine-treated women, oestradiol levels may return to normal values more rapidly than otherwise, within 2 weeks postpartum (Rolland et al., 1975). Following bromocriptine treatment, the mean duration of amenorrhoea is around 35 days, significantly less than in untreated women (Rolland et al.,

1975) whilst ovulation returns by about the 20th postpartum day, as judged by rising progesterone levels.

Postpartum both the gonadal response to gonadotropins (del Pozo *et al.*, 1975) and the gonadotropin response to GRF (Canales *et al.*, 1976) are blunted, and bromocriptine does not immediately restore the normal response pattern in the first few days following delivery. This lack of ovarian responsiveness may not, therefore, entirely be due to high circulating prolactin levels.

Following the use of bromocriptine to suppress lactation, there is no alteration in the involution of the uterus (Benedek-Jaszmann and Sternthal, 1976).

7.5.2 *Suppression of puerperal lactation*

The need to prevent lactation arises if women do not wish to breast feed, after spontaneous or therapeutic abortion, in the presence of mammary infection, and during the administration of drugs that transfer via the milk to the infant. Suppression of lactation can be achieved in a number of ways. Oestrogen and oestrogen–androgen combinations are effective and block the effect of prolactin on the breast. This treatment, however, carries a risk of thrombo-embolism, impaired fertility, and possibly acceleration of neoplastic diseases. The direct inhibition of prolactin production by DA stimulation avoids these hazards. The effect of levodopa is short-lived: in contrast, bromocriptine will suppress lactation throughout the puerperium.

7.5.3 *Suppression of puerperal lactation with bromocriptine*

Bromocriptine, if given in the 24 hours following delivery, will prevent lactation and is also effective in suppressing established lactation later in the puerperium.

Varga *et al.* (1972) compared the effect of bromocriptine, stilboestrol and placebo in inhibiting lactation in mothers who had opted not to breast feed. Bromocriptine 10 mg po was given daily for 6 days, followed by 5 mg daily for 3 days. Bromocriptine was as effective as stilboestrol in suppressing lactation, but breast engorgement occurred in only five of 20 patients on bromocriptine and nine of 20 on stilboestrol.

Many further studies (Table 4) have confirmed that bromocriptine is an effective and safe method to suppress puerperal lactation. Prolactin levels fall with 4–5 hours of initial dosage and return to normal values within 1–7 days of starting treatment (mean 3 days). The prolactin response to suckling is also abolished (Brun del Re *et al.*, 1973). The average bromocriptine dosage necessary to suppress lactation is 5 mg daily; smaller doses may result in breast engorgement. There is no definite relationship between the occurrence of

TABLE 4

Bromocriptine inhibition of puerperal lactation

Authors	Dose (mg) (range, 24 h total)	Period (days)	No. subjects	Effect on plasma prolactin concentration	Clinical effects	Notes
Varga et al. (1972)	10	9	20		Lactation suppressed in all subjects	Bromocriptine as effective as stilboestrol 10–40 mg daily
Brun del Re et al. (1973)	2·5–7·5	13	14	Marked reduction 5 h after first dose	Lactation prevented or established lactation suppressed	Lactation suppression unrelated to prolactin levels or previous milk volume
Rolland and Schellekens (1973)	2·5–7·5	7	27		Response failure in only 1 patient	No side effects
Falzon et al. (1974)	5	14	20		Lactation prevented, no rebound lactation	Bromocriptine as effective as chlorotrianisine

Reference			No.	Prolactin	Lactation	Comments
Goebel et al. (1974)			16	Over 50% reduction in prolactin level in 14 of 16 subjects. Within normal range by 3rd treatment day		Bromocriptine no effect on oestrogens
Seppala et al. (1975a, b)	5	14	20		Lactation suppressed or prevented within 1–7 days starting treatment	Rare postural hypotension
Utian et al. (1975)	5	7	19	Rapid fall to low normal range	Lactation suppressed	
Walker et al. (1975)	5	14	32	100% fall within 4 h of bromocriptine	Lactation suppressed, rebound 7 days after stopping bromocriptine	No relation symptoms; prolactin level
Benedek-Jaszman and Sternthal (1976)	5	14–21	15		Established lactation suppressed in 13 of 15	No side effects
Cooke et al. (1976)	5	14	44	Fall on first treatment day	Lactation, breast congestion suppressed	No effect bromocriptine on clotting factors
Nilson et al. (1976)	5	14	20		Lactation inhibited 18 of 20	No side effects, unlike stilboestrol, no thrombo-embolism

breast discomfort or engorgement, continued slight milk production, and the degree of prolactin suppression caused by bromocriptine. Treatment needs to be continued for 3 weeks to avoid rebound lactation on drug withdrawal (Rolland and Schellekans, 1973). Bromocriptine is effective in the great majority of subjects, and will inhibit lactation when other hormonal treatment has failed.

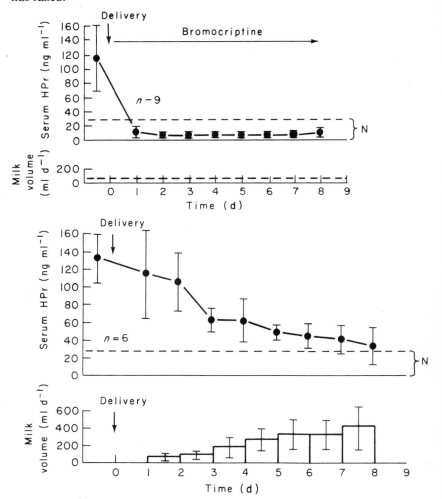

FIG. 3. Suppressive effect of bromocriptine on lactation and serum prolactin in 9 women in the postpartum period. Control: 6 normally breast-feeding women in the postpartum period (M + SD). N, normal range of HPr levels. (After Brun del Re *et al.*, 1973.)

The advantages of bromocriptine suppression of lactation over other treatment is considerable. Bromocriptine results in a short period of postpartum amenorrhoea, does not alter the normal involution of the uterus, and in the low dosage needed to suppress lactation, there is a noticeable absence of side effects (Falzon *et al.*, 1974; Seppala *et al.*, 1975a; Walker *et al.*, 1975). Nausea and hypotension occasionally occur, but abnormal involuntary movements have not been reported following the use of bromocriptine in low dosages (2·5–10 mg daily) to suppress lactation. Unlike oestrogens, there is no risk of vascular complications with bromocriptine.

7.6 BROMOCRIPTINE, HYPERPROLACTINAEMIA AND GALACTORRHOEA

7.6.1 *Hyperprolactinaemia and galactorrhoea*

Hyperprolactinaemia is common. Its main causes are shown below. Franks *et al.* (1975) found that raised prolactin levels (> 15 ng ml^{-1}) occurred in over two-thirds of patients with apparently functionless pituitary tumours. A quarter of these patients had galactorrhoea. Hyperprolactinaemia occurs in approximately a quarter of all patients with acromegaly.

Physiological causes	*Pathological causes*
1 Pregnancy	1 Pituitary-hypothalamic lesions, including pituitary adenomas, craniopharyngiomas, and cysts
2 Following childbirth	2 Persistent hyperprolactinaemia following childbirth
3 Mechanical breast stimulation	3 Drugs:
	a. Blockers of DA synthesis (e.g. reserpine)
	b. DA-receptor antagonists (e.g. chlorpromazine, pimozide)
	c. α-Methyldopa
	4 Myxoedema (excess TRF)
	5 Following oral contraceptive withdrawal (with associated psychological factors)
	6 Idiopathic

In other subjects with hyperprolactinaemia, no evidence of pituitary or neighbourhood tumours can be found. In some of these subjects hyperprolactinaemia persists after lactation has stopped (Chiari–Frommel syndrome) whilst in others no precipitating cause of high prolactin levels can be identified.

The drugs which cause hyperprolactinaemia in the main block DA receptors or interfere with DA synthesis, and include phenothiazines and metoclopramide, butyrophenones, sulpiride, reserpine, and alpha-methyldopa.

Plasma prolactin levels are often elevated in subjects with post-pill galactorrhoea and amenorrhoea. The ingestion of sex steroids is associated with suppression of endogenous gonadotropin secretion. In these patients, ovarian function may be attenuated, and without circulating oestrogen in physiologic concentration, prolactin may induce mammary alveolar function and milk production. However, there is little evidence that the contraceptive pill causes hyperprolactinaemia, and subjects with post-pill galactorrhoea may be either abnormally stressed (causing high prolactin levels) or have an unsuspected pituitary microadenoma.

Increase in TRF levels in some subjects with myxoedema causes an increased pituitary output of prolactin. There are a number of uncommon causes of hyperprolactinaemia. Lung tumours may occasionally secrete prolactin, and in liver disease, normal prolactin breakdown may not occur.

Approximately a third of subjects with hyperprolactinaemia have galactorrhoea. The presence or absence of galactorrhoea is probably dependent largely on the sex steroid status. The crucial factor seems to be the ratio of prolactin to circulating oestradiol (Tyson *et al.*, 1975). This is suggested by the finding that in some women with galactorrhoea and amenorrhoea apparently due to oestrogen treatment, galactorrhoea may persist beyond the return of the menses, although plasma prolactin levels return to normal with bromocriptine treatment.

Possibly a quarter of patients with galactorrhoea have some form of pituitary tumour. This may not be apparent on skull X-ray. A number of tests have been proposed to separate "functional" galactorrhoea from that due to pituitary tumour, although unfortunately none is absolutely reliable.

i. Very high prolactin levels both in plasma and CSF are usually associated with pituitary tumours.

ii. The normal fall in prolactin level following water loading may not occur in subjects with hyperprolactinaemia due to tumours, but is present in those with "functional" galactorrhoea (Board and Bhatnegar, 1975).

iii. Patients with hyperprolactinaemia due to pituitary tumours may show a negligible FSH response to GRF, whilst those with "functional" hyperprolactinaemia often show a greater, although attenuated, response.

iv. In patients with pituitary adenoma or micro adenoma, plasma prolactin level may not vary over a 24-hour cycle (Boyar, 1976) although whether this is also so in those with functional hyperprolactinaemia is uncertain. The response to levodopa or bromocriptine cannot distinguish between "functional" galactorrhoea and that due to tumours.

7.6.2   *Hyperprolactinaemia and hypogonadism*

Hyperprolactinaemia results in hypogonadism in a high proportion of subjects, irrespective of the presence of galactorrhoea. In the female hyperprolactinaemia causes failure of ovulation, amenorrhoea and infertility, and in the male hypospermia and impotence. The relationship between prolactin and gonadotropins is not fully understood. In some women, high prolactin levels causes the full galactorrhoea-amenorrhoea syndrome, whilst in others one symptom, but not the other is present. Irregular or heavy periods rather than amenorrhoea occur in some subjects with hyperprolactinaemia.

Hyperprolactinaemia is one of the major causes of amenorrhoea, responsible in between 13–30 per cent of cases. Other causes of amenorrhoea include hypothalamic or pituitary failure with gonadotropin deficiency and a low LH-FSH output, and ovarian failure.

Why does hyperprolactinaemia cause hypogonadism? There is some evidence that in animals raised prolactin levels are accompanied by lowered FSH and LH levels, and in animals, high prolactin states may cause a central inhibition of FSH and LH release (Horrobin, 1973). Evidence for a central defect is also given by the finding that the hypothalamic response to clomiphene, which normally causes stimulation of FSH and LH-releasing hormone output, is blocked in some patients with hyperprolactinaemia. However, in humans, the main cause of hypogonadism in hyperprolactinaemia is likely to be prolactin blockade of the effects of the gonadotropins on the gonads. In favour of this view is the finding that the majority of subjects with hyperprolactinaemia and hypogonadism are not deficient in gonadotropins (Besser and Thorner, 1976), but rather have a failure of the normal cyclic pattern of gonadotropin secretion (Seki et al., 1955). In these subjects, basal gonadotropin levels are usually in the low normal range and the administration of GRF, which raises LH and FSH levels by a direct action of the pituitary, usually results in normal gonadotropin secretion except when pituitary surgery has been done (Thorner et al., 1974). However, occasionally LH release is impaired (Aono et al., 1976) in the presence of hyperprolactinaemia.

That prolactin blocks the effect of gonadotropins on the gonads is shown by the fact that restoration of normal prolactin levels by bromocriptine is accompanied by restoration of normal gonadal function, although gonadotropin levels are not greatly altered by this treatment. The administration of exogenous gonadotropins is followed by a blunted sex steroid response in the presence of high prolactin levels. Besser and Thorner (1976) described a male with hyperprolactinaemia. He was given three injections of 2000 units human chorionic gonadotropin (HCG) and the plasma testosterone response was measured. This was small and subnormal. However, when prolactin levels were suppressed by bromocriptine, there was a much greater androgen response to HCG. Likewise women with hyperprolactinaemia have a blunted oestrogen response to pituitary gonadotropins, but when prolactin levels are lowered, the oestrogen response is greater.

Suppression of the gonadal response to gonadotropins by prolactin has been shown *in vitro*. If human ovarian follicle cells are cultured in the presence of gonadotropins, the progesterone output in response to gonadotropins is inversely proportional to the amount of added prolactin, high prolactin levels inhibiting progesterone production (McNatty *et al.*, 1974).

Blockade of the gonads by prolactin is usually incomplete, and in the presence of hyperprolactinaemia, sex steroid levels are not grossly depressed or gonadotropin levels grossly elevated, although this occurs occasionally. Prolactin blockade of the action of gonadotropins on the gonads is not entirely responsible for the failure of ovarian responsiveness to FSH immediately postpartum, for there is a lack of oestradiol response to human gonadotropins given 5–10 days following delivery, even when prolactin levels are suppressed by bromocriptine (del Pozo *et al.*, 1975; Canales *et al.*, 1976). Likewise the lack of pituitary response during this period, with failure of LH-FSH output in response to GRF, cannot be attributed to hyperprolactinaemia.

7.6.3 *Bromocriptine in the galactorrhoea-hypogonadal syndrome*

Bromocriptine suppresses galactorrhoea, and restores fertility when these symptoms are the result of hyperprolactinaemia. In the female reduction in elevated prolactin levels results in a return of normal steroidogenesis, cyclical FHS and LH discharge, ovulation and normal menstruation, and in the male, return of potency and spermatogenesis. Other treatments are not so effective as bromocriptine. Clinical experience shows that oestrogens will suppress post-puerperal lactation, but are seldom effective in the suppression of inappropriate lactation. Clomiphene and human chronic gonadotropins, previously used as standard treatment for human infertility, do not lower elevated prolactin levels and have no effect on galactorrhoea. Gonadotropins are now only indicated for the treatment of infertility in patients deficient in gonadotropins, and with normal prolactin levels.

In most females with galactorrhoea, amenorrhoea and hyperprolactin-aemia, irrespective of cause, bromocriptine in average doses of 2·5–10 mg daily causes partial or complete suppression of lactation, and return of ovulation and menses within 8 weeks of commencing treatment.

In most of these subjects bromocriptine reduces prolactin levels to normal, except in some with pituitary tumours (Lutterbeck *et al.*, 1971). The fall in plasma prolactin concentration is greatest in those with the highest basal levels (Tyson *et al.*, 1975). Prolactin levels fall to normal within a few days of starting treatment and remain low as long as treatment is continued. On stopping bromocriptine, there may be a rebound of prolactin levels to higher values than before starting treatment.

Besser *et al.* (1972) described 3 females with galactorrhoea-amenorrhoea, and two males with galactorrhoea and impotence. All initially had high plasma

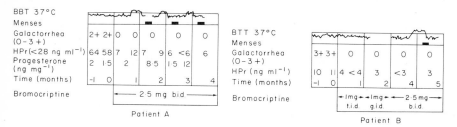

FIG. 4. Effect of treatment with bromocriptine in galactorrhoea-amenorrhoea, showing a different response in two patients. In patient A, prolactin levels returned to normal within the first month of starting treatment with rapid return of ovulatory cycle. In patient B, prolactin levels were suppressed and galactorrhoea ceased on bromocriptine 3 mg daily, but return of the menses only occurred after increasing bromocriptine dosage to 5 mg daily. BBT, basic body temperature; HPr, human prolactin. (After del Pozo *et al.*, 1974.)

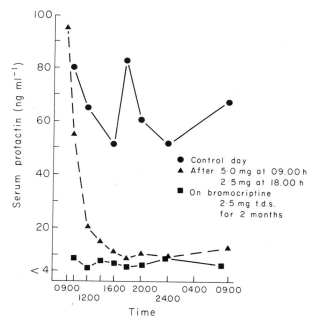

FIG. 5. Serum prolactin levels during the day in a woman with hyperprolactinaemia and amenorrhoea before treatment (control day), after acute administration of bromocriptine (5 mg at 09·00 hours and 2·5 mg at 18·00 hours) and when established on 2·5 mg bromocriptine three times daily. (After Thorner and Besser, 1976.)

prolactin levels. The disease had been established for from 3 months to 6 years. In all subjects, lactation ceased within 1–12 weeks of commencing bromocriptine, menses returned in all the women, and potency in one man. Impotence continued in the other male, who previously had had a partial hypophysectomy for pituitary tumour. Bromocriptine treatment remained effective for up to 10 months.

A surprising feature of bromocriptine treatment is the rapidity with which symptoms resolve on commencing therapy. Overall, in subjects with galactorrhoea treated with bromocriptine, milk production is reduced within 1–2 weeks and completely disappears in 1–3 months. Ovulation and menstruation in the female are restored in 75 per cent of women within 2 months of treatment, and potency regained in the male within a similar period.

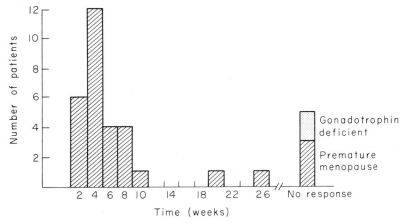

FIG. 6. Interval to resumption of normal menstruation in 34 women with hyperprolactinaemia and gonadal dysfunction. (After Thorner and Besser, 1976.)

However, it can take 8 months to restore normal cyclicity. On stopping treatment symptoms recur in the following order: serum prolactin increases, galactorrhoea then appears, ovulation is missed, and menstruation ceases (Seppala *et al.*, 1976).

Bromocriptine treatment may effect a permanent cure of galactorrhoea-amenorrhoea when this persists postpartum, but in the majority of subjects, symptoms re-emerge on bromocriptine withdrawal (Kunzig, 1975). Recurrence of symptoms may suggest the presence of a previously unsuspected pituitary microadenoma. However, several subjects with pituitary prolactin-secreting tumours have been treated satisfactorily with bromocriptine for several years.

A possible hazard of prolonged bromocriptine treatment is tumour enlargement resulting in optic nerve compression. This is a particular hazard during pregnancy in which normally the pituitary increases markedly in size. It is not yet definitely established if bromocriptine causes any great alteration in pituitary tumour size; a single patient with a pituitary tumour treated with bromocriptine for infertility by Thorner *et al.* (1975a) developed a field defect in the 38th week of pregnancy. Labour was induced and the defect disappeared after delivery (see also section 8.5.1).

A variety of regimes have been devised to avoid the hazard of pituitary compression of the optic nerves leading to blindness during pregnancy. About 3 per cent of cases with pituitary tumours treated with gonadotropin to improve fertility suffer from swelling of the pituitary, and optic nerve compression (Gemzell, 1975). Bromocriptine should not be used to restore

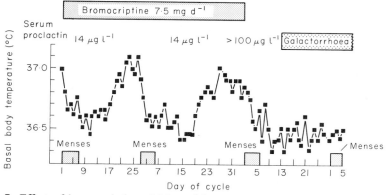

FIG. 7. Effect of bromocriptine withdrawal in women with hyperprolactinaemia and gonadal dysfunction. On stopping bromocriptine galactorrhoea returns and there is cessation of ovulation as judged by the basal body temperature. (After Thorner and Besser, 1976.)

fertility in women with pituitary adenoma who have an established field defect, or in whom there is a suprasellar tumour enlargement. In other subjects, tumours should be irradiated and at least three cycles allowed to occur before attempting conception. If pregnancy does occur, monthly testing of visual fields is vital. Coelingh Bennick *et al.* (1976) suggested that infertile women, treated with bromocriptine to restore fertility, should record basal body temperature as a check on ovulation, and stop bromocriptine as soon as temperature rose. If pregnancy did not occur, bromocriptine was to be recommenced on the first day of the succeeding menstrual cycle.

Bromocriptine treatment of galactorrhoea-amenorrhoea syndromes remains effective for several years, and whilst the drug is continued, prolactin levels remain suppressed. There is no indirect evidence of change of sensitivity of pituitary DA receptors despite continued stimulation. Thorner *et al.* (1974)

TABLE 5

Bromocriptine, galactorrhoea and hypogonadism

Authors	Aetiology Galactorrhoea-hypogonadal syndrome	Bromocriptine Dosage in 24 h (mg)	Period (months)	Prolactin concentration	Effect of bromocriptine on Galactorrhoea	Effect of bromocriptine on Hypogonadism	Notes
Lutterbeck et al. (1971)	Pituitary adenoma	3	1	High levels suppressed	Suppressed	Amenorrhoea reversed	
Besser et al. (1972)		3–9	10	Levels become normal on treatment	Suppressed	Menses returned	Impotence continued in man with hypophysectomy
Thorner et al. (1974)		5	28		Improved all patients	Restoration potency, menstruation	
Lutterbeck et al. (1971)	"Idiopathic"	9	1	Initial high level suppressed by bromocriptine	Suppressed		Side effects nausea and vomiting. Ovulation not restored in one subject with hypophysectomy
Kunzig et al. (1975)	"Idiopathic"				Suppressed	Menstruation, ovulation restored	
Beaumont et al. (1975)	Phenothiazine-induced	5	1	High levels fell in 6 of 7 subjects on bromocriptine	Partial reduction	Return menses in 1 amenorrhoeic patient	Phenothiazines continued
Tyson et al. (1975)	"Post-pill"	7·5	2	Suppressed to normal by return of 1st period	Occasionally persisted beyond 1st period	Menses restored	Stress considered factor in aetiology
Seki and Seki (1974)	Postpartum	7·5	3	Prolactin: fall; LH: no change; FSH: rise; Cyclical FSH/LH excretion restored	Suppressed	Ovulation commenced Pregnancy	5 years duration before treatment

described persistent suppression of lactation with return of menstruation in 11 of 13 patients with amenorrhoea, and retention of normal potency in all of four males for periods of up to 2 years, and Besser and Thorner (1976) reported a male with galactorrhoea impotence treated successfully for 5 years.

Amenorrhoea may occur without hyperprolactinaemia or other well-defined cause. In such women, the role of bromocriptine in restoring menses is uncertain. However, Seppala *et al.* (1976) reported that bromocriptine apparently restored the periods in nine of 18 women with amenorrhoea but normal prolactin levels, and five of these ovulated. In these women, the mean serum prolactin levels fell during bromocriptine treatment. Enthusiasm for restoring periods to all amenorrhoeic women with bromocriptine should, however, be tempered with reasonable caution.

7.6.4   *Bromocriptine treatment of female infertility*

Bromocriptine has been used to restore fertility to a heterogenous group of patients with various symptoms including suspected pituitary tumours, polycystic ovaries, amenorrhoea following contraception, and galactorrhoea. Many, but not all of these subjects have high prolactin levels. The availability of simple treatment for one cause of infertility does not do away with the need to establish that the male is fertile by seminal analysis, and that in women the fallopian tubes are patent. If the woman is not menopausal (sometimes premature) or pregnant, further investigation of infertility can be done. In the presence of normal gonadotropin levels but raised prolactin levels, bromocriptine is normally effective in restoring ovulation.

Thorner *et al.* (1975) reported 13 pregnancies in 12 women treated with bromocriptine for infertility. Five had suspected pituitary tumours, one had polycystic ovaries, and in four, amenorrhoea followed oral contraception or persisted postpartum. Pretreatment prolactin levels were high in eight patients, and fell on treatment. Ten patients conceived within 2 months of starting bromocriptine, and all 13 pregnancies occurred within 6 months. These patients had a normal gonadotropin reserve, as shown by a normal response to GRF. The number of bromocriptine pregnancies now (1977) totals 231, with 191 total live births. Bromocriptine was not teratogenic in these cases.

In infertile patients with normal prolactin levels, since bromocriptine does not alter gonadotropin levels, reduction in prolactin is enough to improve fertility. Alternatively, Thorner *et al.* (1975) suggested the intriguing idea that bromocriptine might act on DA receptors in the gonads. Women with hyperprolactinaemia and amenorrhoea who do not regain menstruation and ovulation on bromocriptine are likely to have a pituitary neoplasm or premature menopause.

8   Bromocriptine growth hormone and acromegaly

8.1   INTRODUCTION

Growth hormone is a polypeptide secreted from the pituitary which has effects on all tissues and organs of the body. Though once thought to be only concerned with growth in infancy and childhood, it is now recognized that GH has profound physiological effects throughout life. The control of GH release from the pituitary depends on many factors, including a GH feedback loop, peptide hormones manufactured in the hypothalamus and carried via the portal blood to the pituitary, glucose-sensitive neurones, and amine neurotransmitter systems inside the brain. The function of this complicated and elegant mechanism is altered by many physiological variables and may be upset by disease. Excess pituitary GH release, commonly due to a pituitary tumour, results in gigantism if occurring before growth has ceased, and in acromegaly in adults. GH deficiency in childhood results in dwarfism.

In normal subjects, levodopa causes GH release from the pituitary and a rise in plasma GH levels. However, in acromegalics, levodopa and DA-stimulants cause a fall and not a rise in plasma GH concentration. Sustained reduction of plasma GH levels by bromocriptine reverses many of the clinical features of acromegaly.

8.1.1   *Growth hormone*

Growth hormone is manufactured in the anterior pituitary, which contains 3–5 mg. The pituitary GH content is higher than that of other individual anterior hypophyseal hormones, and does not decrease with increasing age. The turnover of GH in the plasma is rapid with a half-life of approximately 20–25 minutes. In a single burst of GH secretion sufficient to raise plasma levels to around 30 ng ml^{-1}, only a small proportion of the GH contained in the pituitary is released, and probably the gland is depleted by only 1–2 per cent (Frohman and Bernadis, 1970). The structure of GH has been established; it contains 191 amino acids with two intramolecular S—S bonds (Niall *et al.*, 1971). This is a very similar chemical structure to that of prolactin which has overlapping biological actions to those of GH.

A new era in the understanding of GH opened in the 1960s when Raben, Li and Papkoff reported the isolation and purification of the human hormone (Raben, 1962).

The physiological effects are exerted on all organs of the body. In man, GH causes an increase in body protein, stimulation of protein synthesis, and acceleration of cellular entry of amino acids. There is an increased rate of synthesis and turnover of acid mucopolysaccharides in the skin, mobilization of fat stores, and an increase in fat metabolism. Growth hormone antagonizes the insulin-mediated uptake of glucose, but this diabetogenic effect is masked in the presence of normal pancreatic reserves, and normally prolonged GH administration does not cause diabetes.

Growth hormone causes increased calcium reabsorption from the gut, and increased growth via its action on cartilage formation. This may be due to a component of plasma, somatomedin, which directly stimulates cartilage and increases RNA and DNA synthesis. The plasma hypophysectomized subjects contains little somatomedin; after the administration of GH, somatomedin is usually detectable in the plasma within 4 hours, and is possibly synthesized in the liver.

The biological activity of GH can be assessed by its ability to stimulate body weight in hypophysectomized rats, or to increase the width of tibial epiphysial growth plates. However, this method is not sufficiently sensitive to measure GH in biological fluids. With the development of radioimmunoassay techniques for the determination of GH in 1962 (Utiger et al., 1962), and later modifications of this method, a more sensitive assay became available. Immunological activity of GH does not always correlate well with biological activity, and care has to be taken to exclude cross-reactivity of GH with pro-lactin.

Diamond et al. (1974) showed there were three or more components of immunoreactive GH in the plasma of normal and acromegalic subjects. These components probably differ in molecular size, and behave differently in response to TRF and insulin-hypoglycaemia. The proportion of the active monomeric form to the less active oligomeric form is approximately 4 : 1, and is the same in acromegalic and in normal subjects. Bromocriptine reduces the relative proportions of the monomer to oligomer in acromegalics and thus reduces GH activity and causes an abnormal ratio in bromocriptine-treated acromegalics (Besser and Thorner, 1976).

Nonprimate GH has little physiological effect in man. In contrast, simian and human GH cause major metabolic changes in both hypophysectomized and normal adult subjects, and a greatly increased growth rate in pituitary dwarfs.

8.1.2 Acromegaly and gigantism

The clinical features of acromegaly were described by Marie in 1886. One year later, Minkowski described a case with a pituitary tumour, and in 1895 Brissaud and Meige suggested there was an association between gigantism and acromegaly (see Nelson, 1974). Gigantism and acromegaly are identical disturbances of GH secretion, differing only in the age of onset of the disorder.

In the early years of life, excess GH secretion results in a tall stature. The Alton giant attained a height of 2·7 metres (Fadner, 1944). In adults, increase in length of long bones is no longer possible, but there is a progressive increase in width which in skeletal and facial tissues causes overgrowth of the jaw, orbital ridges, and other parts of the facial skeleton, with an increase in total mass of connective tissue throughout the body. There is also enlargement of many body organs, including the heart, thyroid, spleen, pancreas, parathyroid and kidneys. Profound sweating is common.

Gigantism and acromegaly are commonly caused by pituitary tumours. These may produce prolactin, corticotropin, melanocyte-stimulating hormone, and other hypophyseal hormones in addition to GH, resulting in galactorrhoea, impotence, amenorrhoea, Cushing's syndrome, and hyperpigmentation. In contrast, some pituitary tumours do not secrete hormones, and symptoms of hypopituitarism may develop.

In addition to these hormonal consequences, pituitary neoplasms also cause pressure on the optic nerve, involvement of other cranial nerves and the cavernous sinus, and occasionally compression of the hypothalamus. Rarely the pituitary may burst. The pituitary is situated within the sella turcica of the skull, and pituitary enlargement can be detected on skull X-ray. Specialized neuroradiological techniques, air encephalography or computerized axial tomography of the brain may be necessary to determine exactly the size of a pituitary neoplasm.

In gigantism and acromegaly, plasma GH levels are elevated. In some acromegalics levels are variable over 24 hours, and this may be due to the persistence of a degree of hypothalamic regulation which is not, apparently, suppressed entirely by high plasma GH levels (Cryer and Daughaday, 1969). However, in most acromegalic subjects, sleep-related peaks of plasma GH level, which are present in normal subjects, are attenuated or absent. The responses to other stimuli of GH production, such as arginine and hypoglycaemia, may also be blunted. The response to insulin hypoglycaemia is prevented in normal subjects by glucose infusion, whilst acromegalics fail to suppress serum GH levels below 5 ng ml^{-1} during a glucose tolerance test. Increase in plasma GH level in acromegaly or gigantism is accompanied by impaired glucose tolerance in 50 per cent of subjects, and clinical diabetes mellitus in about 10 per cent. Urinary hydroxyproline excretion is increased in acromegaly due to increased turnover of body collagen which contains large amounts of hydroxyproline.

There is no direct correlation between the degree of elevation of plasma GH levels and the severity of symptoms in acromegaly. However, serum GH levels correlate moderately well with maximum sellar size on lateral tomography (Wright et al., 1969).

8.2   GROWTH HORMONE CONTROL

8.2.1   *Normal variation in growth hormone levels*

Growth hormone secretion is episodic and influenced by many stimuli including psychic factors, endogenous sleep rhythms and exercise. Very high levels of GH are present in the blood in the first few days of life, although there is considerable variability. After 2 weeks of age, lower mean levels are found, and after puberty, plasma GH levels approximate to those of adults, although in children more peaks of GH activity may occur than in adults (Tanner, 1972).

In adults, there is a marked diurnal variation in plasma GH levels. For most of the day, levels are low, below 2–3 ng ml^{-1}. Under normal conditions, small peaks may occur some hours after meals. Major peaks of GH secretion occur during stages III–IV sleep, and with cyclic recurrence of these sleep phases throughout the sleep period, there is a cyclical production of GH. The onset of REM sleep may possibly terminate GH secretion.

In normal subjects, GH secretion is stimulated by hypoglycaemia, inhibition of glucose utilization, prolonged fasting and muscular exercise (Roth *et al.*, 1963a, b; Hunter and Greenwood, 1964). In addition, GH secretion is reduced but not abolished by protein administration. Major or minor stress, as for example, venepuncture, may also cause GH secretion (Lebowitz and Boyd, 1971). Growth hormone levels in man are also affected by levels of circulating thyroid hormone, ACTH, exposure to light or darkness, and the stage of the oestrous cycle. Corticosteroid excess and hypothyroidism both impair the plasma GH response to hyperinsulinism, and corticosteroid excess inhibits the sleep-related peaks of GH secretion. The nonspecific pituitary releasing hormones, TRF and GRF both may cause an increase in circulating GH level, possibly owing to a direct stimulant effect on the pituitary, and progesterone and glucagon will also modify GH responses. Thyrotropin-releasing factor exerts its effect on GH secretion at pituitary level, and causes stimulation of GH release in the hypophysectomized rat, bearing an ectopic pituitary (Udeschini *et al.*, 1976).

8.2.2   *Hypoglycaemia and GH secretion*

In humans, the secretion of GH is an important protection against hypoglycaemia. Small changes in blood sugar concentration that occur naturally have no effect. With larger swings in concentration, the rate of change rather than absolute level of blood glucose is the apparent stimulus for GH secretion. If 0·5–0·1 units of insulin kg^{-1} are given iv, there is a rapid fall in blood sugar to below 50 per cent of initial levels in most normal subjects. Accompanying this fall, there is a rise in plasma GH concentration which is prevented by the administration of glucose with insulin.

Changes in GH levels in man with changes of blood sugar and slow-wave sleep are independent. The increase in GH plasma levels during stages III and IV of sleep is not prevented by glucose iv, although both responses may be prevented by catecholamine receptor blockade.

The insulin-hypoglycaemia GH response is partially or completely abolished by pituitary stalk section, α-adrenergic blockade with phentolamine, or DA receptor blockade with chlorpromazine (Brown and Reichlin, 1972; Martin, 1973), although not greatly modified by DA infusion. These GH responses to changes in blood glucose concentration are probably mediated by glucose sensitive neural structures in animals, sited in the ventromedial hypothalamic nuclei.

8.2.3   *Plasma amino acids and GH levels*

Phenylalanine and other amino acids cause a rise in plasma GH levels in man (Knopf *et al.*, 1965). Arginine is a potent stimulator of GH release, and in children, Bovril, which contains a high arginine content, is used to study pituitary GH responsiveness (Tanner, 1972). Arginine also stimulates the release of insulin, but the increase in plasma GH levels is not due to hypoglycaemia, since arginine also causes a GH response in juvenile diabetics who lack insulin. In nonoestrogenized males, arginine is not an effective stimulus of GH production. Peak plasma GH levels may be higher in women than in men following arginine and other stimuli such as hypoglycaemia, probably owing to the effect of oestrogens in the female.

8.2.4   *Growth hormone-releasing and release-inhibiting factors*

Growth hormone release from the pituitary is under the control of two peptide factors of hypothalamic origin, GH-releasing factor (GHRF) and GH-releasing-inhibiting factor (GHRIF, or somatostatin). Both substances are synthesized in the ventromedial nucleus of the hypothalamus, pass down cell axons, are released at the median eminence, and conveyed by the portal vascular system to the pituitary cell, where they exert their effects. Tissue extracts from the median eminence stimulate the release of GH from the pituitary gland both *in vitro* and *in vivo*, and a potent GH-releasing agent has been isolated from hypophyseal portal blood. Highly purified hypothalamic preparations have a stimulatory effect on the synthesis as well as on the release of GH during incubation of rat pituitary glands (Schally, 1968; Schally *et al.*, 1968; Dickerman *et al.*, 1969). The neurosecretory process involved in the release of these polypeptides is elegantly shown by electron microscopic studies of rat pituitary cells, which reveal an increase in the number of secretory granules being extruded after administration of GHRF (Couch *et al.*, 1969). The nature of the hypothalamic releasing factor for GH is still unknown.

Somatostatin, GHRIF, was first isolated from the hypothalamus and characterized as a polypeptide consisting of 14 amino acids by Guillemin and his colleagues (Brazeau *et al.*, 1973; Lancet, 1974). Like other hypothalamic-releasing factors, somatostatin has a very short half-life, a few minutes only. In man, somatostatin has an acute or chronic inhibitory effect on pituitary GH secretion. It reduces or abolishes GH secretion in normal subjects in response to levodopa and other catecholamine stimuli (Siler *et al.*, 1973). However, in addition to this effect on pituitary GH secretion, somatostatin has separate peripheral effects, and inhibits the secretion of glucagon and insulin from the pancreas.

8.2.5   *Effects of brain amines on GH levels in man and animals*

Growth hormone, unlike other pituitary hormones, stimulates all tissues and organs of the body, and so no specific target-organ hormonal feedback mechanism is possible. Growth hormone itself may regulate GH secretion, as suggested by the finding that the administration of GH before insulin-hypoglycaemia blocks the expected GH plasma rise in the rhesus monkey. This feedback control may be due to interference by GH of the pituitary response to GHRF.

The hypothalamic release of peptide hormones which control pituitary secretion is largely under the control of NA, DA and 5-HT systems in the brain. Dopamine is stimulatory to the release of GHRF and PIF, NA is the major CA neurotransmitter stimulating secretion of GRF and TRF, whilst 5-HT appears to stimulate prolactin release. The secretion of ACTH is inhibited by a CA link in corticotropin-releasing factor control. Drugs which alter the synthesis, storage, release, reuptake or breakdown of brain monoamines cause changes in the levels of many hormones in the blood. Amphetamines, amantadine, levodopa, bromocriptine, apomorphine, monoamine oxidase inhibitors, and catechol-*O*-methyl transferase inhibitors all tend to increase plasma GH levels in normal human subjects, whilst reserpine, phenothiazines, butyrophenones and α-methyl-*p*-tyrosine, lower plasma GH levels (Boyd *et al.*, 1970, Boden *et al.*, 1972). The major metabolic pathway of levodopa is to DA and not to NA, and the rise in plasma GH levels following levodopa (Boyd *et al.*, 1970; Boden *et al.*, 1972) is likely to result from stimulation of TIDA neurones, with secretion of GHRF into the portal circulation. Massara *et al.* (1976) reported that perfusion of DA at 280 μg min^{-1} for 120 minutes did not lead to any significant change in plasma GH in normal subjects, in striking contrast to the increases induced by levodopa, apomorphine, and bromocriptine. Levodopa, but not DA will penetrate to the nervous system in sufficient quantities to influence plasma GH levels, and a central rather than a pituitary effect is likely to be involved in the GH response to levodopa. However, DA may possibly permeate the hypothalamus.

The rise in plasma GH levels after DA stimulants is prevented by pre-

TABLE 6

Drug effects on plasma GH levels in man

Drug	Route	Dose	GH level			Authors
			Normal subjects	Parkinsonism	Acromegaly	
Dopamine	iv	280 μg min^{-1}	Insignificant rise (0·4–4 ng ml) or no change	Insignificant rise (0·4–4 ng ml^{-1})	Fall GH levels	Wilcox et al. (1973), Massara et al. (1976), Verde et al. (1976)
Levodopa	po	500 mg–1 g	Mean peak increase 15–20 ng ml^{-1} at 60–80 min in most subjects	As normals	Around 50% fall in most subjects	Boyd et al. (1970), Eddy et al. (1971), Liuzzi et al. (1972)
Amphetamine	po	20 mg	Mean peak increase 20 ng ml^{-1} in 4 subjects			Parkes et al. (1977)
Amantadine	po	100 mg	No effect singly. Potentiate GH effect levodopa			Massara et al. (1973)
Apomorphine	sc	0·5–1 mg	Mean peak increase 10 ng ml^{-1} in all subjects	Rise in GH levels 1 of 4 subjects	Fall in all subjects	Lal et al. (1973), Brown et al. (1973), Chiodini et al. (1974)

						Reference
Piribedil	po	40–100 mg	No increase 5 of 6 subjects. Rise 1 subject	No increase 4 of 6 subjects. Rise 2 subjects		Debono (1977)
Bromocriptine	po	2.5–20 mg	Mean peak increase 12 ng ml^{-1} 8 of 9 subjects	Rise GH level 1 of 4 subjects	Fall in all subjects	Liuzzi et al. (1974), Camanni et al. (1975), Parkes et al. (1976b)
Noradrenaline	iv		No effect			Roth et al. (1963a), Wilcox et al. (1973)
Phentolamine	iv	0.5 mg min^{-1}	Inhibit GH rise due to levodopa	Inhibit GH rise due to levodopa	GH suppressed to 67% of base line	Kansal et al. (1972), Cryer and Daughaday (1974)
Propranolol	iv	10 mg	Slight mean peak increase. Potentiate GH effect of levodopa			Imura et al. (1971)
Chlorpromazine (also reserpine, α-methyl-p-tyrosine)	po	100 mg	Fasting GH levels reduced		Elevated GH levels reduced	Müller et al. (1967), Sherman et al. (1971), Kolodny et al. (1971)

treatment with DA-receptor blocking drugs. The suppressive effect of chlor-promazine and also reserpine on GH release following insulin appears to be exerted at a CNS, and not a pituitary level, since rates pretreated with these drugs show a normal depletion of pituitary GH content after administration of rat hypothalamic extract (Muller *et al.*, 1967), and reduction in plasma GH levels following chlorpromazine are prevented by pituitary stalk section.

Dopamine appears to be a major stimulant of GH secretion in man. The position in regard to NA is less well defined. Noradrenaline infusion does not cause GH secretion (Roth *et al.*, 1963a), and diethyl dithione carbamate, which prevents NA biosynthesis, does not prevent a rise in plasma GH levels following levodopa (Muller, 1973). However, the levodopa response is partially suppressed by phentolamine and increased by propranolol, which alone causes a modest rise in plasma GH levels (Molinatti *et al.*, 1975; Imura *et al.*, 1971), whilst α-adrenergic blockade with phentolamine causes a fall in level. The β-adrenergic system thus appears to inhibit GH release (Souvatzoglov, 1973).

With regard to 5-HT, increased GH levels have been found in the plasma of patients with excessive serotonin secretion due to the carcinoid syndrome (Feldman and Lebovitz, 1972), or following the administration of the biological precursor, 5-HTP (Imura *et al.*, 1973). However, in normal subjects the stimulatory effects of large amounts of 5-HTP on GH secretion are on the whole slight and erratic (Muller, 1973). There is little evidence for the attractive view that the stimulatory effect of levodopa on GH secretion in man is due to a final activation of a serotoninergic receptor (Ng *et al.*, 1970).

The GH responses in some animal species to manipulation of brain mono-amines is different from man, and in the rat, NA is a hundred times more potent than DA or adrenaline at 0·05 μg per rat in respect of GH release (Müller *et al.*, 1967). In the rat, GH secretion appears to be inhibited by central DA stimulation (Collu *et al.*, 1972), and bromocriptine has no effect on GH production and release in this species (Yanai and Nagasawa, 1974).

In animals, electrical stimulation or direct DA injection into the hypothalamus, hippocampus or amygdala, results in changes in pituitary GH secretion. There are both excitatory and inhibitory inputs from several regions of the limbic system to the hypothalamus (Smith and Root, 1971). Electrical stimulation of the ventromedial hypothalamic nuclei, or of medial basal regions, causes a rise in plasma GH levels, whilst stimulation in other hypo-thalamic regions has no effect. Growth-hormone release after stimulation of the hippocampus and amygdala, is reduced by lowering brain amine levels with α-methyl-*p*-tyrosine, and there may be a CA connection between limbic and hypo-thalamic systems. However, the GH release normally seen after electrical stimulation of ventral hypothalamic nuclei is not inhibited with DA synthesis is prevented (Martin, 1973; Martin *et al.*, 1973). Under these circumstances, electrical stimulation may result in GHRF release.

8.3 EFFECT OF PEPTIDE HORMONES ON BRAIN FUNCTION

Peptide hormones may have profound effects on many different aspects of behaviour and mind (Reichlin, 1974). Somatostatin, TRF and LRF, all have extremely short half-lives, seconds to minutes only, and it is improbable that they exert profound effects on target organs in the distal circulation. However, these peptides have a widespread distribution throughout the brain, and can be obtained from nerve terminal fractions (Winoker and Utiger, 1974; Pelletier *et al.*, 1974a, b). Polypeptide fragments of ACTH are found in the diencephalon, angiotensin II and substance P are found inside as well as outside the brain. The principle of neurosecretion may be widespread throughout the nervous system, and the CNS itself is likely to be a target organ for some releasing-factor peptides. These, fairly universally, cause an inhibition of neuronal excitability in the brain. This is likely to be an important physiological effect, since the affinity constant of individual peptides in causing neuronal inhibition is at least as great as for causing stimulation of target organs.

The physiological action of intracerebral peptide substances has not, at present, been definitely established. They may conceivably have a transmitter function or modulate synaptic responses to amino acids or monoamine neuro-transmitters. In contrast to conventional peripheral hormones, such as thyroid and steroid hormones, which circulate in the bloodstream and have fairly prolonged effects, hypophyseal polypeptides are rapidly degraded by local enzymes, and in view of their characteristic property of conveying local information, have been called cybernins.

In the case of GH, Tang and Cotzias (1976) suggested that the response to levodopa might be altered as a consequence of GH release, and that periodic increases in plasma GH levels might be associated with some of the undesirable effects of long-term levodopa treatment in parkinsonism. The behavioural effects of levodopa, and also of apomorphine, in animals are increased by pre-treatment with GH, and this effect can be prevented by somatostatin. Growth hormone pretreatment causes an increase in the cerebral concentration of dopa and apomorphine (Tang and Cotzias, 1976; Cotzias *et al.*, 1976).

As with GH, TRF will modify the effects of many centrally acting drugs and, in particular, DA (Green *et al.*, 1976). Thyrotropin-releasing factor enhances locomotor activity due to methyl-amphetamine and a monoamine oxidase inhibitor, and may act as an indirect DA-releasing drug in the nigro-striatal pathway (Cohn *et al.*, 1975). Thyrotropin-releasing factor occasionally improves symptoms in parkinsonism (McCaul *et al.*, 1974). In animals, melanocyte-inhibiting factor (MIF) has a similar action to TRF in enhancing the motor response to DA (Plotnikoff *et al.*, 1971) and, in man, has a definite antiparkinsonism action (Barbeau, 1975). Melanocyte stimulating hormone, MSH, causes an increase in parkinsonism tremor (Cotzias *et al.*, 1969), although this tremor may result from a β-adrenergic action of some MSH preparations rather than from a specific effect of MSH on the DA nervous system.

In practice, the consequences of hypothalamic and pituitary hormonal changes due to levodopa or bromocriptine treatment of parkinsonism are slight. Neither drug causes acromegaly, and levodopa, which has occasionally been used to treat movement disorders in childhood, does not cause gigantism. There are isolated reports of goitre, and postmenopausal bleeding in levodopa-treated parkinsonism subjects (Eddy *et al.*, 1971; Kruse-Larsen and Garde, 1971), but these changes have not been definitely attributed to DA stimulation.

8.4   EFFECTS OF DOPAMINE STIMULANTS ON GROWTH HORMONE LEVELS IN MAN

8.4.1   *Normal subjects*

In normal subjects, levodopa, apomorphine, norpropylaporphine, bromocriptine, amphetamines and piribedil cause an increase in plasma GH levels. The rise in plasma GH level caused by levodopa, apomorphine or bromocriptine is antagonized by pretreatment with chlorpromazine (25–100 mg po), pimozide (2–16 mg) or metoclopramide (10–60 mg).

Most normal subjects show an unequivocal rise in plasma GH concentration following levodopa 1 g po. GH levels commence to rise 30–60 minutes following dosage and peak levels occur after 60–120 minutes, at approximately the same time as peak plasma dopa levels. A minimal plasma dopa level of around 400 ng ml^{-1} may be necessary for an unequivocal rise in plasma GH concentration to occur (Mars and Genuth, 1973).

The action of levodopa on GH release in man is likely to result from a *central* action of DA, since the action of levodopa is potentiated and not prevented by peripheral decarboxylase inhibition. Mars and Genuth (1973) demonstrated that, compared with levodopa alone, combined treatment resulted in a five-fold increase in plasma dopa levels, 65 per cent reduction in HVA, and a two-fold rise in plasma GH levels in 10 normal subjects. In contrast to decarboxylase inhibitors, the addition of pyridoxine to levodopa (which results in an enhancement of peripheral dopa metabolism) reduces or abolishes the levodopa-GH response (Mims *et al.*, 1975).

The action of apomorphine on plasma GH levels in normal human subjects is similar to that of levodopa. Apomorphine hydrochloride 0·5–1 mg sc, causes peak GH levels approximately 45–60 minutes following injection (Lal *et al.*, 1973; Brown *et al.*, 1973). Both levodopa and apomorphine cause a greater rise in plasma GH levels in young than in old subjects. The GH response to both drugs is approximately equal in males and in females (Sachar *et al.*, 1972; Maany *et al.*, 1975).

Approximately 95 per cent of normal subjects show an unequivocal rise in plasma GH concentration following levodopa 1 g po, or apomorphine 0·75 mg sc. A slightly lower percentage respond to bromocriptine 2·5–20 mg po. This apparent difference may be due to the fact that bromocriptine causes nausea and vomiting less commonly than levodopa and apomorphine, and the stress of nausea may contribute to the GH response. In some studies, the percentage of normal subjects showing an unequivocal GH response to bromocriptine is as great as to levodopa. Cammani et al. (1975) showed that 8 of 9 normal healthy subjects given bromocriptine 2·5 mg po, had a rise in plasma GH level, peak GH values from 4–31 ng ml^{-1} (mean, 12·5) occurring 90–150 minutes following drug administration and Dammacco et al. (1976) showed that 12 healthy female subjects, aged 17–21, given bromocriptine 2·5 mg po all had a rise in plasma GH concentration, peak levels ranging from 3–46 ng ml^{-1} over baseline values (mean 20).

Direct comparison of the effects of levodopa and different dopaminergic drugs on plasma GH levels in normal subjects is difficult, for plasma drug levels and dose–response curves have seldom been determined. Some of the individual variations in plasma GH level following different drugs may be due to variations in drug absorption or metabolism. However, in normal subjects, and with oral dosage, the order of potency in respect of peak plasma GH levels achieved, and also the number of subjects showing an unequivocal response, appears to be levodopa 1 g > apomorphine 0·75 mg > bromocriptine 25 mg > amphetamine 20 mg > piribedil 80 mg.

The differences in magnitude in GH response following different DA stimulants, is likely to depend on the degree of DA receptor stimulation produced, and also on the separate effects of different DA stimulants on other monoamine systems in the brain. It appears that whilst DA is an extremely potent agonist at DA receptors in GH systems, bromocriptine may be less potent or a partial agonist. The different effects of levodopa and bromocriptine on NA systems may also be relevant; levodopa will slightly increase brain NA levels, whilst bromocriptine acts as a weak NA antagonist. Piribedil has little effect on plasma GH levels in man and also is not a particularly effective anti-parkinsonism drug. Amphetamines, which cause an increase in DA synthesis and release, do not have a direct DA receptor stimulant effect, and have only a modest effect on GH levels in man, whilst amantadine, with broadly similar properties to amphetamines, does not alter plasma GH levels although potentiates the GH effects of levodopa (Massara et al., 1973; Kytömäki et al., 1973).

8.4.2   Growth hormone response in parkinsonism

Fasting GH levels and the GH response to levodopa are possibly abnormal in subjects with parkinsonism, although the data is conflicting. Mena et al. (1973)

showed that plasma GH levels were low in three untreated subjects, at no time during a 24 hour period rising above 7 ng ml^{-1}. However, these flat curves may have been due to age and immobility, with absence of stress, rather than to a specific defect in parkinsonism. Most parkinsonism subjects show an increase in plasma GH levels following DA stimulation, both during initial and chronic levodopa treatment.

The increase in plasma GH levels following DA stimulation in parkinsonism is probably similar in magnitude to that occurring in normal age- and sex-matched controls, although it is difficult to establish this with certainty because of the different effects of levodopa on mobility in both groups (Lebowitz et al., 1974; Parkes et al., 1976a). In 24 of 26 patients with parkinsonism, studied by Debono et al. (1977), treated with levodopa for 1–5 years levodopa 1 g po caused a rise in plasma GH levels greater than 5 ng ml^{-1}, with a mean peak plasma GH level of 21 ng ml^{-1}. Subsequent levodopa dosages at 2 hour intervals result in separate peaks in plasma GH levels in most but not all subjects.

The evidence as to whether the levodopa-GH response in parkinsonism is lost after prolonged levodopa treatment is conflicting. Malarkey et al. (1974), found that only one of 10 subjects with Parkinson's disease treated with levodopa for 1–4 years showed an unequivocal rise in GH to levodopa, whilst the prolactin-suppressive effect of levodopa was maintained. However, in most cases the GH response to levodopa is sustained despite prolonged treatment (Lebowitz et al., 1974; Parkes et al., 1976a).

Following low dosages of bromocriptine (2·5 mg po) in parkinsonism only a minority of subjects show an unequivocal increase in plasma GH levels. This low bromocriptine dosage also does not cause any obvious improvement in parkinsonism. Following higher bromocriptine dosages (25–100 mg) approximately 70 per cent of subjects who respond clinically also show an obvious increase in plasma GH levels. The increase in peak plasma GH levels following bromocriptine 25–100 mg po is dose-related and in subjects who do respond, on the whole those with a good clinical response show high peak plasma GH levels and those with little response, low levels (Parkes et al., 1976b). In parkinsonism the initial therapeutic and peak GH response to bromocriptine occur at approximately the same time, in most cases around 90–120 minutes after oral dosage. The clinical response to bromocriptine is maintained for several hours but GH levels fall to resting levels within 2–4 hours of dosage.

8.4.3   Growth hormone response in acromegaly

Levodopa, apomorphine and bromocriptine all cause a rise in plasma GH levels in normal subjects but a fall in acromegalics. A paradoxical response does not usually occur to other stimuli of GH production. However, occasionally glucose causes a rise and not a fall in GH levels in acromegalics

(Beck and McGarry, 1966; Johnson and Rennie, 1973; Hunter *et al.*, 1974). Abnormal GH responses to levodopa or other physiological stimuli are also seen in a number of other conditions, including renal failure, carcinoma, Turner's syndrome, Huntington's chorea, Wilson's disease, acute porphyria and hypothalamic tumours (Martin, 1973).

Levodopa 500 mg–1 g po causes a consistent fall in plasma GH concentration in most acromegalics (Liuzzi *et al.*, 1972; Mims, 1973; Chiodini *et al.*, 1974). The fall in plasma GH concentration occurs 30–120 minutes following levodopa, and levels remain depressed for 2–4 hours. A few acromegalics have no response (Chiodini *et al.*, 1974). The chronic administration of levodopa does not achieve stable reduction of plasma GH level because of the short period of inhibitory effect, and the combination of levodopa with a decarboxylase inhibitor does not give a more sustained response.

Bromocriptine causes a prolonged (6–8 hour) suppression of plasma GH levels in acromegalics, and if bromocriptine is given at 6- or 8-hour intervals a sustained reduction of raised plasma GH levels over 24 hour results.

How do levodopa and bromocriptine lower plasma GH levels in acromegalic subjects? Several mechanisms seem possible. As already discussed, in normal subjects the elevation in plasma GH levels following DA stimulation is likely to result from activation of TIDA neurones causing GHRF release. Cammani *et al.* (1975) suggested that bromocriptine stimulated GH release in the healthy human by depressing a predominant GHRIF centre, and was inhibitory in acromegalics due to inhibition at prevailing GHRF centres. However, it seems more probable that in acromegalics, but not normal subjects, DA, and DA stimulants have a direct inhibitory effect on the abnormal somatotroph, possibly analogous to the action of DA on the lactotroph in normal subjects.

To investigate why levodopa has the opposite effect on plasma GH concentration in normal and acromegalic subjects Verde *et al.* (1976) gave 10 normal subjects and 20 acromegalic patients levodopa and DA infusion. It was assumed that the blood-brain barrier is impermeable to dopamine (Oldendorf, 1971) and that catecholamines injected systemically are taken up in only a small amount by the hypothalamus (Axelrod, 1965), whilst levodopa will penetrate this brain area freely. In acromegalic patients both levodopa and DA caused inhibition of GH release, whilst in normal subjects levodopa, but not DA caused an increase in plasma GH levels. The inhibitory effect of DA stimulation on GH release in acromegaly may therefore involve DA receptors on GH secreting cells. Dopamine has no effect on normal pituitary cells *in vitro* (MacLeod, 1969) but DA and bromocriptine inhibit the release of GH from rat pituitary tumour cells (Quadri and Meites, 1971; Malarkey and Daughaday, 1972).

Most acromegalic subjects have a rise in GH levels following TRF and GHRF stimulation, although some acromegalics do not respond to either treatment. Thyrotropin-releasing factor and GHRF both appear to stimulate GH release at a pituitary level. Acromegalics who do not respond to these releasing factors also do not respond to levodopa or bromocriptine (Liuzzi *et al.*, 1974; Faglia *et al.*, 1975) and in these subjects the pituitary adenoma cell appears to have been completely autonomous. In acromegalic subjects in whom bromocriptine has caused a partial or complete suppression of GH levels in the blood, TRF will still cause an elevation of plasma GH levels. This effect of TRF on GH levels can be blocked by somatostatin and does not appear to be due to TSH or prolactin release.

The order of potency of different DA stimulants in causing elevation or suppression of plasma GH levels is broadly similar in normal and acromegalic subjects. Thus levodopa causes a large rise in normal subjects and a large fall in most acromegalics, whilst piribedil (2) is comparatively inactive in both groups. Comparing the effects of different DA stimulants in acromegalic subjects, Cammani *et al.* (1975) found that those who responded to bromocriptine 2·5 mg po also responded to levodopa 500 mg po and piribedil 100 mg po although bromocriptine caused a more-frequent striking, and long-lasting effect than the other drugs. Amantadine and the amantadine derivative, 3-dimethyl-5-amino-adamantane, were without effect.

In a group of acromegalics with high resting plasma GH levels (20–90 ng ml^{-1}), Liuzzi *et al.* (1974) found that 60 minutes following bromocriptine 2·5 mg po GH levels had fallen to 16–45 ng ml^{-1}, and after 150 minutes to 6–39 ng ml^{-1}. This time course of reduction in GH levels following bromocriptine corresponds fairly well to the reported time course of activation of DA receptors in animals (Cammani *et al.*, 1975). This is also the case with other DA stimulants; levodopa causes activation of DA receptors in animals for approximately 1–2 hours (Fuxe *et al.*, 1975a) and GH depression in acromegalics for a similar period of time, whilst apomorphine which activates DA receptors in animals for about 1 hour (Andén *et al.*, 1967b), lowers plasma GH levels for the same period (Chiodini *et al.*, 1974).

8.5 BROMOCRIPTINE IN THE TREATMENT OF ACROMEGALY

In both normal and acromegalic subjects, GHRIF will lower plasma GH levels. Growth hormone release-inhibiting factor is, however, ineffective in the treatment of acromegaly since its effects are short-lived, although greater activity may be obtained by combination with an adjuvant (Hall *et al.*, 1973; Besser *et al.*, 1974). As might be expected, the local messenger effect of GHRIF, designed to travel only millimetres in the portal circulation, is largely wasted when diluted in the peripheral blood.

The increase in plasma GH levels in normal subjects due to DA stimulation is prevented by DA antagonists. Both DA agonists and DA antagonists cause a fall in the plasma GH levels in acromegalics, possibly owing to the effect of antagonists on hypothalamic GHRF production and the direct effect of agonists on the pituitary. However, the GH lowering effect of bromocriptine in acromegaly is reduced and not enhanced by the addition of the DA antagonist metoclopramide (Delitala et al., 1976). Chlorpromazine is of little value in the treatment of acromegaly, although it does cause a minor fall in plasma GH levels (Kolodny et al., 1971; Diamond et al., 1973).

Levodopa does not cause a sustained fall in elevated GH levels and is not, therefore, of value in the treatment of acromegaly (Chiodini et al., 1974). The DA-releasing drug, fenfluramine, is no more satisfactory (Sulaiman and Johnson, 1973). Progesterone causes a fall in plasma GH levels, but on account of hormonal and vascular complications is not suitable for long-term treatment of acromegaly (Malarkey and Daughaday, 1971). In contrast to all these drugs, bromocriptine causes prolonged suppression of elevated plasma GH levels and is a safe and effective treatment for the hormonal consequences of acromegaly.

A single dose of bromocriptine 2·5 mg po causes a sustained fall in plasma GH level for 6–10 hours in most acromegalic subjects. To suppress GH levels

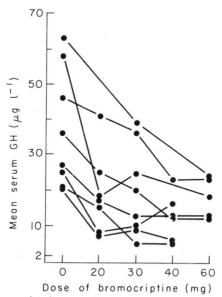

FIG. 8. Effect of progressive increase in the dose of bromocriptine on mean serum growth hormone levels in 8 acromegalic patients. (After Thorner and Besser, 1976.)

over a 24-hour period, it is probably necessary to give bromocriptine 5 mg four times daily (Thorner and Besser, 1976). The bromocriptine dosage necessary to suppress elevated GH levels in acromegaly is greater than that needed to suppress lactation (mean 24-hour dosage 7·5 mg) and less than that usually needed for the treatment of parkinsonism (mean 50 mg daily).

Treatment with bromocriptine causes a significant and sustained fall in the elevated plasma GH levels in approximately 80 per cent of acromegalic subjects. The mean dosage necessary to cause clinical improvement is around 20 mg daily in four divided doses although sometimes dosages as high as 60 mg daily are necessary. Plasma GH levels in most subjects fall within a few days of starting treatment, although levels do not return to the normal range. Plasma GH levels remain low for several years of bromocriptine treatment although on drug withdrawal there is a rebound to levels higher than pretreatment values.

Accompanying bromocriptine treatment there is clinical and biochemical improvement in those symptoms of acromegaly due to an excess of circulating plasma GH. A slow build up of bromocriptine treatment from 2·5 mg daily to that dosage causing obvious clinical improvement and supression of plasma GH levels is necessary to minimize side effects although these, mainly nausea and hypotension, are infrequent and hallucinations and abnormal involuntary movements due to bromocriptine do not occur in acromegaly.

The clinical response is sometimes dramatic and facial features may return to normal. There is a reduction in soft tissue swelling and diminution in sweating also possibly with resolution of long bone thickening. This response is often obvious within 4–8 weeks of starting treatment. Approximately 80 per cent of all acromegalics show a clinical response to bromocriptine. These subjects mainly have initial very high plasma GH levels with a marked fall on bromocriptine. About 20 per cent of subjects do not show a clinical response despite prolonged treatment (up to 6 months), and despite high bromocriptine dosages (60 mg daily). Some of these unresponsive subjects do not have particularly high pretreatment plasma GH levels and also no great suppression of plasma GH levels with bromocriptine. In certain unresponsive subjects, the GH response to TRF and GHRIF is also lost and it is possible that the pathological nature of the pituitary tumour is different from that in bromocriptine-responsive acromegalics.

Biochemical improvement accompanies the clinical improvement due to bromocriptine in acromegaly. Accompanying the fall of plasma GH levels, there is an improvement in glucose tolerance in diabetic subjects, and urinary hydroxyproline levels which are high in untreated acromegalics, return to normal. In subjects in whom bromocriptine does not substantially lower GH levels, urinary hydroxyproline excretion also does not fall (Thorner and Besser, 1976).

TABLE 7

Bromocriptine and acromegaly

Authors	Bromocriptine Dosage in 24 h (mg)	Period	Number of subjects	GH response	Clinical response	Side effects	Notes
Liuzzi et al. (1974)	2·5	Acute	7	GH levels reduced in all patients		Nil	GH levels suppressed 1–7 h
Althoff et al. (1975)	7·5–10	8 weeks	13	GH levels fell by 40% in 9 of 13 subjects	Soft tissue swelling reduced	Nil	Galactorrhoea ceased
Chiodini et al. (1975)	10	12 weeks	12	GH levels fell by 50% in 7 of 12 subjects	Clinical response in those 7 patients with fall in plasma GH. 5 nonresponders	Fall BP	Clinical improvement maintained for over 1 year
Köbberling et al. (1975)	1 7·5	Acute 3 weeks	5	GH levels fell in 4 of 5 subjects	Soft tissue swelling reduced		
Molinatti et al. (1975)	2·5	Acute	15	GH levels fell			GH response to bromocriptine 2·5 mg greater than to levodopa 500 mg
Sachdev et al. (1975)	Maximum 60	46 weeks	21	GH levels fell in 19 of 21 subjects	Soft tissue swelling reduced	Nausea frequent. Constipation	Improvement galactorrhoea, potency, carbohydrate tolerance
Summers et al. (1975)	7·5	4–5 weeks	8	GH levels fell in 2 of 8 subjects		Vomiting 3 subjects	
Thorner et al. (1975)	20	7–11 weeks	11	GH levels fell in 9 of 11 subjects	Soft tissue swelling, sweating reduced in all subjects	Mild constipation only	Improvement in glucose tolerance
Turnbridge et al. (1975)	10–60	26 weeks	21	GH levels fell in 16 of 21 subjects	Soft tissue swelling reduced		Bromocriptine not as effective as hypophysectomy in some subjects
Ueda et al. (1975), Aono et al. (1976)	7·5	8 weeks	1	GH level fell from 72–24 ng ml^{-1}	Soft tissue swelling reduced, ovulation re-established		Bromocriptine more effective than levodopa
Thorner and Besser (1976)	20–60	26 weeks	25	GH levels fell after 4 weeks in 19 of 24 subjects	Improvement soft tissue swelling, glucose tolerance, libido. Reduction sweating	Nausea. Fall BP. Constipation. Dry mouth	Improvement kept for at least 6 months

The reason why plasma GH-levels are only partially suppressed in acromegalics, yet there is a good clinical response, is difficult to determine. Plasma GH levels rarely fall to normal values. As already discussed, bromocriptine alters the ratio of monomeric to oligomeric forms of GH in the plasma, and may reduce physiologically active rather than inactive plasma GH concentration.

The results of different studies of the action of bromocriptine in acromegalic patients are shown in Table 7. In subjects in whom hyperprolactinaemia accompanies acromegaly, both conditions improve on bromocriptine treatment.

8.5.1   Long-term treatment of acromegaly

Wass et al. (1977) described 73 patients with acromegaly treated with bromocriptine 10–60 mg daily for periods of up to 25 months. The dosage of bromocriptine in most subjects was around 10–20 mg daily although increasing the dose above 20 mg daily produced a further improvement in the mean serum GH concentration of 12 of 21 subjects. In individual patients, maximum suppression of GH levels was achieved with bromocriptine 20–60 mg daily.

Seventy-one of these patients with acromegaly showed clinical improvement, with reduction in excessive sweating, hand size and headache, improved facial appearance, increased energy and libedo. On bromocriptine, previously abnormal visual fields became normal in two subjects (one of whom also had radiotherapy). Twenty-three of these acromegalic subjects were diabetic before treatment. On bromocriptine glucose tolerance tests became normal in 15 and improved in a further five.

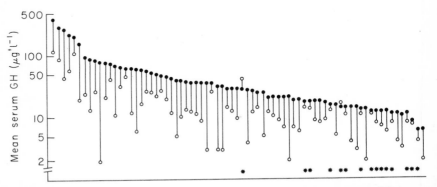

FIG. 9. Change in mean serum growth hormone before (●) and during (O) bromocriptine treatment in 73 patients. Asterisks indicate nonresponders. Growth hormone plotted on a logarithmic scale. (After Wass et al., 1977.)

Mean circulating GH levels fell by more than 7 μg l^{-1} in 57 patients and became undetectable in one patient. However in most subjects GH levels did not fall to normal values. There was some discrepancy between the clinical response and the fall in GH levels, and clinical improvement occasionally occurred in subjects who did not have a fall in plasma GH level. The fall in plasma GH level was maintained throughout treatment in all but three subjects.

There was no evidence of pituitary gland enlargement due to bromocriptine therapy. The size of the pituitary fossa on X-ray did not change in 45 patients after 1 year of bromocriptine treatment, and signs of extra-ocular nerve compression did not occur. Dopamine agonists reduce pituitary cell division and tumour size in rats (MacLeod and Lehmeyer, 1973) and it is possible that bromocriptine causes a reduction and not an increase in the size of pituitary adenomas.

In two subjects a spontaneous remission may have occurred during bromocriptine therapy although the condition of the others deteriorated on drug withdrawal and plasma GH levels rose to their previously elevated values.

9   Bromocriptine and parkinsonism

9.1   INTRODUCTION

In parkinsonism, there is a gross reduction in striatal DA content, in approximate proportion to the degree of cell loss in the pars compacta of the substantia nigra found at postmortem, and also very approximately to the degree of akinesia in life (Olson et al., 1973). Unilateral parkinsonism is accompanied by contralateral DA deficiency. Dopamine deficiency may result from degeneration of pigmented brain stem nuclei (Greenfield and Bosanquet, 1953), and this also results in loss of NA neurones of the locus coeruleus. Hypothalamic CA neurones are not directly involved in parkinsonism.

The concentration of the DA-synthesizing enzyme, L-aromatic acid decarboxylase, is reduced within the striatum in parkinsonism, sometimes to 15 per cent of normal. Despite severe dopa decarboxylase depletion there is apparently always sufficient remaining to enable the enzymic conversion of dopa to dopamine, although nonenzymic conversion may also occur.

Dopamine deficiency occurs in other diseases than parkinsonism, including Wilson's disease, progressive supranuclear palsy, occasional cases of cerebrovascular disease, striato-nigral degeneration, and olivo-ponto-cerebellar atrophy. In all these conditions, there may be a slight clinical response to DA stimulant drugs.

The likely explanation for the therapeutic effect of levodopa in parkinsonism is the conversion of dopa to dopamine, followed by stimulation of intact DA receptors. However, a number of other possibilities have been suggested to account for the delayed initial response to levodopa although the clinical response to levodopa, combined with a peripheral dopa decarboxylase inhibitor, is much more rapid.

Levodopa is a more effective antiparkinsonism drug than any previously available, and causes improvement in akinesia, tremor, rigidity, and postural deformity in most subjects. During long-term levodopa treatment, some degree of benefit is kept for at least 5 years in over half of patients. However, there are many drawbacks to levodopa treatment. Some patients do not respond or develop disabling response swings during treatment. Levodopa causes nausea and vomiting in 80 per cent of subjects, dyskinesias in 80 per cent, hypotension in 95 per cent although this is usually asymptomatic, and mania, acute disorders of awareness and hallucinations in 15 per cent. These unwanted effects may largely result from stimulation of DA receptors at different sites. Peripheral side effects, nausea, vomiting, and the occasional cardiac dysrhythmia can be overcome by the combination of levodopa with a peripheral decarboxylase inhibitor, but combined treatment does not reduce the incidence of centrally mediated unwanted actions of levodopa.

In up to 50 per cent of parkinsonism subjects, response swings develop during levodopa treatment. The most common type of swing is caused by fluctuations in plasma dopa level accompanying intermittent oral dosage (Marsden and Parkes, 1976). Response swings due to freezing occur in both untreated and treated subjects. A rare phenomenon, peak dose akinesia, in which peak dopa levels are accompanied by reduced rather than increased mobility, may also interfere with the steady control of disability.

Dopamine stimulant drugs and, in particular, bromocriptine, have been the greatest advance in the therapy of parkinsonism, since the introduction of dopa and decarboxylase inhibitors.

9.2   BROMOCRIPTINE IN THE TREATMENT OF PARKINSONISM

9.2.1   *Bromocriptine treatment of parkinsonism*

Calne *et al.* (1974a) treated 20 patients with idiopathic Parkinson's disease with bromocriptine in dosages up to 30 mg po daily. This caused about a 20 per cent improvement in functional disability in severely disabled subjects, whilst those who were less disabled improved by a smaller amount. On replacing bromocriptine by placebo, there was a rapid deterioration in mobility. Bromocriptine caused dyskinesias in half these patients, dizziness (possibly related to postural hypotension) in six, hallucinations in three, and emesis in three. These results have been confirmed in several later studies (Calne *et al.*, 1974b; Teychenne *et al.*, 1975a, b; Kartzinel *et al.*, 1976a, b, c). Teychenne *et al.* (1975a) in a double blind study of 28 subjects given bromocriptine 20 mg daily showed this caused a considerable improvement in tremor, rigidity, postural deformity, and akinesia. The side effects of bromocriptine treatment were broadly similar in nature to those seen separately with levodopa, although in addition, bromocriptine occasionally caused erythema, oedema, tenderness in the region of the ankle, burning discomfort in the eyes, double vision, and frequent extrasystoles, all of which were reversed on stopping treatment.

9.2.2   Long-term bromocriptine treatment

The progression of Parkinson's disease is apparently not altered by bromocriptine or any other presently available treatment. However, bromocriptine

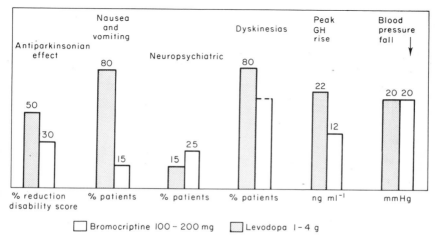

FIG. 10. Comparison of antiparkinsonism and side effects of bromocriptine and levodopa in subjects with parkinsonism.

remains effective in treatment for at least a year with no evidence of loss of response, although bromocriptine has not yet been used for longer periods. In contrast to bromocriptine, resistance to the antiparkinsonism action of propylnorapomorphine (3), and possibly to that of lergotrile (4), develops after some weeks of treatment (Lieberman et al., 1975; Cotzias et al., 1976).

Using bromocriptine alone or combined with anticholinergic drugs, but not levodopa, bromocriptine 20–30 mg daily causes sustained improvement with approximately a 30 per cent reduction in total disability, although the benefit gained by individual patients varies considerably and, on the whole, less disabled patients may show a greater response to bromocriptine than more disabled subjects. Overall, the degree of benefit from bromocriptine approximates to that given separately by levodopa, although Parkes et al. (1976b) in a

TABLE 8

Bromocriptine in parkinsonism

Authors	Bromocriptine Dosage (mg)	Period (weeks)	Other antiparkinsonism treatment	Number of patients	Antiparkinsonism action	Side effects	Notes
Calne et al. (1974a)	Mean 19	12	Levodopa (19), anticholinergics (11)	20	About 20% improvement in disability	As levodopa	Adverse reactions in 17 patients on high dosage
Calne et al. (1974b)	Up to 75		Levodopa (13)	19	Bromocriptine equivalent to levodopa in 6 patients	As levodopa	Bromocriptine well tolerated
Debono et al. (1975)	2·5–40	12	Levodopa (20)	31	Overall 23% reduction in disability	Neuro-psychiatric complications	Dose limiting side effects in 11 patients
Teychenne et al. (1975)	Mean 47	30	Levodopa (14)	28	Significant improvement on bromocriptine compared with placebo	As levodopa	All patients initially on levodopa. 9 bromocriptine failures
Jacobides and Audibert (1975)	7·5	2	Not stated	10	Improvement in gait and tremor	As levodopa	Aetiology of parkinsonism uncertain
Lees et al. (1975)	40	6	Levodopa (4)	12	Striking improvement 3, moderate response 5	Giddiness, constipation, drowsiness	
Gerlach (1976)	30	8	Bromocriptine compared with madopar	20	Varied response. Bromocriptine-response equal to madopar response in some patients	Involuntary movements and psychiatric complications common on both drugs	Ratio of effective dose bromocriptine; levodopa (in madopar) roughly 1 : 10
Parkes et al. (1976d)	26	12	Levodopa (20)	31	20–30% mean reduction in disability	As levodopa: nausea uncommon, confusion frequent	Least disabled patients showed greatest response to bromocriptine
Lieberman et al. (1976)	26	8–40	Levodopa (10)	11	6 responded, 5 no response	As levodopa	
Kartzinel et al. (1976a)	79	26	Levodopa replaced with bromocriptine in all patients	20	All features of parkinsonism improved	As levodopa	Mean 74% reduction in sinemet or levodopa dosage
Kartzinel and Calne (1976)	100	4	Levodopa (9)	9	Unstable diurnal response to levodopa (on–off); response swings less frequent on bromocriptine	Ventricular premature beats 1 patient	Significant advantage of bromocriptine over levodopa in this patient group
Kartzinel et al. (1976b)	100	4	Levodopa (8)	12	26% overall improvement	Transient and dose-dependent	Bromocriptine compared favourably with levodopa

study of 37 parkinsonism subjects concluded that bromocriptine 20–300 mg daily was slightly less potent that levodopa 250–4000 mg daily. A few individual patients may do better on bromocriptine than levodopa.

Bromocriptine, like levodopa, causes improvement in all the cardinal features of parkinsonism, and does not appear to have any preferential effect

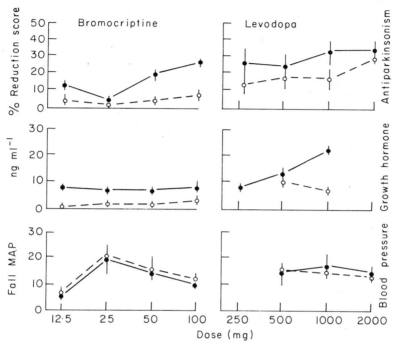

FIG. 11. Dose-response curves to bromocriptine and levodopa. Mean anti-parkinsonism (percentage reduction in total disability score), growth hormone (peak plasma concentration, ng ml^{-1}), and blood pressure (fall in erect mean arterial pressure MAP; mmHg) response ($\pm$ ISEM) to bromocriptine, 12·5, 25, 50, and 100 mg, in seven patients with parkinsonism. Responses in the same patients to levodopa 250, 500, 1000, and 2000 mg, and the effect of metoclopramide 60 mg pretreatment is shown. ———— Bromocriptine or levodopa alone; ------ metoclopramide pretreatment. (After Parkes *et al.*, 1976e.)

on one particular symptom. The response to bromocriptine is obvious within the first week of starting treatment, and when the drug is withdrawn deterioration is equally rapid. The comparative effects of bromocriptine and levodopa in individual parkinsonism subjects are illustrated in Figs 10 and 11. In these subjects, given maximum tolerated drug dosages, the anti-parkinsonism and peak GH response to levodopa were a little greater than to bromocriptine.

9.2.3   Bromocriptine dosage

Average doses of bromocriptine in the treatment of parkinsonism are 20–100 mg po daily, given in three divided doses, although some subjects show an obvious clinical response following bromocriptine 2·5 mg, whilst others require 300 mg daily. Bromocriptine 25–100 mg results in a dose-related improvement in the symptoms of parkinsonism. In six patients described by Debono *et al.* (1976), the mean reduction in disability score following bromocriptine 12·5, 25, 50 and 100 mg was 17, 25, 42 and 48 per cent respectively, although in two subjects, bromocriptine 100 mg had a lesser antiparkinsonism effect than 50 mg. Improvement was first obvious 1–2 hours after the oral administration of bromocriptine, and with the higher dosages, persisted for 6/10 hours.

9.2.4   Combined levodopa-bromocriptine therapy

In parkinsonism subjects with diurnal response swings on levodopa due to fluctuations in plasma dopa levels, the addition of bromocriptine to levodopa causes a smoother response than when levodopa is given alone (Lieberman *et al.*, 1976; Kartzinel *et al.*, 1976a). In this group of patients, bromocriptine has a distinct therapeutic advantage over levodopa. In subjects on combined levodopa-bromocriptine treatment, the dosage of levodopa necessary to control symptoms of parkinsonism can be reduced by approximately half to a third on the addition of bromocriptine 2·5–100 mg daily. Equipotent doses of levodopa and bromocriptine in the treatment of parkinsonism have not definitely been determined, although Gerlach (1976) in a double blind cross-over trial showed that approximate equivalents were 3·5–10 mg bromocriptine; 100 mg levodopa (combined with the decarboxylase inhibitor, benzserazide).

9.2.5   Bromocriptine in the treatment of levodopa-swingers

A third to a half of patients on long-term levodopa therapy develop disabling response swings after 1–5 years of treatment. In most cases, these response swings are primarily due to rapid fluctuations in plasma dopa level although it has not been explained why swings do not occur early in treatment. Response swings may possibly be unmasked by progressive failure of a functional reserve in the striatum.

The addition of bromocriptine to levodopa or, in some patients, replacement of levodopa by bromocriptine often causes a considerable reduction in response swings (Calne *et al.*, 1976). An alternative approach is to give multiple small levodopa dosages at 2-hourly intervals, although this does not always abolish response swings. In this type of patient, bromocriptine possesses a distinct advantage over levodopa (Kartzinel *et al.*, 1976b).

9.2.6 *Factors determining bromocriptine response in parkinsonism*

Approximately one-third of parkinsonism subjects respond well to bromocriptine, one-third show a moderate response, while the remainder respond poorly, if at all. Individual differences in bromocriptine absorption and metabolism may account for good or poor response, although this has not been definitely established. In some subjects, bromocriptine treatment is limited or prevented by unwanted effects. Several conditions closely mimic Parkinson's disease and, as with levodopa, it is probable that the bromocriptine response is limited in disorders such as supranuclear palsy. If subjects with apparent parkinsonism do not respond to levodopa, they are unlikely to respond to bromocriptine (Parkes *et al.*, 1976e) although Lieberman *et al.* (1976) apparently demonstrated that subjects who had become resistant to the action of levodopa would still respond to bromocriptine.

9.2.7 *Bromocriptine and csf amine metabolites*

The csf concentration of homovanillic acid (HVA) is low in most untreated subjects with parkinsonism. Bromocriptine causes a further reduction in HVA concentration (Kartzinel *et al.*, 1976c; Parkes *et al.*, 1976a), maximal 8 hours following oral drug administration. There is no definite correlation between the degree of reduction in concentration and the clinical response to bromocriptine, and a fall in HVA concentration occurs both in subjects with a good clinical response to bromocriptine and those who do not respond. In contrast to bromocriptine, levodopa causes a marked increase in csf HVA concentration. This increase following levodopa is likely to result from an increase in DA metabolism in periventricular areas of the brain, and largely in capillary networks around the caudate nucleus. The fall in csf HVA levels following bromocriptine may result from reduction in both neuronal and vascular DA turnover.

Bromocriptine causes a reduction in the csf concentration of the serotonin metabolite 5-hydroxyindoleacetic acid (5-HIAA; Curzon, 1975). 5-HIAA within the csf appears to be largely derived from both cerebral and spinal 5-HT metabolism, and this fall in csf 5-HIAA concentration is likely to result from a weak stimulant effect of bromocriptine on 5-HT receptors, which is accompanied by a reduction in 5-HT turnover throughout the neuraxis. Levodopa has little or no effect on 5-HIAA concentration in the csf.

9.2.8 *Bromocriptine and dyskinesias*

Dyskinesias occur in approximately 80 per cent of parkinsonism patients treated with levodopa. Choreic tongue and lower facial movements are often the first involuntary movements to appear, followed by choreic movements of the limbs, trunk and limb dystonia, motor restlessness, disturbance of respiratory rhythm, and facial and limb tics. These dyskinesias are dose related, occur mainly at the time of high plasma dopa levels, and occasionally interfere with the therapeutic response. Dyskinesias may be partially or completely prevented by the DA receptor blocking drugs, chlorpromazine and pimozide, although at the expense of a limited therapeutic response to levodopa.

Bromocriptine in dosages greater than 20 mg po daily causes oro-facial dyskinesias, limb chorea and restlessness in approximately 60–80 per cent of subjects with parkinsonism. These movements are exactly similar in appearance to those occurring in the same patients following levodopa. The severity of levodopa dyskinesias is increased on the addition of bromocriptine.

There is a counterpart in animals to bromocriptine dyskinesias in man. In monkeys, a ventral tegmental lesion causes hypokinesis of the opposite limbs and a resting tremor. Bromocriptine causes disappearance of these symptoms, but also causes chorea, restlessness, and various types of stereotyped movement. These dyskinesias in monkeys are of moderate severity and last for a shorter time than does the relief of tremor (Miyamoto *et al.*, 1974). Dopa and piribedil also causes dyskinesias in these animals, of a greater intensity than those due to bromocriptine (Goldstein *et al.*, 1975).

It is not known whether bromocriptine dyskinesias can be prevented in man without interfering with the drug's antiparkinsonism action. However, levodopa dyskinesias in animals can be prevented by DA receptor blocking drugs, such as haloperidol (Goldstein *et al.*, 1975), although this also reduces the effectiveness of levodopa in reducing tremor. Many other drugs affect the severity of dyskinesias in monkeys. The cholinesterase inhibitor physostigmine will ameliorate dyskinesias, whilst drugs that block central acetylcholine receptors potentiate the movements. Amino-oxyacetic acid, an inhibitor of amino transferase (Perry and Hanson, 1973) elevates GABA levels in the brain; this compound diminishes piribedil dyskinesias. In contrast, blockade of GABAminergic receptors by picrotoxin or bicuculline results in a potentiation of piribedil dyskinesias.

The occurrence of bromocriptine dyskinesias in parkinsonism may be partly dependent on pre-existing damage to the motor pathway, and bromocriptine does not cause dyskinesias when used in the treatment of acromegaly or galactorrhoea. However, comparatively low dosages of bromocriptine are used in these disorders.

9.3   COMPARISON OF DOPAMINE STIMULANTS IN THE TREATMENT OF PARKINSONISM

Apomorphine (**3**), propylnorapomorphine (**3**), piribedil (**2**), bromocriptine (**7**), and lergotrile (**8**) have been used in the treatment of parkinsonism (Schwab *et* al., 1969; Vakil et al., 1973; Calne et al., 1974a; Lieberman et al., 1975, 1976; Cotzias et al., 1976).

9.3.1   Apomorphine

Apomorphine causes profound vomiting and, if given orally, absorption is very eratic and there is a high rate of dose-dependent axotemia (Cotzias et al., 1976). On account of these problems, apomorphine is not effective therapy for parkinsonism. However, the apomorphine derivative propylnorapomorphine (NPA) penetrates the brain freely and causes stimulation of mammalian DA receptors for a longer time and with smaller doses than in the case of apomorphine (Mendez et al., 1975). In parkinsonism, NPA causes dose-dependent improvement of tremor, rigidity and akinesia in a similar manner to bromocriptine and levodopa. Improvement of parkinsonism is maximal with doses of 10–15 mg six times daily, and attempts to cause further improvement by increasing the dose to 500 mg daily causes azotemia.

Subjects with severe response fluctuations due to changes in plasma dopa level, intermittent dyskinesias, or both on levodopa, show almost identical behaviour whilst on NPA. As with levodopa, propylnorapomorphine causes neuropsychiatric side effects in 15–20 per cent of subjects, although nausea due to NPA is rare, and vomiting and symptomatic hypotension do not occur.

The clinical response due to NPA is rapid in onset and maximal improvement occurs once stable dosage has been achieved. However, after a period of some 3 weeks, the NPA response gradually declines and, although this tachyphylaxis can be temporarily halted by an increase in NPA dosage or administration of anticholinergic drugs, it can only be abolished by simultaneously giving levodopa (combined with a decarboxylase inhibitor). This drug combination results in a smoother response and less diurnal fluctuations than when levodopa is given as a single drug.

Why does tolerance occur to the antiparkinsonism action of NPA? Different segments of the NPA molecule have radically different postsynaptic effects (Ginos et al., 1976). The dopaminergic effect depends on an intact, non-metabolized, catechol segment whilst the piperidine and the tetrahydro-isoquinoline moiety have antidopaminergic properties, both when tested separately and when connected to an O-methylated catechol. O-Methylation, which occurs readily in the tissues, can thus change NPA into a DA antagonist, and accumulation of such an agent may explain the loss of potency of NPA with the passage of time (Cotzias et al., 1976).

The combination of levodopa and NPA causes a reduced and not increased severity of levodopa dyskinesias. This effect may be due in the long term to the antagonist action of O-methylated catechol fragments.

Like levodopa and bromocriptine NPA causes GH release in parkinsonism subjects, a rise of plasma GH level occurring 1 hour after drug administration.

Growth hormone levels remain elevated in the blood for 45–75 minutes. As with levodopa, GH release due to NPA may modify the transport, uptake, and distribution of this drug, thus changing its cerebral effects.

9.3.2 *Lergotrile*

Lergotrile mesylate (**8**), like bromocriptine, is an ergot-related compound which is a potent inhibitor of prolactin secretion. The antiparkinsonian potency of lergotrile is approximately similar to that of bromocriptine and levodopa (Lieberman *et al.*, 1975, 1976) and, in animals, lergotrile causes a dose-dependent reduction in the intensity of tremor in monkeys with ventro-medial tegmental lesions. However, unlike bromocriptine and levodopa, the anti-tremor effect of lergotrile may diminish after repeated administration, at least in animals.

Lergotrile, in a dosage up to 12 mg daily, is moderately effective for the symptomatic relief of parkinsonism, improvement being rapid in onset and dose-dependent. In some, but not all, subjects tolerance to lergotrile develops. Lergotrile causes involuntary movements similar to those caused separately by levodopa or bromocriptine, and levodopa dyskinesias may be potentiated by the addition of lergotrile. The adverse effects of lergotrile are comparable to those caused by levodopa except that mental changes are more common with lergotrile. Personality changes, paranoid ideas and hallucinations following lergotrile and bromocriptine are not surprising, given the structural similarity of these drugs to LSD. Like bromocriptine, the incidence of nausea and vomiting with lergotrile is extremely low.

If bromocriptine and lergotrile act predominantly as DA receptor stimulants, then their efficacy in parkinsonism might not be dependent upon the number of remaining nigro-striatal DA neurones. These drugs might be effective in some severely disabled patients who conceivably do not respond to levodopa because of their inability to convert it to dopamine. In favour of this idea is the finding of Lieberman *et al.* (1975) that individual severely disabled subjects with parkinsonism have a good clinical response to lergotrile.

Several patients given lergotrile for the possible treatment of hormone-dependent breast cancer have experienced a marked drop in blood pressure, although gradual build-up of dose over a period of several days may avoid this problem. The mechanism of hypotension following lergotrile has not been investigated, but is likely to be similar to that following bromocriptine. Lergotrile has recently come under suspicion of causing hepatic necrosis, and so clinical investigation may be halted.

9.3.3 *Piribedil*

In 1971, Corrodi *et al.* reported a biochemical, histochemical and pharma-cological study of piribedil (**2**), and suggested that this drug stimulated DA receptors in a similar way to apomorphine. However, in animals the action of piribedil was more prolonged and, in addition, high doses had a weak releasing action on DA and NA stores in the brain. Because of these observations, piribedil was used in the treatment of parkinsonism but, although effective in animal models of parkinsonism, little, if any, worthwhile improvement occurs in man. In studies by McLennan *et al.* reported by Shaw and Stern (1973), piribedil in doses of up to 200 mg daily caused little improvement, and drowsiness, confusion and hallucinations were common. Like levodopa, piribedil causes nausea and vomiting in a high proportion of subjects and, given as a single drug, will cause dyskinesias. The DA stimulant effect of piribedil in animals has been shown to result from active metabolites formed by reduction of the methylenedioxy bond.

Differences in piribedil metabolism in animals and man may possibly account for the limited efficacy of piribedil in human parkinsonism. However, piribedil does cause DA receptor stimulation in man as shown by the occurrence of dyskinesias and occasional increase in plasma GH levels.

9.3.4 *Dopamine stimulant and dopamine-releasing drugs in parkinsonism*

Compared with the DA-releasing drugs, amphetamine and amantadine (Schwab *et al.*, 1969; Parkes *et al.*, 1975), bromocriptine, lergotrile and NPA, all have a considerably greater antiparkinsonism action. Dopamine depletion is likely to severely limit the response to DA releasing drugs in parkinsonism, and this may explain the limited clinical efficacy of amphetamine and amantadine. However, both amantadine and amphetamine potentiate the effects of levodopa. All these drugs cause acute confusional states and delusions, often with little change in the sensorium; and all cause a rise in plasma GH level and fall in prolactin level in both normal and parkinsonism subjects. Dyskinesias are produced in up to 80 per cent of subjects given bromocriptine, NPA or lergotrile as single drugs. Amphetamines and amantadine rarely cause dyskinesias in parkinsonism, although amphetamines occasionally cause chorea in addicts on high dosage.

10 Miscellaneous effects of bromocriptine

10.1 CARDIOVASCULAR, EMETIC AND NEUROPSYCHIATRIC EFFECTS

10.1.1 *Bromocriptine and the cardiovascular system*

Bromocriptine, like levodopa, causes a fall in blood pressure in parkinsonism (Calne *et al.*, 1970; Reid *et al.*, 1972; Greenacre *et al.*, 1976), although symptoms of hypotension are uncommon, occurring in only 5 per cent of subjects. In average therapeutic dosages, both bromocriptine and levodopa cause a fall in systolic and diastolic pressure of around 10–20 mmHg. This fall is greater in the erect than the supine posture (Reid *et al.*, 1972). Hypotension is likely to be due to stimulation of DA receptors in renal and mesenteric vascular beds, central DA receptors, and regulatory receptors in autonomic ganglia (Greengard *et al.*, 1973), or possibly presynaptic DA receptors at post-ganglionic sympathetic nerve endings (Langer, 1974).

On standing, normal subjects have a rise in diastolic pressure. This postural compensation is not as great in parkinsonism (Reid *et al.*, 1971; Aminoff and Wilcox, 1971; Gross *et al.*, 1972) and is abolished by bromocriptine treatment. After bromocriptine there is a fall in systolic pressure and an absence in rise of diastolic pressure after prolonged standing (Greenacre *et al.*, 1976). The fall in blood pressure following bromocriptine and levodopa is not altered by metoclopramide pretreatment (Parkes *et al.*, 1976d), and metoclopramide may not cause blockade of peripheral DA vascular receptors.

Bromocriptine may rarely cause cardiac arhythmias. One subject with parkinsonism, treated with bromocriptine 35 mg daily, developed acute ventricular failure with a cardiac dysrhythmia after 8 weeks of treatment (Greenacre *et al.*, 1976). These symptoms resolved on stopping treatment.

10.1.2 *Bromocriptine, nausea and vomiting*

The emetic response to levodopa or apomorphine is abolished in dogs by ablation of medullary chemoreceptor areas. In man, DA-sensitive medullary areas are likely to be outside the blood-brain barrier, since the combination of levodopa with a peripheral decarboxylase inhibitor abolishes the emetic response to levodopa. Tolerance to the emetic action of levodopa slowly develops in some, but not all subjects.

In contrast to levodopa which causes nausea and vomiting in 80 per cent of subjects, bromocriptine causes nausea in only 15 per cent of subjects. Bromo-criptine-induced nausea is seldom accompanied by vomiting, and is of short duration (approximately 15 minutes). The occurrence of both levodopa- and bromocriptine-induced vomiting is not definitely related to the rapidity of increase in plasma drug levels. The latency between drug administration and vomiting is shorter with levodopa (30–60 minutes) than with bromocriptine (60–120 minutes). Nausea and vomiting due to DA stimulants can be prevented by metoclopramide pretreatment; the dosage of metoclopramide (10–20 mg po) sufficient to prevent emesis may be lower than that causing blockade of nigrostriatal DA receptors. However, in high dosage (60 mg), metoclopramide is a competitive antagonist to the antiparkinsonism effects as well as to the emetic effect of both levodopa and bromocriptine (Parkes *et al.*, 1976d).

10.1.3   *Neuropsychiatric effects of bromocriptine*

Lysergic acid derivatives may cause visual and sometimes auditory hallucinatory experiences for 1–6 hours after dosage. All effective antiparkinsonism drugs will also cause hallucinations. This action has not been definitely linked with DA stimulation at any site in the CNS. Levodopa in average therapeutic doses causes hallucinations in between 7–15 per cent of parkinsonian subjects; bromocriptine, in between 10–30 per cent; amantadine, in between 5–10 per cent; and anticholinergics in about 20 per cent. Some of these subjects are on multiple treatments. The greater frequency of hallucinations with bromocriptine as compared with levodopa may be partially accounted for by the effects of the lysergic acid moeity in the bromocriptine molecule. The occurrence of hallucinations with bromocriptine is partly dose related, although many subjects tolerate high dosages without hallucinations.

Visual hallucinations due to bromocriptine are often brightly coloured, and Lilliputian. They may occur in parkinsonian subjects who show no obvious therapeutic response to bromocriptine therapy. They cease on drug withdrawal, although a single case of persistent hallucinations with neuropsychiatric disturbance following bromocriptine withdrawal has been described. However, this subject was also taking levodopa with a decarboxylase inhibitor, the dosage of which was increased after bromocriptine withdrawal. Hallucinations due to bromocriptine do not occur in young subjects with acromegaly⁻ or lactation disorders. Bromocriptine may cause delusions in addition to hallucinations in parkinsonism, and frequently results in disordered awareness resulting in confusion in time and space.

These neuropsychiatric effects of bromocriptine and other drugs used in the treatment of Parkinson's disease can sometimes be prevented by metoclopramide or pimozide in high dosage, although at the expense of increasing parkinsonism.

10.2   MISCELLANEOUS USES OF BROMOCRIPTINE

Bromocriptine has been used in a surprising variety of human diseases, as different as mania and bladder instability. In view of the information this may give about possible central and peripheral roles of the DA nervous systems, these disorders are discussed briefly below.

10.2.1   *Asthma*

Asthma sometimes fails to respond to conventional treatment with steroids and bronchodilators. Three such patients treated with bromocriptine 2·5–20 mg daily by Newman Taylor *et al.* (1976) showed a sustained improvement, with a decrease in bronchodilator requirements. Salbutamol appeared to have a synergistic effect with bromocriptine in preventing airway obstruction. Under these circumstances, bromocriptine may alter the dopaminergic activity of sympathetic ganglia or nerves (Bjorklund et al., 1970). There is no evidence that DA has a direct effect on the human bronchial tree.

10.2.2 Spasmodic torticollis

The cause of spasmodic torticollis is completely unknown. Torticollis or retro-collis is occasionally a side effect of levodopa treatment in parkinsonism, and a few patients with idiopathic torticollis improve following haloperidol or other DA receptor blocking drugs. Bromocriptine 15–80 mg daily had no effect whatsoever on eight of 10 patients with spasmodic torticollis described by Lees et al. (1976). One patient showed a marked deterioration, and one patient with torticollis, previously responsive to levodopa 6 g daily (although at the expense of severe choreoathetosis) on 80 mg of bromocriptine daily was able to stop levodopa gradually without recurrence of retrocollis and with a disappearance in choreoathetoid movements.

10.2.3 Mania

Dorr and Sathanthan (1976) speculated that since the NA metabolite, MOPEG, was in high concentration in the csf in mania, lowering of plasma prolactin level with bromocriptine should prevent the genesis of mania. This surprising concept seemed to be borne out in practice when two manic patients became calm when given bromocriptine 15 mg daily.

10.2.4 Hypertension

In a single hypertensive acromegalic subject reported by Kaye et al. (1976) blood pressure did not respond to propranolol and hydralazine. However, when bromocriptine 20 mg daily was given to control acromegaly, blood pressure fell and later the patient become normotensive on no other therapy than bromocriptine 80 mg daily.

10.2.5 Benign prostatic hypertrophy

In hypophysectomized animals, prolactin causes an increase in prostatic weight (Grayhack and Libowitz, 1967) whilst prolactin antiserum causes a marked reduction in prostatic size (Asano et al., 1971). Farrar and Pryor (1976) therefore studied the possible clinical value of bromocriptine in patients with benign prostatic hypertrophy. The natural history of this disorder is difficult to evaluate and so is any trial of "prostatic pills". However, there appeared to be a real improvement in frequency, nocturia, urgency and urge incontinence. This improvement was possibly due to an action of bromocriptine on bladder instability rather than to improvement in outflow tract obstruction and, in other subjects with unstable bladders, bromocriptine often causes an improvement in micturition symptoms (Farrar and Osborne, 1976).

10.2.6   *Anorexia nervosa*

Anorexia nervosa is a chronic disease characterized by refusal to eat resulting in extreme weight loss and menstrual irregularity. The cause of this syndrome is not known. Barry and Klawans (1976) suggested by analogy with amphetamine-induced anorexia, that in anorexia nervosa there was an increased DA activity at central DA receptors.

One brief trial with levodopa has been reported to be of benefit rather than the reverse in the treatment of anorexia nervosa (Johansson and Knorr, 1974), but it seems improbable that bromocriptine or other DA stimulant drugs will prove of any permanent value in this obscure disorder.

10.2.7   *Myocardial infarction*

Physical and emotional stress increase prolactin secretion. Immediately following cardiac infarction, plasma prolactin levels are high. Such high prolactin levels will greatly increase the responsiveness of cardiovascular smooth muscle to NA and angiotensin (Manku *et al.*, 1973). Also, hyperprolactinaemia can reduce the threshold for electrical excitation of cardiac muscle. Horrobin *et al.* (1973) therefore suggested that following infarction, prolactin inhibition by bromocriptine might make the myocardium less susceptible to arrhythmias.

10.2.8   *Cushing's syndrome*

Ergotamine 0·05 mg given to rats bearing ACTH-secreting pituitary tumours inhibits tumour growth and reverses adrenal enlargement (MacLeod and Lehmeyer, 1974). Because of this, Lamberts and Birkenmayer (1976a, b) investigated the effect of bromocriptine in six patients with pituitary-dependent adrenal overactivity causing Cushing's syndrome. One subject had a pituitary tumour. Bromocriptine 2·5 mg caused a fall in ACTH levels between 4–7 hours after administration. In one patient the clinical effect of bromocriptine was dramatic, with nausea, vomiting, and hypotension. Cortisol 100 mg iv caused a rapid improvement. In pituitary-dependent Cushing's syndrome, there appears to be a central hypothalamic or pituitary DA defect, and many of these subjects have galactorrhoea and high prolactin levels. Bromocriptine will possibly prove an effective treatment. However, levodopa and bromocriptine have little or no effect on plasma ACTH levels under normal circumstances.

10.2.9   *Premenstrual tension*

In patients with premenstrual tension, severe fluid retention and tiredness, depression and lability of mood, Horrobin (1973) suggested that prolactin could play a crucial role in causing these symptoms, because of its effect on fluid and electrolyte balance. Bromocriptine has been used to treat pre-menstrual symptoms, premenstrual migraine, and idiopathic oedema related to the menstrual cycle with apparent success (Benedek-Jaszmann and Hearn-Sturtevant, 1976; Hockaday *et al.*, 1976; Evered *et al.*, 1976) although a clear relation of these symptoms to raised prolactin levels is often lacking. The real need to treat such symptoms must be defined, and there is no evidence, for example, that bromocriptine is of any value whatsoever in the treatment of classic migraine. Addiction to bromocriptine has not yet been reported.

10.2.10   *Hormone-dependent cancer*

Because it appeared that prolactin might play a part in regulating the activity of the prostate and because conventional therapy of prostatic cancer with oestrogens carries a risk of thromboembolism, Coune and Smith (1975) reported a clinical trial of bromocriptine 7·5 mg daily in subjects with prostatic carcinoma. Follow-up for 16 weeks showed bromocriptine had no favourable effect, and did not induce tumour remission.

Bromocriptine inhibits tumour growth of carcinogen-induced mammary cancer in the rat, which is prolactin dependent (Pearson *et al.*, 1969; Heuson *et al.*, 1970). However, in human breast cancer bromocriptine 15 mg daily does not inhibit tumour progression (European Breast Cancer group, 1972).

10.2.11   *Hepatic encephalopathy*

In patients with chronic portasystemic encephalopathy it has been suggested that there is a defect in dopaminergic neurotransmission (Fischer and Baldessarini, 1971). This evidence is largely based on the alerting action of levodopa in this disorder, which is possibly successful by causing replenish-ment of catecholamine stores which are depleted by accummulated amine products, acting as false neurotransmitters. Although levodopa does have a brief alerting effect it often causes vomiting in patients with liver disease and hence is of little value in long-term treatment. Bromocriptine has been successfully used in one patient previously incapacitated by chronic portasystemic encephalopathy and in whom levodopa caused a severe gastro-intestinal disturbance and postural hypotension (Morgan *et al.*, 1977). This patient was given bromocriptine by mouth in maximum dosage of 15 mg daily for a 3-month period during which there was a very considerable clinical and psychometric improvement. He became alert, his recent memory improved and speech and gait disorders virtually disappeared. On replacing bromocriptine with placebo his speech became so slurred as to be incomprehensible and his ataxia returned. On psychometric testing, cognitive function improved on bromocriptine and deteriorated when the drug was withdrawn. No side effects from the drug were experienced. The dramatic improvement in this patient remains to be confirmed in others, although it seems probable that bromo-criptine may have a role in the treatment of portasystemic encephalopathy, particularly if the response to more conventional methods has been poor.

Acknowledgements

I owe an enormous debt of gratitude to many people. First and foremost this review could not have been written without the expert advice and encouragement of Miss Joyce Parker. She gave constant help throughout the preparation of this article and was an invaluable source of references.

Secondly I am most grateful to Professor Flückiger, Dr Graham Kennedy and other members of the staff of Sandoz who read the manuscript and made many helpful suggestions. The mistakes are all mine.

Thirdly I acknowledge the secretarial help of Mrs I. Jebson and Mrs P. Asselman. Dr P. Jenner and Dr P. Price gave considerable advice about the biochemical and clinical effects of bromocriptine.

References

Abuzzahab, F. X. (1971). *Federation Proceedings*, **30**, 381.
Aghajanian, G. K. and Bunney, B. S. (1973). *In* "Frontiers in Catecholamine Research" (Eds E. Usdin and S. Snyder), p. 643. Pergamon Press, Oxford.
Ahren, K., Hamberger, L. and Perklev, T. (1971). *Acta physiologica Scandinavica*, **82**, 191.
Althoff, P-H., Neubauer, M., Handzel, R., Bechstein, V. and Schoffling, K. (1975). *Acta Endocrinologia (Kharkov)* Supplement, **199**, 119.
Aminoff, M. J. and Wilcox, C. S. (1971). *British Medical Journal*, iv, 80.
Amsler, C. (1923). *Naunyn-Schmiedebergs Archiv für Experimentelle Pathologie und Pharmakologie*, **97**, 1.
Andén, N. E. and Strombom, U. (1974). *Psychopharmacologia (Berlin)*, **38**, 91.
Andén, N. E., Corrodi, H., Fuxe, K. and Hökfelt, T. (1967a). *European Journal of Pharmacology*, **2**, 59.
Andén, N. E., Fuxe, K., Hökfelt, T. and Rubensson, A. (1967b). *Journal of Pharmacy and Pharmacology*, **19**, 335.

Andén, N. E., Rubensson, A., Fuxe, K. and Hökfelt, T. (1967c). *Journal of Pharmacy and Pharmacology*, **19**, 627.

Andén, N. E., Stromberg, U. and Svenson, T. H. (1973). *Psychopharmacologia (Berlin)*, **29**, 289.

Anlezark, G., Meldrum, B. and Trimble, M. (1975). Abstracts of the Sixth International Congress of Pharmacology, Helsinki, 20–25 July, p. 301.

Aono, T., Miyake, A., Shioji, T., Kinugasa, T., Onishi, T. and Kurachi, K. (1976). *Endocrinology and Metabolism*, **42**, 696.

Arnfred, T. and Randrup, A. (1968). *Acta Pharmacologia et Toxicologia*, **26**, 384.

Asano, M., Kanzaki, S., Sekiguchi, E. and Tasa, T. (1971). *Journal of Urology*, **106**, 248.

Axelrod, J. (1965). *Recent Progress in Hormone Research*, **21**, 597.

Barbeau, A. (1975). *Lancet*, **ii**, 683.

Barger, G., Carr, F. H. and Dale, H. (1906). *British Medical Journal*, **ii**, 1792.

Barry, V. C. and Klawans, H. L. (1976). *Journal of Neurological Transmission*, **38**, 107.

Beaumont, P., Bruwer, J., Pimstone, B. and Vinik, A. (1975). *South African Medical Journal*, **49**, 476.

Beck, J. C. and McGarry, E. E. (1966). *Proceedings of the Royal Society of Medicine*, **59**, 25.

Benedek-Jaszmann, L. J. and Hearn-Sturtevant, M. D. (1976). *Lancet*, **i**, 1095.

Benedek-Jaszmann, L. J. and Sternthal, V. (1976). *Practitioner*, **216**, 450.

Berle, P. and Apostolakis, M. (1971). *Acta Endocrinologia (Kharkov)*, **67**, 63.

Besser, G. M. and Thorner, M. O. (1976). *Postgraduate Medical Journal*, **52**, Supplement 1, 64.

Besser, G. M., Parke, L., Edwards, C. R. W., Forsythe, I. A. and McNeilly, A. S. (1972). *British Medical Journal*, **iii**, 669.

Besser, G. M., Mortimer, C. H., Carr, D., Schally, A. V., Coy, D. H., Evered, D., Kastin, A. J., Tunbridge, W. M. G., Thorner, M. O. and Hall, R. (1974). *British Medical Journal*, **i**, 354.

Birkmayer, W. and Hornykiewicz, O. (1962). *Acta Psychiatrica Nervenkranke*, **203**, 560.

Bjorklund, A., Cegrell, L., Falck, B., Ritzen, M. and Rosengren, E. (1970). *Acta Physiologica Scandinavica*, **78**, 334.

Board, J. S. and Bhatnegar, A. S. (1975). *American Journal of Obstetrics and Gynecology*, **123**, 41.

Boden, G., Lundy, L. and Owen, O. (1972). *Neuroendocrinology*, **10**, 309.

Bonnar, J., Franklin, M., Nott, P. N. and McNeilly, A. S. (1975). *British Medical Journal*, **iv**, 82.

Bowers, C. Y. and Folkers, K. (1973). *Biochemical and Biophysical Research Communications*, **51**, 512.

Bowers, C. Y., Friesen, H. G., Hwang, P., Guyda, H. J. and Folkers, K. (1971). *Biochemical and Biophysical Research Communications*, **45**, 1033.

Boyar, R. M. (1976). *New England Journal of Medicine*, **294**, 905.

Boyd, A. F., Lebovitz, H. E. and Pfeiffer, J. B. (1970). *New England Journal of Medicine*, **283**, 1425.

Boyd, A. E., Spencer, E., Jackson, I. M. and Reichlin, S. (1976). *Endocrinology*, **99**, 861.

Brazeau, P., Vale, W., Burgus, R., Ling, N., Butcher, M., Rivier, J. and Guillemin, R. (1973). *Science*, **179**, 77.

Brown, J. H. and Makman, M. (1972). *Proceedings of the National Academy of Sciences, USA*, **69**, 539.

Brown, G. M. and Reichlin, S. (1972). *Psychosomatic Medicine*, **34**, 45.

Brown, W. A., van Woert, M. H. and Ambani, L. M. (1973). *Journal of Clinical Endocrinology*, **37**, 463.

Brown, G. M., Garfinkel, P. E., Warsh, J. J. and Stancer, H. C. (1976). *Journal of Clinical Endocrinology*, **43**, 236.

Brun del Re, R., del Pozo, E., Grandi, P., Friesen, H., Hinselmann, M. and Wyss, H. (1973). *Obstetrics and Gynecology*, **41**, 884.

Burt, D. R., Enna, S. J., Creese, I. and Snyder, S. H. (1975). *Neuroscience Abstracts*, **1**, 404.

Butcher, R. W. and Sutherland, E. W. (1962). *Journal of Biological Chemistry*, **237**, 1244.

Calne, D. B., Brennan, J., Spiers, A. S. D. and Stern, G. M. (1970). *British Medical Journal*, **i**, 474.

Calne, D. B., Teychenne, P. F., Claveria, L. E., Eastman, R., Greenacre, J. K. and Petrie, A. (1974a). *British Medical Journal*, **iv**, 442.

Calne, D. B., Teychenne, P. F., Leigh, P. N., Bamji, A. N. and Greenacre, J. K. (1974b). *Lancet*, **ii**, 1355.

Calne, D. B., Kartzinel, R. and Shoulson, I. (1976). *Postgraduate Medical Journal*, **52**, 81.

Camanni, F., Massara, F., Belforte, L. and Molinatti, G. M. (1975). *Journal of Clinical Endocrinology*, **40**, 363.

Canales, E. S., Soria, J., Zarate, A., Mason, M. and Molina, M. (1976). *British Journal of Obstetrics and Gynaecology*, **83**, 387.

Carenzi, A., Guidotti, A., Revuelta, A. and Costa, E. (1975). *Journal of Pharmacology and Experimental Therapeutics*, **194**, 311.

Carlsson, A. (1975a). *In* "Pre- and Post-synaptic Receptors" (Eds E. Usdin and W. Bunney), p. 49. Marcel Dekker, New York.

Carlsson, A. (1975b). *In* "Proceedings of the Association for Research in Nervous and Mental Diseases". 5–6 December, New York (Discussion), Raven Press, New York.

Carlsson, A., Lindquist, M. and Magnusson, T. (1957). *Nature*, **180**, 1200.

Carlsson, A., Fuxe, K., Hamberger, B. and Lindquist, M. (1966). *Acta Physiologica Scandinavica*, **67**, 481.

Cegrell, L. (1967). *Life Sciences*, **6**, 2491.

Chase, T. N. (1974). *Advances in Neurology* (Eds F. McDowell and A. Barbeau), vol. 5, p. 31. Raven Press, New York.

Chiodini, P. G., Liuzzi, A., Botalla, L., Cremascoli, G. and Silvestrini, F. (1974). *Journal of Clinical Endocrinology*, **38**, 200.

Chiodini, P. G., Liuzzi, A., Botalla, L. Oppizzi, G., Muller, E. E. and Silvestrini, F. (1975). *Journal of Clinical Endocrinology*, **40**, 705.

Clement-Cormier, Y. C., Kebabian, J. W., Petzold, G. L. and Greengard, P. (1974). *Proceedings of the National Academy of Sciences, USA*, **71**, 1113.

Coelingh-Bennick, H. J. T., Haspels, A. A. and Snuiverink, H. (1976). *Lancet*, **i**, 1117.

Cohn, M. L., Cohn, M. and Taylor, F. H. (1975). *Brain Research*, **96**, 134.

Collu, R., Fraschini, F., Visconti, P. and Martini, L. (1972). *Endocrinology*, **90**, 1231.

Connor, J. D. (1970). *Journal of Physiology (London)*, **208**, 691.

Cooke, I., Foley, M., Lenton, E., Preston, E., Millar, D., Jenkins, A., Obiekwe, B., McNeilly, A., Parsons, J. and Kennedy, G. (1976). *Postgraduate Medical Journal*, **52**, 75.

Cools, A. R., Hendriks, G. and Korten, J. (1975). *Journal of Neurotransmission*, **36**, 91.

Cools, A. R. and van Rossum, J. M. (1976). *Psychopharmacologia (Berlin)*, **45**, 243.

Cooper, J. R., Bloom, F. E. and Roth, R. H. (1974). "The Biochemical Basis of Neuropharmacology", p. 152. Oxford University Press, London and New York.

Corrodi, H., Fuxe, K., Ljungdahl, Å. and Ögren, S-O. (1970). *Brain Research*, **24**, 451.

Corrodi, H., Fuxe, K. and Ungerstedt, U. (1971). *Journal of Pharmacy and Pharmacology*, **23**, 989.

Corrodi, H., Fuxe, K., Hökfelt, T., Lidbrink, P. and Ungerstedt, U. (1973). *Journal of Pharmacy and Pharmacology*, **25**, 409.

Corrodi, H., Farnebo, L-O., Fuxe, K. and Hamberger, B. (1975). *European Journal of Pharmacology*, **30**, 172.

Costall, B. and Naylor, R. J. (1976). *Journal of Pharmacy and Pharmacology*, **28**, 592.

Costall, B. and Olley, J. E. (1971). *Neuropharmacology*, **10**, 297.

Costa, E., Groppetti, A. and Naimzada, K. M. (1972). *British Journal of Pharmacology*, **44**, 742.

Costall, B., Naylor, R. J. and Pycock, C. (1975). *Journal of Pharmacy and Pharmacology*, **27**, 943.

Cotzias, G. C., Papavasiliou, P. S. and Gellene, R. (1969). *New England Journal of Medicine*, **280**, 337.

Cotzias, G. C., Papavasiliou, P. S., Tolosa, E. S., Mendez, J. S. and Bell-Midura, M. (1976). *New England Journal of Medicine*, **294**, 567.

Couch, E. F., Arimura, A. and Schally, A. V. (1969). *Endocrinology*, **85**, 1084.

Coune, A. and Smith, P. (1975). *Cancer Chemotherapy Abstracts*, **59**, 209.

Creese, I., Burt, D. R. and Snyder, S. H. (1975). *Life Sciences*, **17**, 993.

Creese, I., Burt, D. R. and Snyder, S. H. (1976). *Life Sciences*, **17**, 1715.

Cryer, P. E. and Daughaday, W. H. (1969). *Journal of Clinical Endocrinology*, **29**, 386.

Cryer, P. E. and Daughaday, W. H. (1974). *Journal of Clinical Endocrinology*, **39**, 658.

Curzon, G. (1975). *In* "Advances in Neurology" (Eds D. Calne, T. Chase and A. Barbeau), vol. 9, p. 349. Raven Press, New York.

Dale, H. H. (1906). *Journal of Physiology*, **34**, 163.

Dammacco, F., Rigillo, N., Tafaro, E., Gagliardi, F., Chetri, G. and Dammacco, A. (1976). *Hormone and Metabolism Research*, **8**, 247.

Debono, A. G. (1977). Personal communication.

Debono, A. G., Donaldson, I., Marsden, C. D. and Parkes, J. D. (1975). *Lancet*, **ii**, 987.

Debono, A. G., Jenner, P., Marsden, C. D., Parkes, J. D., Tarsy, D. and Walters, J. (1977). *Journal of Neurology, Neurosurgery and Psychiatry*, **40**, 162.

Delitala, G., Masala, A., Alagna, S. and Devilla, L. (1976). *IRCS Medicine and Science*, **3**, 82.

del Pozo, E. and Fluckiger, E. (1973). Proceedings of the International Symposium on Human Prolactin, Brussels, June 1973. p. 291. Excerpta Medica, Amsterdam.

del Pozo, E., Varga, L., Wyss, H., Tolis, G., Friesen, H., Wenner, R., Vetter, L. and Uettwiller, A. (1974). *Journal of Clinical Endocrinology*, **39**, 18.

del Pozo, E., Varga, L., Schulz, K. D., Kunzig, H. J., Marbach, P., Lopez del Campo, G. and Eppenbeger, U. (1975). *Obstetrics and Gynaecology*, **46**, 539.

Diamond, R. C., Brammer, S. R., Atkinson, R. J. Jr., Howard, W. J. and Earl, J. M. (1973). *Journal of Clinical Endocrinology*, **36**, 1189.

Diamond, R. C., Wartofsky, L. and Rosen, S. W. (1974). *Journal of Clinical Endocrinology*, **39**, 1133.

Dickerman, E., Negro-Vilar, A. and Meites, J. (1969). *Endocrinology*, **84**, 814.

Dickey, R. P. and Stone, S. C. (1976). *Obstetrics and Gynecology*, **48**, 84.

Dodart, M. (1976). *Journal des Savants*, p. 76.

Donaldson, I. M., Dolphin, A., Jenner, P., Marsden, C. D. and Pycock, C. (1976). *Brain*, **99**, 427.

Dorr, C. and Sathananthan, K. (1976). *British Medical Journal*, i, 1342.

Dray, A., Fowler, L. J., Oakley, N. R., Simmonds, M. A. and Tanner, T. (1975). *British Journal of Pharmacology*, **55**, 288P.

Dray, A. and Oakley, N. R. (1976). *Journal of Pharmacy and Pharmacology*, **28**, 586.

Duvoisin, R. C. (1967). *Archives of Neurology (Chicago)*, **17**, 124.

Duvoisin, R. C. (1976). *Lancet*, **ii**, 204.

Eddy, R. L., Jones, A. L., Chakmakjian, Z. H. and Silverthorne, M. C. (1971). *Journal of Clinical Endocrinology*, **33**, 709.

Edwards, C. R. W. and Jeffcoate, W. J. (1976). *In* "Pharmacological and Clinical Aspects of Bromocriptine (Parlodel)", p. 43. Proceedings of a Symposium held at The Royal College of Physicians, London, 14 May, 1976.

Edwards, C. R. W., Miall, P. A., Hamker, J. P., Thorner, M. O., Al-Dujaili, E. A. S. and Besser, G. M. (1975). *Lancet*, **ii**, 903.

Elkhawad, A. O. and Woodruff, G. N. (1975). *British Journal of Pharmacology*, **54**, 107.

Ernst, A. M. (1967). *Psychopharmacologia (Berlin)*, **10**, 316.

Evered, D. C., Horrobin, D. F., Vice, P. A., Cole, E. N. and Nassar, B. A. (1976). *Proceedings of the Royal Society of Medicine*, **69**, 421.

Fadner, F. (1944). Biography of Robert Wadlow. Bruce Humphries. Cited in R. H. Williams (Ed.) "Textbook of Endocrinology", 5th Edition. 1974. p. 70. W. B. Saunders Co, Philadelphia.

Faglia, G., Paracchi, A., Beck-Pecco, Z. P. and Ferrari, C. (1975). *Acta Endocrinologia (Kharkov) Supplement*, **199**, 323.

Falck, B. and Hellman, B. (1964). *Acta Endocrinologia (Kharkov)*, **45**, 133.

Falzon, D. M., Galea, R. and Camilleri, A. P. (1974). *Gynaecologic Investigations*, **5**, 133.

Farrar, D. J. and Osborne, J. L. (1976). *British Journal of Urology*, **48**, 235.

Farrar, D. J. and Pryor, J. S. (1976). *British Journal of Urology*, **48**, 73.

Feldman, J. M., and Lebowitz, H. E. (1972). *In* "Abstracts 4th International Congress of Endocrinology", p. 35. Excerpta Medica, Amsterdam.

Fischer, J. E. and Baldessarini, R. J. (1971). *Lancet*, **ii**, 75.

Flückiger, E. (1976). *In* "Pharmacological and Clinical Aspects of Bromocriptine (Parlodel)", p. 12. Proceedings of a Symposium held at The Royal College of Physicians, London, 14 May, 1976.

Flückiger, E. and Wagner, H. R. (1968). *Experientia*, **24**, 1130.

Flückiger, E., Doepfner, W., Marko, M. and Niederer, W. (1976). *Postgraduate Medical Journal*, **52**, Supplement 1, 57.

Franks, G., Murray, M. A. F., Jequier, A. M., Steele, S. J., Nabarro, J. D. N. and Jacobs, H. S. (1975). *Clinical Endocrinology*, **4**, 597.

Frohman, L. A. and Bernadis, L. L. (1970). *Endocrinology*, **86**, 305.

Fuxe, K. and Hökfelt, T. (1969). *In* "Frontiers in Neuroendocrinology" (Eds W. F. Ganong and L. Martini), p. 47. London. Oxford University Press, New York.

Fuxe, K. and Ungerstedt, U. (1970). *In* "Symposium on Amphetamine and Related compounds" (Eds E. Costa and S. Garattini), p. 83. Tamburini, Milan.

Fuxe, K. and Ungerstedt, U. (1974). *Medical Biology*, **52**, 48.

Fuxe, K., Hökfelt, T. and Nilsson, O. (1967). *Life Sciences*, **6**, 2057.

Fuxe, K., Corrodi, H., Hökfelt, T., Lidbrink, P. and Ungerstedt, U. (1974a). *Medical Biology*, **52**, 121.

Fuxe, K., Goldstein, M., Hökfelt, T., Jonsson, G. and Lidbrink, P. (1974b). *In* "Advances in Neurology" (Eds F. McDowell and A. Barbeau), vol. 5, p. 405. Raven Press, New York.

Fuxe, K., Agnati, L. F., Corrodi, H., Everett, B. J., Hökfelt, T., Loestrom, A. and Ungerstedt, U. (1975a). *In* "Advances in Neurology" (Eds D. B. Calne, T. Chase, and A. Barbeau), vol. 9, p. 223. Raven Press, New York.

Fuxe, K., Agnati, L. F., Hökfelt, T., Johnsson, G., Lidbrink, P., Ljungdahl, Á., Lofstrom, A. and Ungerstedt, U. (1975b). *Journal of Pharmacology (Paris)*, **6**, 117.

Gautvik, K. M., Hoyt, R. F. and Tashjian, A. H. (1973). *Journal of Cellular and Comparative Physiology*, **82**, 401.

Gemzell, C. (1975). *American Journal of Obstetrics and Gynecology*, **121**, 311.

Gerlach, J. (1976). *Acta Neurological Scandinavica*, **53**, 189.

Ginos, J. Z., Cotzias, G. C. and Tolosa, E. S. (1976). Reported in Cotzias *et al.*, 1976.

Glass, M., Shaw, R. W., Williams, J. W., Butt, W. R., Logan Edwards, R. and London, D. R. (1976). *Clinical Endocrinology*, **5**, 551.

Goebel, R., Rjosk, H. K., and Werder, K. V. (1974). *Acta Endocrinologia (Kharkov) Supplement*, **184**, 113.

Goldberg, L. I. (1972). *Pharmacological Reviews*, **24**, 1.

Goldstein, M., Battista, A. F. and Miyamoto, T. (1975). *In* "Advances in Neurology" (Eds D. B. Calne, T. N. Chase and A. Barbeau), vol. 9, p. 299. Raven Press, New York.

Gourdji, D., Morin, A. and Tixier-Vidal, A. (1973). *In* "Human Prolactin" (Eds J. L. Pasteels and C. Robyn), p. 163. Excerpta Medica, Amsterdam.

Grauwiler, J. and Griffith, R. W. (1974). *IRCS Medicine and Science*, **2**, 1516.

Grayhack, J. T. and Libowitz, J. M. (1967). *Investigative Urology*, **5**, 87.

Green, A. R. and Graheme-Smith, D. C. (1974). *Neuropharmacology*, **13**, 949.

Green, A. R., Heal, D. J., Graheme-Smith, D. G. and Kelly, P. H. (1976). *Neuropharmacology*, **15**, 591.

Greenacre, J. K., Teychenne, P. F., Petrie, A., Calne, D. B., Leigh, P. N. and Reid, J. L. (1976). *British Journal of Clinical Pharmacology*, **3**, 571.

Greenfield, J. S. and Bosanquet, F. D. (1953). *Journal of Neurology, Neurosurgery and Psychiatry*, **16**, 213.

Greengard, P. and Kebabian, J. W. (1974). *Federation Proceedings*, **33**, 1059.

Greengard, P., McAfee, D. A. and Kebabian, J. W. (1972). *In* "Advances in Cyclic Nucleotide Research" (Eds P. Greengard and G. A. Robison), vol. 1, p. 337. Raven Press, New York.

Greengard, P., Nathanson, J. A. and Kebabian, J. W. (1973). *In* "Frontiers in Catecholamine Research" (Eds E. Usdin and S. Snyder), p. 377. Pergamon Press, Oxford.

Griffith, R. W. (1974). *IRCP Medicine and Science Library Compendium*, **2**, 1661.

Griffith, R. W. and Richardson, B. P. (1975). *IRCP Medicine and Science Library Compendium*, **3**, 298.

Gross, M., Bannister, R. and Godwin-Austen, R. (1972). *Lancet*, **i**, 174.

Guillemin, R. (1976). *Triangle*, **15**, 1.

Hakanson, R. (1970). *Acta Physiologica Scandinavica Supplement*, **340**, 1.

Hakanson, R. and Owman, C. H. (1967). *Life Sciences*, **6**, 759.

Hakanson, R., Owman, C. H., Sjöberg, N-O. and Sporrong, B. (1970). *Histochemie*, **21**, 189.

Hall, R., Besser, G. M., Schally, A. V., Coy, D. H., Evered, D., Goldie, D. J., Kastin, A. J., McNeilly, A. S., Mortimer, C. H., Phenekos, C., Tunbridge, W. M. G. and Weightman, D. (1973). *Lancet*, **ii**, 581.

Heuson, J. C., Waelbroeck-van Gauer, C. and Legros, N. (1970). *European Journal of Cancer*, **6**, 353.

Hockaday, J. M., Peet, K. M. S. and Hockaday, T. D. R. (1976). *Headache*, **16**, 109.

Hökfelt, T. and Fuxe, K. (1972). *In* "Brain–Endocrine Interaction, Median Eminence, Structure and Function" (Ed. K. M. Knigge), p. 181. Karger, Basel.

Hökfelt, T., Ljungdahl, Å., Fuxe, K. and Johansson, O. (1974). *Science*, **184**, 177.

Horn, A. S., Cuello, A. C. and Miller, R. J. (1974). *Journal of Neurochemistry*, **22**, 2.

Hornykiewicz, O. (1976). Reported in Kelly and Moore, 1976.

Horrobin, D. F. (1973). "Prolactin: Physiology and Clinical Significance". M.T.P. Lancaster.

Horrobin, D. F., McNeilly, A. S., Jackson, F. S., Reid, D. S., Tynan, M., Nassar, B. A., Manku, M. S. and Elliott, K. (1973). *Lancet*, **ii**, 1261.

Hunter, W. M. and Greenwood, F. C. (1964). *British Medical Journal*, **1**, 804.

Hunter, W. M., Gillingham, F. J., Harris, P., Kanis, J. A., McGurk, F. M., McLelland, J. and Strong, J. A. (1974). *Journal of Endocrinology*, **63**, 21.

Imura, H., Kato, Y., Ikeda, M., Morimoto, M., Yawata, M. and Fukase, M. (1971). *Journal of Clinical Endocrinology*, **28**, 1079.

Imura, H., Nakai, I. and Yoshimi, T. (1973). *Journal of Clinical Endocrinology*, **36**, 204.

Iversen, L. L. (1975). *Science*, **188**, 1084.

Jacobides, G. B. and Audibert, A. (1975). *Therapeutische Umschau und Medizinische Bibliographie*, **32**, 469.

Jacobowitz, D. M. and Greene, L. A. (1974). *Journal of Neurobiology*, **5**, 65.

Johansson, A. J. and Knorr, N. J. (1974). *Lancet*, **ii**, 591.

Johnson, R. H. and Rennie, M. J. (1973). *Clinical Science*, **44**, 63.

Johnson, A. M., Vigouret, J. M. and Loew, D. M. (1973). *Experientia*, **29**, 763.

Johnson, A. M., Loew, D. M. and Vigouret, J. M. (1976). *British Journal of Pharmacology*, **56**, 59.

Kamberi, I. A., Mical, R. S. and Porter, J. C. (1971). *Endocrinology*, **88**, 1012.

Kansal, P. C., Buse, J., Talbert, O. R. and Buse, M. G. (1972). *Journal of Clinical Endocrinology*, **34**, 99.

Kartzinel, R. and Calne, D. B. (1976). *Neurology (Minneapolis)*, **26**, 508.

Kartzinel, R., Eng, N. and Calne, D. B. (1976a) cited in Kartzinel *et al.* (1976).

Kartzinel, R., Perlow, M., Teychenne, P., Gielen, A. C., Gillespie, M. M., Sadowsky, D. A. and Calne, D. B. (1976b). *Lancet*, **ii**, 272.

Kartzinel, R., Shoulson, I. and Calne, D. B. (1976c). *Neurology (Minneapolis)*, **26**, 511.

Kaye, S. B., Shaw, K. M. and Ross, E. J. (1976). *Lancet*, **i**, 1177.

Kebabian, J. W., Clement-Cormier, Y. C., Petzold, G. L. and Greengard, P. (1975). *In* "Advances in Neurology" (Eds D. B. Calne, T. N. Chase and A. Barbeau), vol. 9, p. 1. Raven Press, New York.

Kebabian, J. W., Petzold, G. L. and Greengard, P. (1972). *Proceedings of the National Academy of Sciences, USA*, **69**, 2145.

Kehr, W., Carlsson, A., Lindquist, M., Magnusson, T. and Atack, C. (1972). *Journal of Pharmacy and Pharmacology*, **24**, 744.

Kelly, P. H. (1975). *Brain Research*, **100**, 163.

Kelly, P. H. and Moore, K. E. (1976). *Nature (London)*, **263**, 695.

Knopf, R. F., Conn, J. W., Fajans, S. S., Floyd, J. C., Guntsche, E. M. and Rull, J. A. (1965). *Journal of Endocrinology*, **25**, 1140.

Kobberking, J., Juppner, H., Volkmann, B., Unger, K., Schwinn, G. and Dirks, H. (1975). *Acta Endocrinologia (Kharkov) Supplement*, **193**, 93.

Kolodny, H. D., Sherman, L., Singh, A., Kim, S. and Benjamin, F. (1971). *New England Journal of Medicine*, **284**, 616.

Kurse-Larsen, C. and Garde, K. (1971). *Lancet*, i, 707.

Künzig, H. J., Geiger, W., Schulz, K. D. and Lose, K. H. (1975). *Archiv für Gynaekologie*, **218**, 85.

Künzig, H. J., Schulz, K. D. and Geiger, W. (1977). *Acta Endocrinologia Supplement*, **208**, 40.

Kytomaki, O., Mousiainen, R., Pekkarinen, A., Rinne, U. K. and Viljanen, M. (1973). *Journal of Neurotransmission*, **34**, 145.

Lal, S., De la Vega, C. E., Sourkes, T. L. and Friesen, H. G. (1973). *Journal of Clinical Endocrinology*, **37**, 719.

Lamberts, S. W. J. and Birkenhager, J. C. (1976a). *Journal of Endocrinology*, **70**, 315.

Lamberts, S. W. J. and Birkenhager, J. C. (1976b). *Lancet*, ii, 811.

Lancet (1974). Editorial: *Lancet*, i, 1148.

Langer, S. Z. (1974). *Biochemical Pharmacology*, **23**, 1793.

Lebowitz, H. E. and Boyd, A. E. (1971). *New England Journal of Medicine*, **284**, 61.

Lebowitz, H. E., Skyler, J. S. and Boyd, A. E. (1974). *In* "Advanced in Neurology" (Eds McDowell, F. and Barbeau, A.), vol. 5, p. 461. Raven Press, New York.

Lees, A. J., Shaw, K. M. and Stern, G. M. (1975). *Lancet*, ii, 709.

Lees, A. J., Shaw, K. M. and Stern, G. M. (1976). *British Medical Journal*, i, 1343.

Leighton, P. C., McNeilly, A. S. and Chard, T. (1976). *Journal of Endocrinology*, **68**, 177.

Libet, B. and Owman, C. (1974). *Journal of Physiology (London)*, **237**, 635.

Lieberman, A., Miyamoto, T., Battista, A. F. and Goldstein, M. (1975). *Neurology (Minneapolis)*, **25**, 459.

Lieberman, A., Zolfaghari, M., Boal, D., Hassouri, H., Vogel, B., Battista, A., Fuxes, K. and Goldstein, M. (1976). *Neurology (Minneapolis)*, **26**, 405.

Liuzzi, A., Chiodini, P. G., Botalla, L., Cremascoli, G. and Silvestrini, F. (1972). *Journal of Clinical Endocrinology*, **35**, 941.

Liuzzi, A., Chiodini, P. G., Botalla, L., Cremascoli, G., Muller, E. and Silvestrini, F. (1974). *Journal of Clinical Endocrinology*, **38**, 910.

Lloyd, K. G., Davidson, L. and Hornykiewicz, O. (1973). *In* "Advances in Neurology". Progress in the treatment of Parkinsonism. (Ed. D. B. Calne), vol. 3, p. 173. Raven Press, New York.

Lloyd, K. G., Mohler, H., Heitz, P. and Bartholini, G. (1975). *Journal of Neurochemistry*, **25**, 789.

Loew, D. M., Vigouret, J. M. and Jaton, A. L. (1976). *Postgraduate Medical Journal*, **52** (Supplement 1), 40.

Lutterbeck, P. M., Pryor, J. S., Varga, L. and Wenner, R. (1971). *British Medical Journal*, iii, 228.

Lyons, W. R., Li, C. H. and Johnson, R. E. (1958). *Recent Progress in Hormone Research*, **14**, 219.

Maany, A., Frazier, A. and Mendels, J. (1975). *Journal of Clinical Endocrinology*, **40**, 162.

McCaul, J. A., Cassell, K. J. and Stern, G. M. (1974). *Lancet*, **i**, 735.

McCune, R. W., Gill, T. H., von Hungen, K. and Roberts, S. (1971). *Life Sciences*, **10**, 443.

MacLeod, R. M. (1969). *Endocrinology*, **85**, 916.

MacLeod, R. M. (1976). *Frontiers in Neuroendocrinology*, **4**, 169.

MacLeod, R. M. and Lehmeyer, J. E. (1974). *Endocrinology*, **94**, 1077.

McNatty, K. P., Sawers, R. S. and McNeilly, A. S. (1974). *Nature*, **250**, 653.

McNeilly, A. S. (1974). *British Journal of Hospital Medicine*, **ii**, 57.

McNeilly, A. S. (1975). *Postgraduate Medical Journal*, **51**, 231.

McNeilly, A. S. and Chard, T. (1974). *Clinical Endocrinology*, **3**, 105.

Magrini, G., Ebiner, J. R., Buckharat, P. and Felber, J. P. (1976). *Journal of Clinical Endocrinology*, **43**, 944.

Mahajan, K. K., Horrobin, D. F. and Robinson, C. J. (1957). *Journal of Endocrinology*, **64**, 587.

Malarkey, W. B. and Daughaday, W. H. (1971). *Journal of Clinical Endocrinology*, **33**, 424.

Malarkey, W. B. and Daughaday, W. H. (1972). *Endocrinology*, **91**, 1314.

Malarkey, W. B., Cyrus, J. and Paulson, G. W. (1974). *Journal of Clinical Endocrinology*, **39**, 229.

Manku, M. S., Nassar, B. A. and Horrobin, D. F. (1973). *Lancet*, **ii**, 991.

Marko, M. and Flückiger, E. (1974). *Experentia*, **30**, 1174.

Mars, H. and Genuth, S. M. (1973). *Clinical Pharmacology and Therapeutics*, **14**, 390.

Marsden, C. D. and Parkes, J. D. (1976). *Lancet*, **i**, 292.

Martin, J. B. (1973). *New England Journal of Medicine*, **288**, 1384.

Martin, J. B., Kontor, J. and Mead, P. (1973). *Endocrinology*, **92**, 1357.

Massara, F., Camanni, F., Belforte, L. and Molinatt, G. M. (1976). *Lancet*, **i**, 913.

Massara, F., Camanni, F. and Molinatti, G. M. (1973). *Hormone and Metabolism Research*, **2**, 454.

Meier-Ruge, W. and Iwangoff, P. (1976). *Postgraduate Medical Journal*, **52** (Supplement 1), 47.

Meites, J. (1974). *Journal of Investigative Dermatology*, **63**, 119.

Mena, I., Cotzias, G. C., Brown, F. B., Papavasiliou, P. S. and Miller, S. (1973). *New England Journal of Medicine*, **288**, 320.

Mendez, J. S., Cotzias, G. C. and Finn, B. W. (1975). *Life Sciences*, **16**, 1737.

Menon, M. K., Clark, W. G. and Cannon, J. G. (1976). *Journal of Pharmacy and Pharmacology*, **28**, 778.

Meyer, M. B., McNay, J. L. and Goldberg, L. I. (1967). *Journal of Pharmacology and Experimental Therapeutics*, **156**, 186.

Miller, R. J. and Iversen, L. L. (1974). *Naunyn-Schmiedebergs Archiv für Experimentelle Pathologie und Pharmakologie*, **282**, 213.

Miller, R. J., Horn, A. S., Iversen, L. L. and Pinder, R. M. (1974). *Nature (London)*, **250**, 238.

Milson, J. A. and Pycock, C. J. (1976). *British Journal of Pharmacology*, **56**, 77.

Mims, R. B. (1973). *Journal of Clinical Endocrinology*, **37**, 34.

Mims, R. B., Scott, C. L., Modebe, O. and Bethune, J. E. (1975). *Journal of Clinical Endocrinology*, **40**, 256.

Mishra, R. K., Gardner, E. L., Katzman, R. and Makman, M. H. (1974). *Proceedings of the National Academy of Sciences, USA*, **71**, 3883.

Miyamoto, T., Battista, A., Goldstein, M. and Fuxe, K. (1974). *Journal of Pharmacy and Pharmacology*, **26**, 452.

Modigh, K. (1974). *Acta Physiologica Scandinavica, Supplement*, **403**, 1.

Moir, C. (1932). *British Medical Journal*, **1**, 1119.

Molinatti, G. M., Camanni, F., Massara, F. and Isaia, G. C. (1975). *Panminerva Medicine*, **17**, 101.

Morgan, M. Y., Jakobovits, A., Elithorn, A., James, I. M. and Sherlock, S. (1977). *New England Journal of Medicine*, **296**, 739.

Morpurgo, C. (1962). *Archiv für Experimentelle Pathologie und Pharmakologie*, **137**, 84.

Muller, E. E. (1973). *In* "Frontiers in Catecholamine Research" (Eds E. Usdin and S. Snyder), vol. 1, p. 839. Pergamon Press, Oxford.

Muller, E. E., Saito, T., Arimura, A. and Schally, A. V. (1967). *Endocrinology*, **80**, 109.

Nader, S., Kjeld, J. M., Blair, C. M., Tooley, M., Gordon, H. and Fraser, T. R. (1975). *British Journal of Obstetrics and Gynaecology*, **82**, 750.

Nader, S., Mashiter, K., Doyle, F. H. and Joplin, G. F. (1976). *Clinical Endocrinology*, **5**, 245.

Nagasawa, H., Yanai, R. and Flückiger, E. (1973). *In* "Human Prolactin" (Eds J. L. Pasteels and C. Robyn), p. 314. *Excerpta Medica*, Amsterdam.

Nandi, S. (1959). *University of California Publications in Zoology*, **65**, 1.

Nelson, D. H. (1974). *In* "Harrison's Principles of Internal Medicine", p. 449. 7th Edition, McGraw-Hill, New York.

Newman Taylor, A. J., Soutar, C., Shneerson, J. and Turner Warwick, M. (1976). Paper read at the Thoracic Society Meeting, Liverpool, July 15–16.

Ng, K. Y., Chase, T. N., Colburn, R. W. and Kopin, I. J. (1970). *Science*, **170**, 76.

Niall, H. D., Hogan, M. L. and Sauer, R. (1971). *Proceedings of the National Academy of Sciences, USA*, **68**, 866.

Nicholl, C. S. and Bern, H. A. (1972). *In* "Lactogenic Hormones" (Eds G. E. W. Wolstenholme and J. Knight), p. 299. Churchill Livingstone, London.

Nilson, P. A., Meling, A-B. and Abildgaard, U. (1976). *Acta Obstetrica Gynecologia Scandinavica*, **55**, 39.

Nobin, A. and Bjorklund, A. (1973). *Acta Physiologica Scandinavica Supplement*, **388**, 1.

Oldendorf, W. H. (1971). *American Journal of Physiology*, **221**, 1629.

Olson, L., Fuxe, K. and Hökfelt, T. (1971), cited in Hökfelt and Fuxe, 1971.

Olson, L., Nystrom, B. and Seiger, A. (1973). *Brain Research*, **63**, 231.

Parkes, J. D. (1975). *In* "Recent Advances in Drug Research" (Ed. A. B. Simmonds), vol. 8, p. 11. Academic Press, London and New York.

Parkes, J. D., Bedard, P. and Marsden, C. D. (1976c). *Lancet*, **ii**, 155.

Parkes, J. D., Debono, A. G. and Jenner, P. (1977). *British Journal of Clinical Pharmacology*. **4**, 343.

Parkes, J. D., Debono, A. G. and Marsden, C. D. (1976a). *Lancet*, **i**, 483.

Parkes, J. D., Debono, A. G. and Marsen, C. D. (1976b). *Journal of Neurology, Neurosurgery and Psychiatry*, **38**, 1101.

Parkes, J. D., Debono, A. G. and Marsden, C. D. (1976e). *Journal of Neurology, Neurosurgery and Psychiatry*, **39**, 1101.

Parkes, J. D., Marsden, C. D., Donaldson, I., Debono, A. G., Walters, J., Kennedy, G. and Asselman, P. (1976d). *Journal of Neurology, Neurosurgery and Psychiatry*, **39**, 184.

Pasteels, J. L., Danguy, A., Frerotte, M. and Ectors, F. (1971). *Annals of Endocrinology* (*Paris*), **32**, 188.

Pearson, O. H., Llerena, D., Llerena, L., Molina, A. and Butler, T. (1969). *Transactions of the Association of American Physicians*, **82**, 225.

Pelletier, G., Labrie, F., Arimura, A. and Schally, A. V. (1974a). *American Journal of Anatomy*, **140**, 445.

Pelletier, G., Labrie, F., Puviani, R., Arimura, A. and Schally, A. V. (1974b). *Endocrinology*, **95**, 314.

Perez-Lopez, F. R. (1975). *Obstetrics and Gynaecology*, **46**, 621.

Perry, T. L. and Hansen, S. (1973). *Journal of Neurochemistry*, **21**, 1167.

Pijneburg, A., Woodruff, G. and van Rossum, J. (1973). *Brain Research*, **59**, 289.

Plotnikoff, N. P., Kastin, A. J., Anderson, M. S. and Schally, A. V. (1971). *Life Sciences*, **10**, 1279.

Pontiroli, A. E., Castegnaro, E., Vettaro, M. P., Viberti, G. C. and Pozza, G. (1977). *Acta Endocrinologia* (*Kharkov*), **84**, 36.

Powell, E. W. and Leman, R. B. (1976). *Brain Research*, **105**, 389.

Puech, A., Fichelle, J., Chermat, R., Simon, P. and Boissier, J. (1975). *In* Abstracts of the Sixth International Congress of Pharmacology, p. 262. Helsinki, July 20–25.

Pycock, C. J. and Marsden, C. D. (1977). *Journal of Neurological Science*, **31**, 113.

Pycock, C. J., Donaldson, I. and Marsden, C. D. (1975). *Brain Research*, **97**, 317.

Pycock, C. J., Jenner, P. G. and Marsden, C. D. (1977). *Naunyn-Schmiedebergs Archiv für Experimentelle Pathologie und Pharmakologie*, **297**, 133.

Quadri, S. K. and Meites, J. (1971). *Proceedings of the Society for Experimental Biology and Medicine*, **138**, 999.

Raben, M. S. (1962). *New England Journal of Medicine*, **266**, 31.

Reichlin, S. (1974). *In* "Textbook of Endocrinology", 5th Edition (Ed. R. H. Williams), p. 826. W. B. Saunders, Philadelphia.

Reid, J. L., Calne, D. B., George, C. F., Pallis, C. and Vakil, S. D. (1971). *Clinical Science*, **41**, 63.

Reid, J. L., Calne, D. B., George, C. F. and Vakil, S. D. (1972). *Clinical Science*, **43**, 851.

Rioch, D. M. (1931). *Journal of Comparative Neurology*, **53**, 319.

Rochette, L. and Bralet, J. (1975). *Journal of Neurological Transmission*, **37**, 259.

Rolland, R. and Schellekans, L. (1973). *British Journal of Obstetrics and Gynaecology*, **80**, 945.

Rolland, R., de Jong, F. H., Schellekans, L. A. and Lequin, R. M. (1975). *Clinical Endocrinology*, **4**, 27.

Roth, J., Glick, S. M., Yalow, R. S. and Berson, S. A. (1963a). *Metabolism*, **12**, 577.

Roth, J., Glick, S. M., Yalow, R. S. and Berson, S. A. (1963b). *Science*, **140**, 987.

Saameli, K. (1976). *Postgraduate Medical Journal*, **52** (Supplement 1), 7.

Sachar, E. J., Mushrush, G., Perlow, M., Weitzman, E. D. and Sassin, J. (1972). *Science*, **178**, 1304.

Sachdev, Y., Gomez-Pan, A., Tunbridge, W. M. G., Duns, A., Weightman, D. R. and Hall, R. (1975). *Lancet*, **ii**, 1164.

Sassin, J. F., Frantz, A. G., Kapen, S. and Weitzman, E. D. (1973). *Journal of Clinical Endocrinology*, **37**, 436.

Schally, A. V. (1968). *Science*, **160**, 1137.

Schally, A. V. (1976). *In* "Basic Applications and Clinical Uses of Hypothalamic Hormones" (Eds A. L. Charro Salgado, R. Fernandez-Durango and J. G. Lopez del Campo), p. 1. Excerpta Medica, Amsterdam, Oxford.

Schally, A. V., Muller, E. E. and Sawano, S. (1968). *Endocrinology*, **82**, 271.

Schally, A. V., Arimura, A., Takahara, J., Redding, T. W. and Dupont, A. (1974). *Federation Proceedings*, **33**, 237.

Schnieden, H. and Cox, B. (1976). *European Journal of Pharmacology*, **39**, 133.

Schorderet, M. (1976). *Neuroscience Letters*, **2**, 87.

Schwab, R. S., Amador, L. V. and Lettvin, J. Y. (1969). *Transactions of the American Neurological Association*, **76**, 251.

Seki, K. and Seki, M. (1974). *Journal of Clinical Endocrinology*, **38**, 508.

Seki, K., Seki, M. and Okumura, T. (1975). *Acta Endocrinologia (Kharkov)*, **79**, 25.

Seppala, M., Ylinen, O., Sternthal, V., Soiva, K. and Vara, P. (1975a). *International Journal of Gynaecology and Obstetrics*, **13**, 1.

Seppala, M., Hirvonen, E., Ranta, T. and Virkkunen, P. (1975b). *Acta Endocrinologia (Kharkov)*, **78**, Supplement, **199**, 349.

Seppala, M., Hirvonen, E. and Ranta, T. (1976). *Lancet*, **i**, 229.

Shaw, K. M. and Stern, C. M. (1973). Quoted in Vekil *et al.*, 1973.

Shelesnyak, M. C. (1954). *American Journal of Physiology*, **179**, 301.

Shelesnyak, N. C. (1957). *Recent Progress in Hormone Research*, **13**, 269.

Sherman, L., Kim, S., Benjamin, F. and Kolodny, H. D. (1971). *New England Journal of Medicine*, **284**, 72.

Siler, T. M., Vandenberg, G., Yen, S. S. C., Brazeau, P., Vale, W. and Guillemin, R. J. (1973). *Journal of Clinical Endocrinology*, **37**, 632.

Smith, G. P. and Root, A. W. (1971). *Neuroendocrinology*, **8**, 235.

Smith, O. C. (1930). *Journal of Comparative Neurology*, **51**, 65.

Snider, S., Hutt, C., Stein, B. and Fahn, S. (1975). *Neuroscience Letters*, **4**, 237.

Snider, S. R., Hutt, C., Stein, B., Prasad, A. L. N. and Fahn, S. (1976). *Journal of Pharmacy and Pharmacology*, **28**, 563.

Souvatzoglou, A. (1973). *Acta Endocrinologia (Kharkov)*, **73**, 259.

Stromberg, U. (1970). *Psychopharmacologia*, **18**, 58.

Stromberg, U. and Svensson, T. H. (1971). *Acta Pharmacologia (Kharkov)*, **30**, 161.

Struyker-Boudier, H., Gielen, W., Cools, A. and van Rossum, J. (1974). *Archives Internationales de Pharmacodynamie et Thérapie*, **202**, 62.

Sulaiman, W. R. and Johnson, R. H. (1973). *British Medical Journal*, **ii**, 329.

Summers, V. K., Hipkin, L. J., Diver, M. J. and Davis, J. C. (1975). *Journal of Clinical Endocrinology*, **40**, 904.

Svensson, T. H., Bunney, B. S. and Aghajanian, G. K. (1975). *Brain Research*, **92**, 291.

Takahara, J., Arimura, A. and Schally, A. V. (1974). *Endocrinology*, **95**, 462.

Tang, L. C. and Cotzias, G. C. (1976). *Archives of Neurology*, **33**, 131.

Tanner, J. M. (1972). *Nature*, **237**, 433.

Tarsy, D. and Baldessarini, R. J. (1973). *Nature New Biology*, **245**, 262.

Tarsy, D., Parkes, J. D. and Marsden, C. D. (1975). *Archives Neurology*, **32**, 134.

Tashjian, A. H. and Hoyt, R. F. (1972). *In* "Molecular Genetics and Developmental Biology" (Ed. M. Sussman), p. 353. Prentice Hall Inc., Englewood Cliffs, New Jersey.

Teychenne, P. F., Clane, D. B., Leigh, P. N., Greenacre, J. K., Reid, J. L., Petrie, A. and Bamji, A. N. (1975). *Lancet*, **ii**, 473.

Thierry, A. M., Blane, G., Sobel, A., Steimes, L. and Glowinski, J. (1973). *Science*, **182**, 499.

Thornburg, J. E. and Moore, K. E. (1972). *Neuropharmacology*, **66**, 675.

Thorner, M. O. (1975). *Lancet*, **i**, 662.

Thorner, M. O. and Besser, G. M. (1976). *Postgraduate Medical Journal,* **52,** *Supplement,* **1,** 71.

Thorner, M. O., McNeilly, A. S., Hagan, C. and Besser, G. M. (1974). *British Medical Journal,* **i,** 419.

Thorner, M. O., Chait, A., Aitken, M., Benker, G., Bloom, S. R., Mortimer, C. H., Sanders, P., Stuart Mason, A. and Besser, G. M. (1975a). *British Medical Journal,* **ii,** 299.

Thorner, M. O., Besser, G. M., Jones, A., Dacie, J. and Jones, A. E. (1975b). *British Medical Journal,* **iv,** 694.

Trabucchi, M., Spano, P. F., Tonon, G. C. and Frattola, L. (1976). *Life Sciences,* **19,** 225.

Trendelenberg, U. (1963). *Pharmacological Reviews,* **15,** 225.

Turkington, R. W. (1971). *Journal of Clinical Endocrinology,* **33,** 210.

Turnbridge, W. M. G., Sachdev, Y., Gomez-Pan, A., Duns, A. and Hall, R. (1975). *Acta Endocrinologia (Kharkov), Supplement,* **199,** 302.

Tyson, J. E., Andreasson, B., Huth, J., Smith, B. and Zacur, H. (1975). *Obstetrics and Gynaecology,* **46,** 1.

Tyson, J. E., Khojandi, M., Huth, J., Smith, B. and Thomas, P. (1975b). *American Journal of Obstetrics and Gynecology,* **121,** 375.

Udeschini, G., Cocchi, D., Panerai, A. E., Gil-Ad, I., Rossi, G. L., Chiodini, P. G., Liuzzi, A. and Muller, E. E. (1976). *Endocrinology,* **98,** 807.

Ueda, G., Sato, Y., Yamasaki, M., Shioji, T., Aono, T. and Kurachi, K. (1975). *Endocrinology (Japan),* **22,** 265.

Ungerstedt, U. (1971). *Acta Physiological Scandinavica Supplement,* **367,** 69.

Utian, W. H., Begg, G., Vinik, A. I., Paul, M. and Shuman, L. (1975). *British Journal of Obstetrics and Gynaecology,* **82,** 755.

Utiger, R. D., Parker, M. L. and Daughaday, W. (1962). *Journal of Clinical Investigation,* **41,** 254.

Vakil, S. D., Calne, D. B., Reid, J. L. and Seymour, C. A. (1973). *In* "Progress in the Treatment of Parkinsonism" (Ed. D. B. Calne), p. 121. Raven Press, New York.

van der Gugten, A. A., Sahuleka, P. C., van Galen, G. H. and Kwa, H. G. (1976a). *Journal of Endocrinology,* **68,** 369.

van der Gugten, A. A., Sahuleka, P. C., van Galan, G. H. and Kwa, H. G. (1976b). *Journal of Endocrinology,* **68,** 355.

van Rossum, J. (1970). *International Journal of Neurobiology,* **12,** 307.

Varga, L., Lutterbeck, P. M., Pryor, J. S., Wenner, R. and Erb, H. (1972). *British Medical Journal,* **ii,** 743.

Verde, G., Oppizzi, G., Colussi, G., Cremascoli, G., Botalla, L., Muller, E. E., Silvestrini, F., Chiodini, P. G. and Liuzzi, A. (1976). *Clinical Endocrinology,* **5,** 419.

Vigouret, J. M., Johnson, A. M. and Loew, D. M. (1973). *Archives of Pharmacology, Supplement,* **277,** 84.

Voigtlander, P. F. von and Moore, K. E. (1973). *Neuropharmacology,* **12,** 451.

Voigtlander, P. F. von, Boukma, S. J. and Johnson, G. A. (1973). *Neuropharmacology,* **12,** 1081.

Walker, S., Groom, G., Hibbard, B. M., Griffiths, K. and Davis, R. H. (1975). *Lancet,* **ii,** 842.

Walters, J. and Roth, R. H. (1976). *Naunyn-Schmiedebergs Archives für Experimentelle Pathologie und Pharmakologie,* **296,** 5.

Wass, J. A. H., Thorner, M. O. and Besser, G. M. (1976). *Lancet,* **i,** 1135.

Wass, J. A. M., Thorner, M. O., Morris, D. V., Rees, L. H., Mason, A. S., Jones, A. E. and Besser, G. M. (1977). *British Medical Journal*, i, 875.

Wayne, A. R., Gill, J. R., Yamaba, H., Lovenberg, W. and Keiser, R. (1974). *Journal of Clinical Investigation*, **54**, 194.

Wilcox, C. S., Aminoff, M. J., Keenan, J., Millar, J. G. B. and Kremer, M. (1973). *Journal of Endocrinology*, **58**, vi.

Winokur, A. and Utiger, R. D. (1974). *Science*, **185**, 265.

Wright, A. D., McLachlan, M. S. F., Doyle, F. H. and Russell Fraser, T. (1969). *British Medical Journal*, iv, 582.

Wuttke, W., Dohler, K. D. and Gelato, M. (1976). *Journal of Endocrinology*, **68**, 391.

Yanai, R. and Nagsawa, H. (1974). *Hormone Research*, **5**, 1.

Yeh, B. K., McNay, J. L. and Goldberg, L. I. (1969). *Journal of Pharmacology and Experimental Therapeutics*, **168**, 303.

York, D. M. (1970). *Brain Research*, **5**, 263.

Subject Index

Cumulative Index of Authors

Cumulative Index of Titles

DATE DUE

		261-2500	Printed in USA